Measurement-Based Care in Child and Adolescent Psychiatry

Editors

RAJEEV KRISHNA
JESSICA JEFFREY
EUGENE GRUDNIKOFF
BARRY SARVET

CHILD AND ADOLESCENT PSYCHIATRIC CLINICS OF NORTH AMERICA

www.childpsych.theclinics.com

Consulting Editor
TODD E. PETERS

October 2020 • Volume 29 • Number 4

ELSEVIER

1600 John F. Kennedy Boulevard • Suite 1800 • Philadelphia, Pennsylvania, 19103-2899

http://www.theclinics.com

CHILD AND ADOLESCENT PSYCHIATRIC CLINICS OF NORTH AMERICA Volume 29, Number 4
October 2020 ISSN 1056–4993, ISBN-13: 978-0-323-76029-4

Editor: Lauren Boyle
Developmental Editor: Kristen Helm

Child and Adolescent Psychiatric Clinics of North America (ISSN 1056-4993) is published quarterly by Elsevier Inc., 360 Park Avenue South, New York, NY 10010-1710. Months of issue are January, April, July, and October. Business and Editorial Offices: 1600 John F. Kennedy Boulevard, Suite 1800, Philadelphia, PA 19103-2899. Periodicals postage paid at New York, NY and additional mailing offices. Subscription prices are $338.00 per year (US individuals), $661.00 per year (US institutions), $100.00 per year (US & Canadian students), $388.00 per year (Canadian individuals), $804.00 per year (Canadian institutions), $446.00 per year (international individuals), $804.00 per year (international institutions), and $200.00 per year (international students). International air speed delivery is included in all *Clinics* subscription prices. All prices are subject to change without notice. **POSTMASTER:** Send address changes to *Child and Adolescent Psychiatric Clinics of North America*, Elsevier Health Sciences Division, Subscription Customer Service, 3251 Riverport Lane, Maryland Heights, MO 63043. **Customer Service: 1-800-654-2452 (U.S. and Canada); 314-447-8871 (outside U.S. and Canada). Fax: 314-447-8029. E-mail:** JournalsCustomer Service-usa@elsevier.com **(for print support) or** journalsonlinesupport-usa@elsevier.com **(for online support).**

Reprints. For copies of 100 or more of articles in this publication, please contact the Commercial Reprints Department, Elsevier Inc., 360 Park Avenue South, New York, New York 10010-1710 Tel.: 212-633-3874; Fax: 212-633-3820, E-mail: reprints@elsevier.com.

Child and Adolescent Psychiatric Clinics of North America is covered in *MEDLINE/PubMed (Index Medicus), ISI, SSCI, Research Alert, Social Search, Current Contents,* and *EMBASE/Excerpta Medica.*

Contributors

CONSULTING EDITOR

TODD E. PETERS, MD, FAPA
Vice President/Chief Medical Officer (CMO), Chief Medical Information Officer (CMIO), Sheppard Pratt Health System, Baltimore, Maryland

EDITORS

BARRY SARVET, MD
Professor and Chair, Department of Psychiatry, University of Massachusetts Medical School-Baystate, Baystate Medical Center, Statewide Medical Director, Massachusetts Child Psychiatry Access Program, Springfield, Massachusetts

JESSICA JEFFREY, MD, MPH, MBA, FAPA, DFAACAP
Associate Clinical Professor of Psychiatry, UCLA Department of Psychiatry and Biobehavioral Sciences, Associate Medical Director of Ambulatory Psychiatry Services, Associate Director, Division of Population Behavioral Health, University of California, Los Angeles, UCLA Jane & Terry Semel Institute of Neuroscience & Human Behavior, Nathanson Family Resilience Center, Los Angeles, California

EUGENE GRUDNIKOFF, MD
Assistant Professor of Psychiatry, New York City Health + Hospitals/Elmhurst, Icahn School of Medicine at Mount Sinai, Elmhurst, New York

RAJEEV KRISHNA, MD, PhD, MBA
Big Lots Behavioral Health Service Line, Medical Director of Inpatient Services, Nationwide Children's Hospital, The Ohio State University Wexner Medical Center, Assistant Professor, Clinical, Department of Psychiatry and Behavioral Health, The Ohio State University College of Medicine, Columbus, Ohio

AUTHORS

ARTHUR REESE ABRIGHT, MD
Professor of Psychiatry, New York City Health + Hospitals/Elmhurst, Icahn School of Medicine at Mount Sinai, Elmhurst, New York

ALAN AXELSON, MD
Distinguished Life Fellow, AACAP and APA, Principal, InterCare Solutions Ltd, Technology and Strategic Consulting, Pittsburgh, Pennsylvania

DAVID AXELSON, MD
Department of Psychiatry, Big Lots Behavioral Health Service Line, Nationwide Children's Hospital, The Ohio State University Wexner Medical Center, Columbus, Ohio

RACHEL BALLARD, MD
Pritzker Department of Psychiatry and Behavioral Health, Ann and Robert H. Lurie Children's Hospital of Chicago, Chicago, Illinois

JOSEPH BLADER, PhD
The University of Texas Health Science Center at San Antonio, San Antonio, Texas

MARK S. BORER, MD, DLFAPA, DFAACAP
Private Practice and Consulting Child and Adolescent Psychiatrist, Co-Chair of AACAP's Healthcare Access and Economics Committee, Psychiatric Access for Central Delaware, Dover, Delaware

DAVID BRENT, MD
Distinguished Professor of Psychiatry, Pediatrics, Epidemiology, and Clinical and Translational Science and Endowed Chair in Suicide Studies, University of Pittsburgh, School of Medicine, Pittsburgh, Pennsylvania

OSCAR G. BUKSTEIN, MD, MPH
Department of Psychiatry, Boston Children's Hospital, Department of Pediatrics, Harvard Medical School, Boston, Massachusetts

CRISTEN COLLINS, MD
Department of Psychiatry and Behavioral Health, Nationwide Children's Hospital, Department of Psychiatry and Behavioral Health, The Ohio State University Wexner Medical Center Harding Hospital, Columbus, Ohio

MICHAEL ENENBACH, MD
Associate Clinical Professor, Department of Psychiatry and Biobehavioral Sciences, Division of Child and Adolescent Psychiatry, UCLA Jane & Terry Semel Institute of Neuroscience & Human Behavior, Division of Population Behavioral Health, UCLA, Nathanson Family Resilience Center, Los Angeles, California

VICTOR M. FORNARI, MD, MS
Donald and Barbara Zucker School of Medicine at Hofstra/Northwell, Glen Oaks, New York

MARY A. FRISTAD, PhD
Department of Psychiatry, Big Lots Behavioral Health Service Line, Nationwide Children's Hospital, The Ohio State University Wexner Medical Center, Columbus, Ohio

EUGENE GRUDNIKOFF, MD
Assistant Professor of Psychiatry, New York City Health + Hospitals/Elmhurst, Icahn School of Medicine at Mount Sinai, Elmhurst, New York

SION KIM HARRIS, PhD, CPH
Center for Adolescent Behavioral Health Research, Division of Adolescent/Young Adult Medicine, Department of Medicine, Boston Children's Hospital, Department of Pediatrics, Harvard Medical School, Boston, Massachusetts

CLAUDINE HIGDON, MD
Donald and Barbara Zucker School of Medicine at Hofstra/Northwell, Glen Oaks, New York

CODY A. HOSTUTLER, PhD
Department of Pediatric Psychology and Neuropsychology, Nationwide Children's Hospital, Department of Pediatrics, The Ohio State University Columbus, Ohio

JESSICA JEFFREY, MD, MPH, MBA, FAPA, DFAACAP
Associate Clinical Professor of Psychiatry, UCLA Department of Psychiatry and Biobehavioral Sciences, Associate Medical Director of Ambulatory Psychiatry Services,

Associate Director, Division of Population Behavioral Health, University of California, Los Angeles, UCLA Jane & Terry Semel Institute of Neuroscience & Human Behavior, Nathanson Family Resilience Center, Los Angeles, California

VAMSI K. KALARI, MD
Donald and Barbara Zucker School of Medicine at Hofstra/Northwell, Glen Oaks, New York

ANNA KERLEK, MD
Department of Psychiatry and Behavioral Health, Nationwide Children's Hospital, Department of Psychiatry and Behavioral Health, The Ohio State University Wexner Medical Center Harding Hospital, Columbus, Ohio

ALEXANDRA KLOMHAUS, MS
Department of Biostatistics, Division of Population Behavioral Health, Fielding School of Public Health, UCLA, UCLA Jane & Terry Semel Institute for Neuroscience & Human Behavior, Nathanson Family Resilience Center, Los Angeles, California

RAJEEV KRISHNA, MD, PhD, MBA
Big Lots Behavioral Health Service Line, Medical Director of Inpatient Services, Nationwide Children's Hospital, The Ohio State University Wexner Medical Center, Assistant Professor, Clinical, Department of Psychiatry and Behavioral Health, The Ohio State University College of Medicine, Columbus, Ohio

JOHN LAVIGNE, PhD
Pritzker Department of Psychiatry and Behavioral Health, Ann and Robert H. Lurie Children's Hospital of Chicago, Chicago, Illinois

PATRICIA LESTER, MD
Division of Population Behavioral Health, Director, Nathanson Family Resilience Center, Nathanson Family Professor of Psychiatry, University of California, Los Angeles, Los Angeles, California

ANDREW S. LUSTBADER, MD, FAAP
Associate Clinical Professor, Yale Child Study Center, New Haven, Connecticut; Director, Therapeutic Center for Children and Families, Westport, Connecticut

SARAH MOHIUDDIN, MD
University of Michigan, Ann Arbor, Michigan

AMIT PARIKH, MD
Department of Psychiatry, Big Lots Behavioral Health Service Line, Nationwide Children's Hospital, The Ohio State University Wexner Medical Center, Columbus, Ohio

PARESH D. PATEL, MD, PhD
Clinical Professor of Psychiatry, Ambulatory Care Clinical Chief and Director of Health IT in Psychiatry, Michigan Medicine, Ann Arbor, Michigan

ADAM C. POWELL, PhD
Payer+Provider Syndicate, Boston, Massachusetts

UJJWAL RAMTEKKAR, MD, MPE, MBA
Department of Child and Adolescent Psychiatry, Nationwide Children's Hospital, Department of Psychiatry, The Ohio State University Columbus, Ohio

ELENA RODRIGUEZ-VILLA, BS
Department of Psychiatry, Beth Israel Deaconess Medical Center, Harvard Medical
School, Boston, Massachusetts

COURTNEY ROMBA, MD
Pritzker Department of Psychiatry and Behavioral Health, Ann and Robert H. Lurie
Children's Hospital of Chicago, Chicago, Illinois

BARRY SARVET, MD
Professor and Chair, Department of Psychiatry, University of Massachusetts Medical
School-Baystate, Baystate Medical Center, Statewide Medical Director, Massachusetts
Child Psychiatry Access Program, Springfield, Massachusetts

LYDIA A. SHRIER, MD, MPH
Center for Adolescent Behavioral Health Research, Division of Adolescent/Young Adult
Medicine, Department of Medicine, Boston Children's Hospital, Department of Pediatrics,
Harvard Medical School, Boston, Massachusetts

KEVIN M. SIMON, MD
Department of Psychiatry, Boston Children's Hospital, Harvard Medical School,
Adolescent Substance Use and Addiction Program, Division of Developmental Medicine,
Department of Pediatrics, Boston Children's Hospital, Boston, Massachusetts

JOHN TOROUS, MD, MBI
Department of Psychiatry, Beth Israel Deaconess Medical Center, Harvard Medical
School, Boston, Massachusetts

JOHN WALKUP, MD
Pritzker Department of Psychiatry and Behavioral Health, Ann and Robert H. Lurie
Children's Hospital of Chicago, Chicago, Illinois

BONNIE T. ZIMA, MD, MPH
Professor-in-Residence, UCLA Jane & Terry Semel Institute for Neuroscience & Human
Behavior, University of California, Los Angeles, UCLA Center for Health Services and
Society, Los Angeles, California

Contents

Measurement-based care (MBC) is recognized as a valuable component to maximize quality in psychiatric care; however, actual use of MBC by practitioners is poor. A host of implementation barriers have been noted, and are likely significant contributors to this poor adoption. Many of these barriers are related to work-flow issues that can be managed or mitigated by appropriate infrastructure considerations. This article offers an overview of the continuum of infrastructures to support MBC in clinical practice, delineating the tradeoffs between these infrastructures, and then identifying specific experience-based strategies for addressing several major patient-, provider-, and organization-level barriers to MBC implementation.

Measurement-based care (MBC) is the routine collection of data using standardized, validated measures and use of these data to guide treatment. MBC has been implemented throughout medicine to improve patient outcomes, but its use in mental health care remains low. This article summarizes the evidence of MBC's efficacy in adults then reviews the sparser data in youth mental health care. The literature indicates that MBC must be administered immediately before or during every encounter, results must be available to and reviewed by providers immediately, results must be shared with the patient, and results must be used to guide treatment.

Measurement-based care involves the practice of systematically administrating rating scales to patients in order to use the collected information to enhance clinical evaluation, monitor treatment progress, and directly inform decisions relating to each patient's treatment. Rating scales must be psychometrically validated and efficiently administered within the practice setting. Brief rating scales that are available within the public domain may help to optimize workflows and prevent response fatigue. Clinicians should also have a sufficient understanding of the underlying psychometric properties of rating scales to accurately interpret changes in scores over time and use these results to appropriately direct care.

Section II: Clinical Applications

Measurement-based care is a helpful adjunct to clinical assessment in improving outcomes in depression in adults and adolescents. Measurement-based care principles are incorporated in current regulatory requirements for use of standardized instruments in efforts to improve care and prevent suicide. Challenges for child and adolescent psychiatrists and other clinicians in implementing measurement-based care include concerns about time and expense involved in administration and interpretation of results from rating scales and other instruments. Implementation can be facilitated by selection of instruments that are brief, easy to administer and score, compatible with electronic health record systems, and available in the public domain.

Treatment of pediatric anxiety disorders is complicated by their number, comorbidity, and the differential impact of a child's anxiety on the child and parents. Measurement-based care, using patient-level rating scales, can guide clinical decisions, track symptom improvement, and monitor treatment response. We review instruments for measurement-based care in pediatric anxiety. Measures used to track pediatric anxiety should be brief, accessible, sensitive to change, and reliable. Because parent–child agreement about a child's anxiety tends to be low, measures from both should be obtained. Measurements can also track functional improvement, expectancy related to treatment, and readiness to change.

Attention-deficit/hyperactivity disorder (ADHD) is one of the most common childhood psychiatric diagnoses. The core symptoms of ADHD include inattention, impulsivity, and hyperactivity. ADHD entails impairments that have extensive and profound detrimental effects on many critical developmental areas. As a valid neurobiologic condition that causes significant impairments in those affected, it is one of the best-researched disorders in medicine. Measurement-based care in treatment of ADHD is critical in establishing a diagnosis, determining a treatment target, and assessing treatment response. This article highlights the rationale for measurement-based care in ADHD, how to implement measurement-based care in clinical practice, and common challenges encountered.

Measurement-based care in adolescent substance use is an important element of the evidence-based framework of Screening, Brief Intervention, and Referral to Treatment (SBIRT). Use of a validated measure for detecting substance use, misuse, and substance use disorders is significantly more effective than the use of unvalidated tools or clinician intuition. There are now a variety of established and new validated screening tools that are available for use with adolescents and that capture the range of adolescent substance use behaviors. This area, however, continues to evolve rapidly.

Challenges associated with the integration of pediatric mental health care in the primary care setting include limitations of training and time, high volume of patients, need for coordination with external specialists, limited infrastructure, and limited funding. All of these issues can negatively influence the quality of mental health service delivery. Measurement-based care (MBC) processes have the potential to mitigate many of these challenges and generate data, allowing practices to evaluate and improve the performance of integrated mental health processes. Implementing MBC requires initial investment of staff resources for planning and training and information technology resources.

Section III: Special Considerations

Measurement-based care is conceptualized as a driver for quality improvement. The triple aim in the National Quality Strategy purposively muddles the population levels to provide a health policy goal that is encompassing, transactional, and will stimulate change. Specification of the population level has implications for the purpose, proposed target mechanisms that drive quality improvement, methodologic challenges, and implications for program evaluation and data interpretation. To demonstrate, population levels are conceptualized at the individual (tier 1), clinical aggregate (tier 2), and national level (tier 3).

Although screening can significantly improve the identification of youth with mental health needs in primary care, there is no evidence that screening improves outcomes. Measurement-based care using clinical mental health registries has been shown to improve screening outcomes in adult primary care populations and pediatric physical health needs; however, there is limited attention to pediatric mental health registries in

a research role in generating aggregated data. Psychiatric illnesses are multifactorial and not uniform in nature, patient distress/suffering have a complex etiology, and appropriate treatments are varied. Measures commonly used in measurement-based care are subjective ratings of symptom severity. In clinical mental health settings, measurement-based care may contribute more of a qualitative role as part of the psychiatric input to the identification and severity of illness. Psychiatrists must limit the use of measurement-based care in assisting the assessment of patient progress.

CHILD AND ADOLESCENT PSYCHIATRIC CLINICS

FORTHCOMING ISSUES

January 2021
Sleep Disorders in Children and Adolescents
Argelinda Baroni and Jessica Lunsford-Avery, *Editors*

April 2021
Emotion Dysregulation in Children: Part I
Gabrielle A. Carlson and Manpreet K. Singh, *Editors*

July 2021
Emotion Dysregulation in Children: Part II
Gabrielle A. Carlson and Manpreet K. Singh, *Editors*

RECENT ISSUES

July 2020
Autism Spectrum Disorder Across the Lifespan: Part II
Robert W. Wisner-Carlson, Scott R. Pekrul, Thomas Flis, and Robert Schloesser, *Editors*

April 2020
Autism Spectrum Disorder Across the Lifespan: Part I
Robert W. Wisner-Carlson, Scott R. Pekrul, Thomas Flis, and Robert Schloesser, *Editors*

January 2020
Psychosis in Children and Adolescents: A Guide for Clinicians
Ellen M. House and John W. Tyson, *Editors*

SERIES OF RELATED INTEREST

Psychiatric Clinics of North America
https://www.psych.theclinics.com/
Pediatric Clinics of North America
https://www.pediatric.theclinics.com/
Neurologic Clinics
https://www.neurologic.theclinics.com/

AACAP Members: Please go to www.jaacap.org for information on access to the Child and Adolescent Psychiatric Clinics. *Resident* Members of AACAP: Special access information is available at www.childpsych.theclinics.com.

THE CLINICS ARE AVAILABLE ONLINE!
Access your subscription at:
www.theclinics.com

Preface
The Time Has Come for Measurement-Based Care in Child and Adolescent Psychiatry

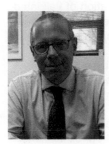
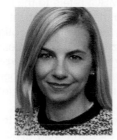
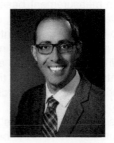

Barry Sarvet, MD   Jessica Jeffrey, MD, MPH, MBA   Eugene Grudnikoff, MD

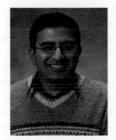

Rajeev Krishna, MD, PhD

Editors

For generations, children's mental health services have been undervalued within the health care system. This has been exemplified by inadequate funding, interminable persistence of inadequate access to care for everyone, insured and uninsured, and significant disparities in mental health care for people of color, people living in poverty, and disenfranchised, marginalized communities. A pervasive belief justifying this state of affairs is that mental health care is like a "black hole"—the idea that no matter what we do to address mental health conditions, it will never be enough. We all know that stigma against people with mental health conditions underlies this idea, particularly the notion that mental health conditions are intrinsic flaws in the essential nature of human beings, and a cynical view of the effectiveness of treatment, despite mountains of

Child Adolesc Psychiatric Clin N Am 29 (2020) xiii–xvi
https://doi.org/10.1016/j.chc.2020.07.001
1056-4993/20/© 2020 Published by Elsevier Inc.

evidence to the contrary. Related to this is a belief that mental health conditions are essentially subjective and not as "real" as physical health conditions. Parents frequently wish there could be a lab test to confirm their child's psychiatric diagnosis. This wish belies a desire, not only for precision but also for validation of what they already know in the face of widespread implicit bias against the objective reality of the child's mental health condition. Most mental health professionals are antistigma warriors; however, our reluctance to incorporate quantitative measurement in the process of clinical practice may reinforce stigma by appearing to buy in to the belief that mental health is essentially unmeasurable and by implication not objectively real.

The term measurement-based care (MBC) refers to the incorporation of validated quantitative clinical measures, usually in the form of patient-reported outcome measures, into the process of mental health treatment. With optimal implementation, the measures are tailored to the individualized goals of the treatment plan. The results and trending of the measures are jointly reviewed and interpreted by both providers and patients in order to inform the assessment of patient progress, and in turn, collaborative decision making regarding ongoing modification of interventions in the treatment plan.

The reasons for psychiatrists' reluctance to adopt MBC in the process of psychiatric care are manifold. One is the belief that we don't really need it, that our clinical interviewing skills are much more accurate than a brief questionnaire in judging patient progress. It's certainly tempting to believe this, if only it were true. A study by Hatfield and colleagues[1] demonstrated surprisingly poor concordance of informal ratings of progress by mental health clinicians with independent assessments. Given that widespread erosion of professional satisfaction among physicians is often attributed to increasing administrative burdens within clinical practice, the question of whether or not measures add value is extremely pertinent indeed. Another reason for limited adoption of MBC is a concern that patients will be annoyed by filling out questionnaires and that patients would have less confidence in their clinician for using these tools to gauge progress. In contradiction to this view, a study by Dowrick and colleagues[2] demonstrated that the use of clinical measures was well received by patients, that patients most commonly considered the process to signify increased thoroughness of their care, and that the measures helped them to express themselves to their provider.

In this issue, the article by Parikh and colleagues summarizes an accumulating body of evidence that MBC is clinically valuable and associated with improved outcomes. The discussion by Axelson and Brent addresses the importance of MBC in improving funding and increasing the parity of mental health treatment in relation to other health care services. A significant portion of the issue is devoted to implementation of MBC for various applications within child and adolescent psychiatry practice, including the article by Jeffrey and colleagues regarding measure selection, and separate articles on the use of MBC for specific children's mental health syndromes as well as the utilization of MBC in the primary care setting. Making MBC a part of routine care will require health information technology resources to facilitate the administration, scoring, and interpretation of clinical measures. The article by Torous and colleagues discusses innovations in mobile health technology in support of MBC.

There is an inverted common sense argument in support of MBC that has been made, which goes something like this: "Not using quantitative measures in the context of psychiatric practice is analogous to a primary care doctor prescribing insulin to a patient with insulin-dependent diabetes without measuring blood glucose." This is a somewhat specious argument because quantitative measures of mental health status are arguably not as precise as blood glucose measurement, and mental health treatments do not have nearly as dynamic a dose/response relationship as that of insulin. Nonetheless, as argued by Fortney and colleagues,[3] we appear to be at a "tipping point" in regard to MBC with growing scientific consensus of its value, prompting recent moves by The Joint Commission and other regulators of health care delivery to treat the adoption of MBC as an expectation rather than an exhortation for mental health providers.

Regardless of the opinions of rank and file psychiatrists, it does appear that the time for widespread adoption of MBC has come, and in this context it is important that we acknowledge that MBC has a "dark side," related primarily to the potential for its misuse and incorrect application. In their counterpoint article at the end of the issue, Lustbader and Borer explore the potential harms of MBC, notably associated with the reductionistic use of clinical measurement as a substitute rather than a complement to a traditional clinical interview, as well as the concern that insurance companies would withhold authorization of payment for the care of patients who are not demonstrating linear progress in their treatment. Some children's mental health professionals have seen this before in the education sector associated with the dramatic expansion in standardized educational testing from the No Child Left Behind Act of 2001, resulting in erosion of the quality of public education stemming from "teaching to the test" and linkage of federal funding of public schools with performance on standardized testing. This underscores the importance of articulating clinically sound applications of MBC and ongoing advocacy for improved funding for children's mental health services.

Barry Sarvet, MD
Department of Psychiatry
University of Massachusetts
Medical School–Baystate
WG703, 759 Chestnut Street
Springfield, MA, USA

Jessica Jeffrey, MD, MPH, MBA
Department of Psychiatry and
Biobehavioral Sciences
University of California Los Angeles
760 Westwood Plaza, A7-372
Los Angeles, CA 90024, USA

Eugene Grudnikoff, MD
Icahn School of Medicine at Mount Sinai
New York City Health + Hospitals/Elmhurst
79-01 Broadway
Elmhurst, NY 11373, USA

Rajeev Krishna, MD, PhD
Nationwide Children's Hospital
Psychiatry and Behavioral Health
T5 700 Children's Drive
Columbus, OH 43205, USA

E-mail addresses:
barry.sarvet@baystatehealth.org (B. Sarvet)
JJeffrey@mednet.ucla.edu (J. Jeffrey)
grudnikoffe@nychhc.org (E. Grudnikoff)
Rajeev.Krishna@nationwidechildrens.org (R. Krishna)

REFERENCES

1. Hatfield D, McCullough L, Frantz SH, et al. Do we know when our clients get worse? An investigation of therapists' ability to detect negative client change. Clin Psychol Psychother 2010;17(1):25–32.
2. Dowrick C, Leydon G, McBride A, et al. Patients' and doctors' views on depression severity questionnaires incentivised in UK quality and outcomes framework: qualitative study. BMJ 2009;338:b663.
3. Fortney JC, Unutzer J, Wrenn G, et al. A tipping point for measurement-based care. Psychiatr Serv 2017;68(2):179–88.

Section I: Overarching Principles

Implementing Measurement-Based Care in Various Practice Settings

Rajeev Krishna, MD, PhD, MBA[a,b,*], Jessica Jeffrey, MD, MPH, MBA[c,d],
Paresh D. Patel, MD, PhD[e]

KEYWORDS

- Measurement feedback system • Implementation barriers • Psychiatric care
- Work flow

KEY POINTS

- Implementation challenges create significant barriers to the adoption of measurement-based care (MBC).
- Multiple MBC infrastructure frameworks exist and can impact the barriers and complexities of adoption and uptake.
- Recognition and management of specific structural and infrastructure barriers can help support a successful implementation.

INTRODUCTION

Measurement-based care (MBC) is the health care process of identifying clear and measurable treatment targets for a given disorder, regularly monitoring current treatment progress against this target, and continuing treatment adjustments until the desired target is reached. In psychiatry and mental health care, it is the use of validated, standardized, self-reported measures of pathology and impairment that can be used to mark these treatment goals and establish progress.[1] Although the value of MBC in psychiatry has been recognized for years, the difficulty of implementing systems to achieve consistent use of MBC in psychiatry has been an ongoing and vexing problem for the field, with actual use persistently under 20% of practitioners.[2] As is often the case in situations in which it has been difficult to translate evidence-based care into effective practice, a host of implementation barriers impedes progress.[3]

[a] Big Lots Behavioral Health Service Line, Nationwide Children's Hospital, Columbus, OH, USA; [b] Department of Psychiatry and Behavioral Health, The Ohio State University College of Medicine, Columbus, OH, USA; [c] Department of Psychiatry and Biobehavioral Sciences, Division of Population Behavioral Health, UCLA Jane and Terry Semel Institute of Neuroscience and Human Behavior, 760 Westwood Plaza, A7-372, Los Angeles, CA 90024, USA; [d] Nathanson Family Resilience Center, Los Angeles, CA 90024, USA; [e] Department of Psychiatry, The University of Michigan College of Medicine, 4250 Plymouth Road, Ann Arbor, MI 48109, USA
* Corresponding author.
E-mail address: Rajeev.Krishna@nationwidechildrens.org

Child Adolesc Psychiatric Clin N Am 29 (2020) 573–586
https://doi.org/10.1016/j.chc.2020.06.007
1056-4993/20/© 2020 Elsevier Inc. All rights reserved.

childpsych.theclinics.com

Although there is little formal literature around implementation of MBC to guide organizations and providers, there is a growing body of case studies, implementation experience, and anecdotal knowledge that can be valuable. This article attempts to capture experiences of several institutions in the implementation of MBC systems, distilling common themes and strategies that may be applicable across the spectrum of psychiatric practice. The authors begin by providing some background on the major implementation barriers to MBC, then offer a framework for considering major implementation infrastructures, and close by exploring more individual considerations that span infrastructures but must be considered in any MBC implementation effort.

BACKGROUND AND SCOPE

The use of MBC methodology has been demonstrated to lead to improved treatment outcomes in psychiatric patients in a variety of settings.[1,4–6] Despite evidence in support of this practice, it remains challenging to implement the infrastructures necessary to consistently acquire and track outcome measures in patients. Indeed, the implementation challenge around MBC is felt to be among the greatest barriers to adoption of this otherwise evidence-based methodology. A recent review article discusses the burden of implementation and the impact on adoption of MBC.[3] Specifically, barriers to the implementation of MBC are divided into groups with key barriers in each.

Patient-level barriers include

- Motivation to complete measures
- Time to complete measures
- Concerns about confidentiality
- Comfort and facility with applicable technologies

Provider-Level barriers include

- Preference for own clinical assessment/lack of recognition of value
- Administrative burden/impact on flow
- Impact on payments and coverage
- Lack of training

Organizational-Level barriers include

- Data infrastructure constraints and integration with existing health records
- Fear of liability in unmonitored systems
- Technology management and integration

System-Level barriers include

- Reimbursements
- Systemic incentives versus costs

Although this provides a useful framework for understanding the source of overall resistance, the authors are only able to offer high-level insights into conceptual strategies to alter these trends, ultimately concluding the need for added research in this regard. Unfortunately, there is limited literature dedicated to describing practical solutions to the implementation barriers posed.

Given the limited information available on practical strategies to address implementation barriers, this article attempts to provide a framework for considering these barriers combined with anecdotal implementation experience from the authors, who have been working in large systems to implement MBC infrastructures for many years. This article will specifically discuss strategies for addressing patient-, provider-, and organizational-level barriers to MBC at the infrastructure and implementation level. System-level barriers, including the impact of reimbursements and larger systemic effects are notably highlighted in other articles of this issue, as are extensive discussions around the clinical utility and use of measures. Thus this article will discuss the practical question of how a provider's choice of measures for a patient can be conveyed to the follow-up visit and appropriately administered, rather than the clinical question of how to select those measures.

INFRASTRUCTURE SELECTION

One of the most significant decisions to be made with respect to the implementation of MBC is infrastructure that will be utilized. There are a range of infrastructure options, from simple paper-and-pencil assessment tools to fully automated systems that provide longitudinal and aggregate views of data. These options fall along a continuum that trades off simplicity, automation, human factors, and cost along multiple dimensions. As the selection of infrastructure will largely impact the effect of other barriers, consideration of these infrastructure options is the first step in approaching MBC implementation.

To understand the impact of infrastructure selection, it is important to consider the process flow that is being affected. **Fig. 1** depicts an overview of the implementation and flow of MBC, from the implementation decision itself, through the cycle of actions representing the care of an individual patient across multiple encounters. These steps represent a framework for considering intervention points and potential barriers that impact the adoption of MBC in a given practice setting:

- Provider decides to implement MBC. This step represents the process a provider or organization goes through to determine that MBC is useful and worth implementing. Many of the cognitive barriers (recognizing the evidence and value) of MBC are addressed in other articles of this issue.
- Measure acquisition. This represents the process of acquiring the appropriate measures. These may be proprietary or public domain. Although the measures themselves are discussed elsewhere, the infrastructure selected impacts the availability of such measures in a given context.
- Measure selection. This step represents the actual selection of appropriate measures for a given patient.

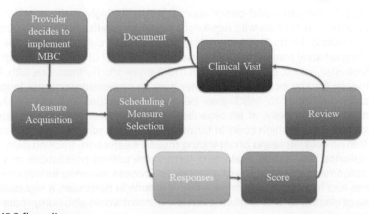

Fig. 1. MBC flow diagram.

- Responses. This represents the process of administering selected measures to a particular patient or family.
- Score. This step represents the need to score and report on the responses provided.
- Review. This step represents the review of results by the provider in preparation for the clinical visit.
- Clinical visit. This step represents the clinical visit, with use of data from longitudinally collected measures to help inform and guide interactions and treatment decisions.
- Document. This step represents the process of documenting the results of the clinical visit, including the results of collected measures. It captures, in particular, the need to document these results whether using paper or electronic health record systems, and the potential time and complexity consumed in this process.

The cycle of MBC ends once again in scheduling and measure selection, as the determination of which measures are appropriate is continuously revised to match the current needs of a given patient.

With this framework in place, one can consider several of the various broad infrastructure choices involved in launching an MBC program, and in particular can consider the components of the MBC process cycle that are positively or negatively impacted by each option.

Paper and Pencil

Perhaps the easiest and most straightforward approach to the implementation of MBC is the use of paper measures administered at the time of assessment and manually scored. Consideration of how this impacts the flow diagram is depicted in **Fig. 2**. This is the obvious traditional model used in the absence of electronic resources, and has been available for decades. It offers the clear advantage of immediate access, low infrastructure cost, and high flexibility. Individual providers can simply access public domain measures online and administer them to patients on an as-needed basis. This model similarly offers access to a range of copyrighted measures that are easily available through purchase of the actual measure and scoring rubric. This all serves to lower the entry bar for implementing MBC from an infrastructure standpoint. Two easy sources of paper measures that can be immediately implemented include those shown in **Box 1**.

Unfortunately, the paper-and-pencil approach incurs a high overall cost despite the low entry barrier and clashes with regulatory inertia for digitization and sharing of the entire health record. Formally, the monetary cost saved through use of a paper based system is immediately traded off against the monetary cost of provider or staff time to select, administer, score, and document in this framework. Furthermore, although the review process for any individual encounter may be straightforward, the longitudinal data tracking essential to MBC also becomes a manual and potentially time-consuming process. Finally, at an organizational and system level, the paper-and-pencil approach creates high costs in terms of data management, integrity, and verifiability. With no central means of organizing measure selection, tracking data, or verifying compliance, use of aggregate data to manage patient populations or evaluate provider outcomes becomes at best a laborious process requiring further investment of staff time and resources. For larger health systems in particular, a regulatory drive toward use of electronic data capture and management would also complicate the use of this methodology.

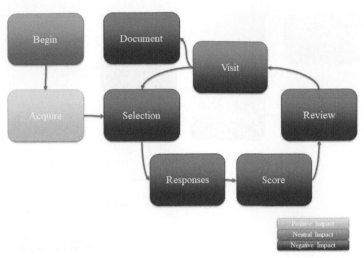

Fig. 2. Paper and Pencil implementation impacts.

Basic Automation

The first step along the continuum from paper-and-pencil to full automation is to automate some of the core processes of MBC. The administration, scoring, and reporting of specific outcome measures is a natural target for this type of automation, and this is what is offered by basic automation systems. Consideration of how this impacts the flow diagram is depicted in **Fig. 3**. Rather than acquiring and administering a paper-and-pencil assessment, the provider or staff presents patients with an electronic device (iPad or kiosk computer) that is configured to administer a specific set of assessments, and score and report on the results. The intent is to literally replicate the paper-and-pencil process, while eliminating the most laborious steps that gain the least from human intervention. To that end, such systems can significantly lower the workflow and staff time complexity of implementing MBC. The PROMIS question bank noted earlier for paper-and-pencil forms also offers several computer-administered testing options, and is a good resource for this domain of functionality. More broadly, online tools for administering certain individual measures can be found by Internet search, although the validity and security may vary. Several professional organizations also provide resources in this domain, including the ePRO app from the National Network of Depression Centers, and the PsychPRO system by the APA, although scope and capabilities vary. Some such systems are integrated with federal payers to submit MIPS (Merit-based Incentive Payment System) data, which can be financially beneficial to participating practices.

Box 1	
Sources of paper measures	
APA Online Assessment Measures	https://www.psychiatry.org/psychiatrists/practice/dsm/educational-resources/assessment-measures
PROMIS measures[7]	http://www.healthmeasures.net/explore-measurement-systems/promis

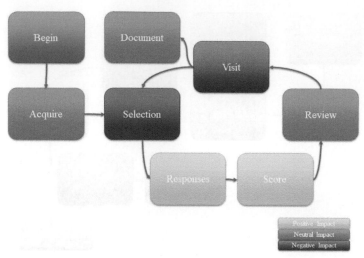

Fig. 3. Basic Automation implementation impacts.

Although basic automation systems provide a notable step up from paper and pencil, and have the advantage of still being relatively cheap, their limited focus also means that many of the same challenges of paper-and-pencil systems remain. The biggest impact of these systems is on administration and scoring, and because the results can be reported in a consistent way and are already in electronic form, review and documentation are also simplified. Lack of integration with health record systems can cause a significant barrier, particularly in larger health systems where system and regulatory pressure mandates that this information then be manually transferred to the electronic health record. Also, while these systems may make the acquisition of valid assessments in the public domain easier, proprietary assessments are unlikely to be available, and depending on system architecture, individual measures may need to be manually assigned at each visit.

Full Automation

There are several commercial products available that offer full automation and management of patient measures to allow for implementation of MBC. Consideration of how this impacts the flow diagram is depicted in **Fig. 4**. These systems allow for automated administration, scoring, and reporting of selected measures as with basic automation, but now add longitudinal tracking of data and individuation of patients. This means that these systems can not only track data for a particular patient or guardian independently and collate these data together as part of an easy-to-review reporting system, but they are also able to remember the assessments a particular patient might need, and automatically administer them at specific intervals without provider or staff intervention. These systems can even be used to collect assessment information from home, or from third-party individuals such as teachers or grandparents. Some offer automated screening and selection of appropriate measures with subsequent provider refinement. Various degrees of electronic health record integration are also available depending on the vendor.

The process for utilizing such a commercial system involves signing up with a vendor and training on that vendor's system. A patient caseload must then be loaded into the system, with necessary contact information and assessment requirements

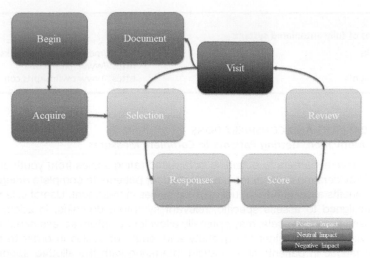

Fig. 4. Full automation implementation impacts.

that can be managed in an ongoing way. In large part, the system will then manage the work of prompting for assessment completion, collecting and scoring the results, and presenting organized results with longitudinal data for review.

Although this is all highly valuable functionality, it does come with a price. As of this writing, there are no free options for acquiring this level of sophistication. Prices and functionality vary across vendors and must be explored to determine the best fit for a particular provider, practice, or institution. In general, such systems are also constrained to public domain measures, or measures that have a specific licensing arrangement with the vendor. The costs involved do trade off against staff and provider time needed for the other options. Examples of such systems include those shown in **Box 2**.

Electronic Health Record Integrated Systems

The final category of MBC infrastructure that must be considered is something of a lateral move from the fully automated systems just described, and those are the integrated patient-reported outcome tools that are built into most modern electronic health record (EHR) systems. Consideration of how this impacts the flow diagram is depicted in **Fig. 5**. Perhaps the biggest advantage of these systems is that if an institution is utilizing an EHR with such functionality, this capability is already present and likely already deployed. Furthermore, some assessment measures may already be present in the system (eg: the PROMIS question banks are integrated into several EHR systems). A potential down-side of these systems compared with independent fully automated products is that patient outcome measures are a small component of the scope of EHR systems, and thus particularly for behavioral health are generally not as carefully considered or sophisticated as the dedicated commercial systems focusing solely on this population. For child psychiatrists, a notable failing is the limited ability to capture data from third-party respondents such as teachers, although this is less of a problem in the adult domain. Given the unique conflict of considering a custom versus integrated solution for an institution that already has an EHR with patient reported outcome measures, a more detailed exploration of this can be found later in this article.

Box 2	
Examples of fully automated systems	
BH-Works	https://mdlogix.com/bhworks-page/
Mirah	https://www.mirah.com/
OWL Insights	https://www.owlinsights.com/

PATIENT BARRIERS AND CONSIDERATIONS
Creating Motivation: Getting Patients to Complete Measures

There are several barriers to obtaining completed rating scales from youth and their parents. Providers must weigh the time needed for patients to complete rating scales with the benefits associated with using rating scales in treatment. Use of select rating scales, designed to assess specific, relevant symptom domains, in addition to a broad-based symptom scale, may optimally allow for symptom assessment;[8] however, a provider must consider the quantity and length of scales in order to prevent response fatigue in patients and to avoid interfering with the allotted appointment time.[9]

In addition to the challenges of optimally designing an effective clinical workflow, it is essential that patients have an awareness that obtaining rating scale results is important to their providers and that the results will be used to guide treatment and monitor outcomes. Ultimately, patients will only complete rating scales if it is clear both in messaging and in behaviors that these scales are important to their care, and that the results are actively used by the treatment team. Implementation of rating scales within clinical settings requires clear messaging to administrative staff and patients that rating scales are a component of standard clinical care, as administrative staff may be asked to introduce and administer rating scales to youth and their caregivers. Thus, staff must appreciate the clinical importance of rating scales and receive training to introduce rating scales. Staff may be trained to explain that rating scales are used to measure behavioral health vital signs, analogous to how primary care physicians measure vital signs such as height, weight, blood pressure, and pulse.[9] They

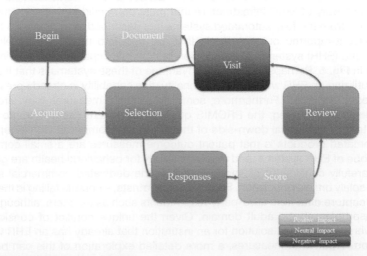

Fig. 5. EHR implementation impacts.

should also provide patients with information about the approximate time needed to complete rating scales and inform patients of the confidentiality and security of their responses.[9] When a provider discusses rating scale results with a patient during the appointment, this reinforces the importance of the rating scale scores to guide care and, thus, may increase patients' willingness to complete rating scales prior to subsequent appointments.

As a final practical strategy, creating time prior to appointments in order to complete rating scales is helpful, and in some populations vital. Pursuant to the concept of behavioral health vital signs, time should be allocated prior to the start of the face-to-face encounter to complete scales, just as it is for height, weight, and blood pressure. In practice, it is useful to explicitly schedule patients to arrive at the clinic prior to their actual provider face-to-face time (as allocated on the provider's schedule) to complete these tasks. The authors' experience has been that explicitly scheduling patients to arrive before their formal visit so that there is 1 clear scheduled time and the visit time with the provider is essentially hidden is more effective even than providing a traditionally scheduled time and requesting/reminding patients to arrive early, as is the more common practice.[10]

Creating Time: the Tradeoffs of Completing Measures at Home

The ability to deploy and administer assessments from home has several potential advantages and is a major selling point for automated and commercial systems. Foremost, the ability to have patients and families complete assessments before coming to the office reduces the workflow and clinic flow management needs during clinic visits. Theoretically, this eliminates not only the need to arrange for patients to present early for visits to complete assessments, but also eliminates the need to deploy and manage the technology to support this activity during the check-in process. This functionality also introduces an entirely new realm of clinical management strategies, allowing a provider to remotely assess and follow up with some patients between clinic visits, or potentially even reduce the frequency of visits for certain patient classes (eg, stable monitoring) without increasing the related risk of interval unrecognized decompensation. Importantly, this functionality is also generally seen as a preferred option by patients and families.

Despite these advantages, there are several clinical challenges that arise and must be considered and accounted for. From a practical workflow standpoint, although it is theoretically possible to avoid the infrastructure and clinic flow issues associated with completing measures in the office, a significant fraction of any given patient population is likely to forget or be unable to complete assessments prior to arrival. Thus, if the intent is to ensure completion of measures before all visits (to achieve true clinical utility), a backup system must be in place to capture this subpopulation. Perhaps the more vexing clinical questions are how to manage a greater time separation between data collection and review, and which questions are appropriate to ask outside of a clinical encounter. For example, one would find general agreement that a set of measures completed in the morning for an afternoon visit are likely valid for that encounter, but less agreement for the same measures completed a week prior. Similarly, one might find general agreement that a suicidality assessment is appropriate in the office just prior to a clinical encounter, but the same assessment completed at home the evening prior (after the clinic has closed) is immediately fraught with legal, ethical, and potentially infrastructure implications (eg, whether positive critical patient responses are immediately addressed by on-call staff).

Managing Confidentiality and Security

One of the identified challenges of electronic collection of mental health outcome measures is patient concern about confidentiality of responses. This spans the range from family members concerned about confidentiality against other family members (eg, pediatric patient and a parent), to broader concern about others in health care accessing mental health information. Traditionally, the option to make mental health data sensitive and separate from the general medical record has been part of the solution, but this trades confidentiality for a perpetuation of the stigma of mental health treatment and also prevents needed information from being accessible to other providers. In many instances, confidentiality concerns can be addressed by direct disclosure and communication. In the authors' practices, mental health records are not segregated, with little concern from patients and few related errors. When considering infrastructures, however, a separate system from the primary medical record with capabilities to segregate information and provide confidentiality within the family unit may be of value.

PROVIDER BARRIERS AND CONSIDERATIONS
Overcoming Provider Perception and Training

One of the notable and unfortunate facts about MBC in psychiatry is the degree to which providers have not adopted or accepted the process despite a growing body of evidence demonstrating value. This creates a major barrier to overall engagement, because patients will quickly identify that a provider is not interested in the data they are producing, and will themselves disengage from the process. The key barriers to this acceptance tend to revolve around the sense that MBC is not as valuable as a clinical examination, or quite to the contrary fear that MBC will essentially replace their clinical examination (at least in the eyes of administrators and payers). By contrast, the authors' experience has been that once providers become used to the idea of MBC and see that their key concerns do not bear out, feedback about such systems is quite positive.[10] Although the issue of demonstrating the evidence and value is left to other articles, this supports the notion that pushing forward with a well thought out MBC implementation supplemented with education about the value of MBC can be successful at altering perception and increasing buy-in.

Managing Workflows

Building and maintaining provider buy-in can be a challenge, but this is increased by negative or perceived negative impacts on work-flow. One way of reducing this initial activation energy is by setting up the infrastructure to explicitly provide value beyond the measures themselves. Infrastructure selection affects this, with greater value to be gained from automated systems that minimize the added work for the provider and report outcomes in a way that can be easily integrated into documentation. Similarly, although not formal MBC, the collection of useful history information (eg, psychiatric history, medication history, and medication compliance) prior to a visit can reduce the time during the visit to collect basic information and reduce subsequent documentation time. In effect, as depicted in **Fig. 6**, the provider's work can be broken down into the patient interaction and documentation, which can be further broken down into alliance building, history collection/history documentation, and treatment planning/plan documentation. An infrastructure that can reduce the data collection and documentation burden creates more time to extract the actual value of the face-to-face interaction (alliance building, diagnostic clarification, and treatment planning) and reduce the overall documentation burden. These benefits accrue to the provider almost immediately and help bridge the gap to consistent MBC usage, so long as careful consideration is given to these opportunities as part of the implementation and roll-out plan, including early discussions with billing and compliance representatives to ensure smooth integration of MBC data and minimum need for repeat documentation.

ORGANIZATIONAL BARRIERS AND CONSIDERATIONS
Managing Risk in Unmonitored Systems

One of the frequent considerations for both large and small practice organizations when deploying a MBC framework is concern about risk and liability if a patient offers critical responses to an assessment in an unmonitored situation (eg, completed from home between visits, or missed by the provider for other reasons). There is legal uncertainty around the effectiveness of disclaimers and other warnings to seek higher levels of care when using such systems in mental health. Although there are currently no final answers to this question, empiric evidence suggests the medicolegal fear may be exaggerated. At one of the author's institutions (Michigan Medicine), self-injury and suicide questions have been asked electronically, days before an upcoming appointment, for over 15 years, with health system legal approval of disclaimer language, without active monitoring of responses, and without adverse events attributable to unreviewed responses. This experience suggesting patients may be trusted to use the portal responsibly and follow instructions to seek a higher level of care when warranted.

Electronic Health Record Integration

Given the degree to which EHR systems are a part of modern medical and mental health care, the authors consider here the tradeoffs in using an existing EHR system as the infrastructure tool for MBC implementation, versus the potential downsides of this option.

Advantages of deploying MBC through an existing EHR system include

- Data consolidation. All aspects of the outcome measures workflow are maintained in the EHR and within the patient's record, including when they are assigned, who assigned them, when the patient completed them, and all associated responses and comments. Among other things, this limits the data breach security risk to that associated with the EHR.
- Automation of measure assignment. Access to the EHR permits various degrees of automation ranging from manual assignment to fully unsupervised assignment

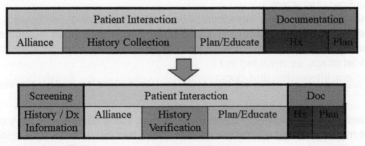

Fig. 6. History collection impact on provider workflow.

based on scheduling department, chief complaint, visit type, or even individual provider name.

- Alignment with other workflows. Integration can leverage the full breadth of the EHR, including but not limited to scheduled visits, scheduling notes, provider notes, visit diagnoses, problem lists, review of systems, orders, and clinical decision support. For example, responses to a screening measure in primary care can trigger an alert or queue up orders for specialty service referral.
- Decreases the technology burden to patients, by leveraging the patient's EHR portal, which is already supported by most EHRs and the tool of choice for patient engagement self-care. In the authors' experience, each additional Web login adds a cognitive load that erodes compliance. Some elderly are particularly wary of or taxed by digital tools. Integration with the EHR inherently confers credibility and (in enabled systems) permits outcome measure collection without the burden of logging in to a Web interface.
- Avoids redundancy. For example, when Meaningful Use, now called the Merit-based Incentive Payment System (MIPS) drove the deployment of depression screening throughout large health systems, only system-wide solutions avoided the risk of the same measure being pushed by different departments at a frequency inconsistent with the psychometric properties of the measure.
- Aligns with enterprise reports and strategic goals. Modern EHRs have a robust data reporting infrastructure that is used for a variety of goals, including individual provider performance metrics, enterprise quality metrics, automated reporting to payers, and regulatory compliance where other events in the patient timeline are important.
- Aligns with strategic goals. Integration of measures with the EHR permits a richer dataset for research studies. Moreover, participation in population health initiatives, such as the American Psychiatric Association's PsychPRO registry, is facilitated by parallel abstraction of key data that are already part of the EHR, such as visit diagnoses, medications prescribed, and comorbid illnesses.
- Provider satisfaction. Increasing provider burnout is partly attributed to the challenges of working with EHRs. Integration with the EHR permits seamless access to results in the clinical workflow and effortless inclusion of results into clinical documentation.
- Low barrier to implementation. In most cases, outcome measure functionality is included in the cost of an EHR, so there is no additional licensing or subscription cost. Moreover, with minimal effort, well established psychometric tools can become almost turnkey implementations. For example, the National Network of Depression Centers has worked with Epic Systems to incorporate its Mood Disorders Program measures into Epic's foundation system, making it available to all Epic customers.
- Health data portability. Interoperability is a major focus of Medicare's hospital prospective payment system. Integrating behavioral health outcomes measures with the EHR permits more efficient sharing through interoperability standards.

There are, however, potential tradeoffs and limitations to EHR integrated MBC systems:

- Patient privacy concerns. As previously noted, some patients are wary of having their mental health data treated the same as other health data. This is inherently more difficult in a common infrastructure, though most EHRs provide options for segregating sensitive documentation. A decision to segment behavioral health outcomes measures must be balanced against the perpetuation of stigma and fragmentation of the patient's health record.

- EHR lacks outcome measure functionality. As mentioned earlier, not all EHRs have integrated outcomes measures.
- EHR functionality is not fully mature or optimized for behavioral health. This is perhaps the biggest challenge. As mentioned earlier, measures are only a small scope of EHR functionality and, when available, are good, but not ideal. For example, Epic systems does not offer a mechanism for caregiver-reported measures. EHRs are patient-centric, so parent or teacher measures are only available in the minor's portal, raising privacy concerns. As another example, EHRs are good at accepting patient data, but not so good at reflecting results for patient consumption. Patient experience representatives have reported that the ability to see trended results in the patient portal is a strong promoter of patient engagement. Fortunately, vendors are recognizing the need and are addressing these and other noncritical deficiencies.

SUMMARY

MBC methodology has been recognized to add value and improve quality and consistency of care in mental health services. Despite a decade of literature supporting this, practical challenges to the implementation of this methodology frequently prevent individual providers and health systems from adopting MBC as part of their practice. Ultimately, a final decision on the local MBC infrastructure and implementation strategy must take into account the nature of the clinical environment, existing infrastructures, resource and workflow considerations, and patient population. Although no single solution will reach the sweet spot for all potential practitioners and practice settings, this article attempts to offer a general framework for consideration of the infrastructure and implementation needs to facilitate the adoption of MBC. The authors believe that appropriate consideration of a base infrastructure, supplemented by early consideration of known barriers and active use of mitigation strategies, can dramatically lower the impact of these barriers, and smooth the adoption of MBC techniques throughout mental health.

DISCLOSURE

The authors have nothing to disclose.

REFERENCES

1. Scott K, Lewis CC. Using measurement-based care to enhance any treatment. Cogn Behav Pract 2015;22(1):49–59.
2. Zimmerman M, McGlinchey J. Why don't psychiatrists use scales to measure outcome when treating depressed patients. J Clin Psychiatry 2008;69:1916–9.
3. Lewis C, Boyd M, Puspitasary A. Implementing measurement-based care in behavioral health: a review. JAMA Psychiatry 2019;76:324–35.
4. Trivedi M, Rush A, Wisniewski S, et al. Evaluation of outcomes with citalopram for depression using measurement-based care in STAR*D: implications for Clinical Practice. Am J Psychiatry 2006;163:26–40.
5. Krägeloh CU, Czuba KJ, Billington DR, et al. Using feedback from patient-reported outcome measures in mental health services: a scoping study and typology. Psychiatr Serv 2014;66(3):224–41.

6. Fortney JC, Unützer J, Wrenn G, et al. A tipping point for measurement-based care. Psychiatr Serv 2016;68(2):179–88.

7. Ader DN. Developing the patient-reported outcomes measurement information system (PROMIS). Med Care 2007;45(5):S1–2.

8. Meyers K, Winters N. Ten-year review of rating scales. I: overview of scale functioning, psychometric properties, and selection. J Am Acad Child Adolesc Psychiatry 2002;41:114–22.

9. Jeffrey J, Hajal NJ, Klomhaus A, et al. The use of behavioral health rating scales for primary care providers. Ment Health Fam Med 2019;15:884–92.

10. Krishna R, Valleru J, Smith W. Implementing outcome-based care in pediatric psychiatry: early results and overcoming barriers. Pediatr Qual Saf 2019;4(1): e132.

Evidence Base for Measurement-Based Care in Child and Adolescent Psychiatry

Amit Parikh, MD[a,b], Mary A. Fristad, PhD[a,b], David Axelson, MD[a,b],
Rajeev Krishna, MD, PHD[a,b],*

KEYWORDS

- Measurement-based care • Patient-reported outcomes • Feedback-informed care
- Measurement feedback systems • Routine outcome monitoring
- Child and adolescent psychiatry

KEY POINTS

- Measurement-based care (MBC) is the routine collection of data using standardized and validated measures and subsequent use of data collected to guide treatment.
- There is strong evidence to support MBC in adult mental health care.
- There is a growing body of evidence to support the implementation of MBC in youth mental health care.
- The literature supports that, to be effective, MBC must be implemented immediately before or during every patient encounter, results must be available and reviewed by providers immediately, results must be shared with the patient, and results must be used to guide treatment.

INTRODUCTION

The prevalence of behavioral health disorders in youth is increasing worldwide. Data from the 2016 National Survey of Children's Health show that the prevalence of at least 1 mental health disorder in youth aged 0 to 17 years is 16.5%.[1] Most (75%) adult mental illness emerges before age 25 years, and 45% of the total burden of disease among people between 10 and 24 years old is attributed to mental illness.[2] These statistics underscore the importance of finding modalities to improve the care of this vulnerable population.

Measurement-based care (MBC) has been proposed as a means to improve clinical outcomes. An increasing number of original studies and review articles show its effectiveness in the adult population. This article briefly reviews these studies, then examines the evidence for use of MBC in clinical practice with children and

a Department of Psychiatry and Behavioral Health, The Ohio State University College of Medicine, Columbus, OH, USA; b Big Lots Behavioral Health Service Line, Nationwide Children's Hospital, 444 Butterfly Gardens Drive, Columbus, OH 43215, USA
* Corresponding author.
E-mail address: Rajeev.Krishna@nationwidechildrens.org

Child Adolesc Psychiatric Clin N Am 29 (2020) 587–599
https://doi.org/10.1016/j.chc.2020.06.001
1056-4993/20/© 2020 Elsevier Inc. All rights reserved.

adolescents. It concludes with a recommendation for implementation of MBC in behavioral health care for youth.

DEFINING MEASUREMENT-BASED CARE

A significant challenge in developing an evidence base for MBC is variability in the definition and meaning of the term and the concepts surrounding it. MBC was applied to mental health care by Trivedi and colleagues[3] in 2006 as "the routine measurement of symptoms and side effects at each treatment visit and the use of a treatment manual describing when and how to modify medication doses based on these measures." It was further broadly defined by The Joint Commission as "using objective data to track the impact of care, treatment, or services."[4] Later, Aboroya and colleagues[5] expanded the definition of MBC to include "the use of validated clinical measurement instruments to objectify the assessment, treatment and clinical outcomes, including efficacy, safety, tolerability, functioning, and quality of life, in patients with psychiatric disorders." This definition is in contrast with usual care, or treatment as usual, in which providers typically use clinical interviews alone to assess mental disorder. Furthermore, although the term MBC has been adopted in this article, other terms to describe similar procedures continue to be used in the literature, including continuous assessment, feedback-informed treatment, monitoring treatment progress, outcome assessment, outcomes measures, patient-focused research, patient-level feedback, patient-reported outcomes, progress monitoring, and routine outcome monitoring.[6] Ultimately, a wide variety of patient-reported outcome measures (PROMs) are reported in the literature, with variations in timing, scope, and frequency of feedback. They are all categorized under the umbrella of MBC or a related term, because of a lack of clarity regarding goals and mechanisms of using patient-reported outcomes.[7]

Given this, it is important to define clearly the terminology used in this article. MBC has 2 main components (1) routine (ie, every visit), meaning collection of data using standardized and validated measures; and (2) use of these collected data to guide treatment (ie, feedback-informed care). MBC is used routinely throughout other fields in medicine. For example, blood pressure reading, glucose levels, and lipid values are routinely used to measure symptoms and subsequently guide treatment. Just as these measures are considered standard of care in other fields, some groups have begun to conceptualize measures in mental health care as psychiatric vital signs to reinforce their importance.[8,9]

Well-known tools such as the Patient Health Questionnaire, 9 Item[10] (PHQ-9) and the Generalized Anxiety Disorder, 7 Item[11] (GAD-7) are examples of tools currently used in clinical care. In mental health research, the routine use of validated measures is well established. Landmark studies that now are used to guide clinical practice, such as the Sequenced Treatment Alternatives to Relieve Depression[12] (STAR-D) in adults and The Treatment for Adolescents with Depression Study[13] (TADS) in youth, both used standardized assessment tools to track outcomes. Although these studies provide useful clinical guidelines that are frequently used, a gap remains between research and clinical outcomes. Some investigators have attributed this to the lack of standardized assessment tools in clinical care.[14] A recently conducted national survey indicated 14% of behavioral health clinicians reported using standardized measures at least monthly, whereas 62% had never used them.[14,15] Another survey found that fewer than 20% of behavioral health providers used MBC.[16] Thus, although the idea of MBC is not new, it continues to be adopted by a minority of clinicians.[17]

STANDARDIZED MEASURES

MBC is based on the use of psychometrically strong measures that can be implemented routinely. Psychometrically strong measures have 3 primary components: reliability, validity, and sensitivity to change.[18] These measures must be consistent across time and observers (reliability), measure what they are supposed to (validity), and be able to capture clinically relevant changes (sensitivity to change). These measures are used in research (as discussed) including drug trials that are required to prove efficacy of their compounds to the Food and Drug Administration.[14] However, the measures used in these types of trials typically are time intensive and disease specific. With the push toward MBC, a large number of tools are now available; however, there is considerable variability in their quality. Review articles have compared available tools in disease-specific models such as depression[18] and bipolar disorder.[19] There are also tools that have been used extensively in the psychotherapy literature to measure broader constructs than a specific disease's symptoms, from the more comprehensive Outcomes Questionnaire 45 (OQ-45) to the ultrabrief Outcome Rating Scale/Session Rating Scale (ORS/SRS), both of which are a part of the Partners for Change Outcome Management System (PCOMS).[7] A recent systematic review found that, although 29 different outcomes measures have been used in the literature pertaining to young people (aged 12–25 years), none had been specifically designed for young people.[20] Ensuring the strength of measures chosen is important.

The measures that are implemented can be completed by patients, observers (parent or guardian), or both. Although some literature indicates that observer-provided (rather than patient-reported) scales more accurately reflect symptoms,[21,22] conflicting evidence suggests that patients' reports of symptoms are more accurate (particularly in adolescents).[23] This difference from the adult population is key, because many youth do not enter into therapy voluntarily and adolescence is a developmental phase that includes an increased need for autonomy.[24] The implementation of standardized intake questionnaires has allowed adolescents to believe their concerns are being heard directly, fostering improved therapeutic alliance, which has been linked to improved treatment outcomes.[25–28]

IMPLEMENTATION

Once a measure that captures the relevant data from the appropriate sources is selected, it must be implemented in a specific manner. The implementation standard of MBC adopted in this article is more rigorous than what is reported in much of the literature. Ineffective approaches to data collection include administration only during the initial encounter or sporadically during treatment, as well as not administering immediately before or during the encounter.[14] Once measures are obtained, they need to be appropriately managed. Krägeloh and colleagues[7] reviewed 27 studies using PROMs and described 5 levels of feedback: (1) PROM with no feedback; (2) PROM reported back to the clinician; (3) PROM reported back to the clinician and client; (4) PROM reported back to the clinician and client, with opportunities for discussion; (5) PROM reported back to the clinician and client with a formal procedure in which a discussion of PROMs can affect subsequent treatment.[7]

To be effective and fit the model of MBC proposed in this article, administration must be completed immediately before or during every patient encounter, with the data available to the provider and patient in real time so it can be reviewed with the patient and guide treatment strategies (levels 4 and 5).

Advancements in the electronic health record (EHR) and emergence of many digital measurement feedback systems (MFSs) have made the administration, review, and implementation of these measures simpler. A recent review article evaluated 49 different MFSs that are now available.[29] These systems can automatically tailor assessments to be completed based on patient attributes, then measure, score, norm, and graph the results. Incorporating these systems into the EHR allows the ability to monitor and track results efficiently.[30] Specifically, use of electronic methods of data collection has been shown to be accepted by patients and providers as having minimal impact on daily clinical routines.[31]

CLINICAL JUDGMENT

When discussing the use of standardized measures, one frequent counterpoint cited is clinical judgment and expertise. A survey of mental health professionals based in the United States in 2012 (eg, psychiatrists, psychologists, counselors) showed that providers estimate 80% of their clients improve and 90% rated themselves in the upper quartile for competence.[32] The reliance of providers on clinical judgment alone has proved to be less effective than clinical judgment combined with relevant measures. The accuracy of clinical diagnosis without the use of standardized assessment tools also has been questioned.[33] Studies have shown that mental health providers are historically poor at detecting deterioration among patients[34] and therefore struggle to recognize treatment failure.[35] Providers are also poor at identifying patients stagnating in care,[36] which can lead to clinical inertia, which has been defined as the "overestimation of care provided; use of 'soft' reasons to avoid intensification of therapy; and lack of education, training, and practice organization aimed at achieving therapeutic goals."[37] Taken together, this leads to suboptimal patient outcomes. Use of MBC is not to replace clinical judgment and clinician experience; however, it is intended to provide further data to improve the accuracy of diagnosis and efficacy of treatments.[38]

CLINICAL EFFICACY IN ADULTS

At least 12 review articles or meta-analyses have been published regarding MBC in adults.[6,7,14,35,39–46] Although a full review of the adult literature is outside the scope of this article, it briefly summarizes the evidence as a tool to extrapolate into the sparser data in child and adolescent psychiatry. Overall, the cumulative findings from 12 reviews indicate the evidence is strong enough to recommend implementation of MBC, with the major findings summarized here.

Compared with care as usual, these reviews found that MBC:

1. Improved clinical outcomes
2. Reduced patient deterioration
3. Increased patient retention
4. Improved identification of patients who were on track and those not on track
5. Improved communication between providers and patients
6. Was more beneficial when feedback was provided to patients and providers rather than solely to providers
7. Was more beneficial when feedback provided to patients included past measurement rather than only results obtained during the current clinical encounter
8. Increased rates of improvement and treatment adjustments (in those with substance use disorder)

All but 2 of the reviewed reports found evidence favoring use of MBC. A 2018 meta-analysis by Østergard and colleagues[46] did not conclude that MBC was beneficial, although its validity has been called in to question because of shortcomings in the quality of studies allowed in the analysis, which could have led to inappropriate conclusions.[47] A 2016 Cochrane Review conducted by Kendrick and colleagues[43] did not reach significance; however, that review did not include studies that used measurement data to enhance care, an integral part of how effective MBC is currently conceptualized.[6]

CLINICAL EFFICACY IN CHILDREN AND ADOLESCENTS

With mounting evidence of the benefits of MBC in adults, more groups have been attempting to translate these positive results into the child and adolescent population. However, studies in this age group are still are lacking in number and strength compared with the adult literature.

Four review articles have discussed components of MBC in youth.[18,20,24,48] Two of these reviews discussed tools that can be used in MBC, rather than the efficacy of MBC itself. The other 2 discussed implementation of MBC in psychotherapy. Tam and Ronan[24] reviewed 12 studies in 2017 and concluded there were promising early findings to support MBC (Hedges g = 0.28). By contrast, Bergman and colleagues[48] published a Cochrane Review in 2018 covering 6 studies (5 of which were included in Tam and Ronan's[24] study) and were unable to conclude that feedback from clients improved client outcomes. In their view, the studies had a high risk of bias and inconsistent results. Although the inconsistency in these review articles is concerning, the authors believe that they are more reflective of a very limited and heterogeneous underlying literature base that may not be ripe for gaining added insight through the meta-analysis process. As such, this article presents much of the underlying literature for direct consideration.

Fourteen published studies to date have evaluated the effectiveness of MBC. These studies are heterogeneous in their clinical settings, measures used, how and when measures were collected, and how and when data were provided to providers and patients. The literature is largely falls in 1 of 3 domains: those conducted in school settings,[49–51] those focused on individual therapy,[17,52–59] and those focused on group therapy.[60,61] Note that no available research evaluated the efficacy of MBC in medication management in youth.

Given the amount of time children spend in school,[62] it is not surprising that school is a common setting in which services are provided.[63] Three studies have considered the benefits of implementing MBC in individual therapy conducted in a school setting (**Table 1**). Melendez[49] examined patient-reported outcomes in 69 children aged 12 to 18 years seen in a school therapy setting. Participants completed measures during each session, but feedback was only provided to therapists of those in the experimental group. Youth in this group had significantly lower symptoms reported over an extended period. When feedback was discontinued, their trajectory converged with that of the control group despite the fact that implementation was less than ideal, with therapists only receiving weekly postsession feedback.[49] Cooper and colleagues[50,51] conducted 2 studies using PCOMS in the United Kingdom. In each study, measures were completed at the start of each session and immediately reviewed with the patient, a child aged 7 to 11 years who had been referred for therapy. In their first study of 288 children, implementation of MBC led to a significant decrease in psychological distress (particularly in children with physical or mental disabilities, older children, and when cognitive behavior therapy was used), with an effect size (d) of 1.49.[50] In their second study of 38 children, only parents scores showed significant improvement in the MBC group compared with the control group over time; however, all other measured outcomes showed a trend toward MBC being beneficial. This

Table 1
Study findings based on settings

Source	Population Age (y)	Result of MBC Implementation
School-Based Psychotherapy		
Melendez,[49] 2002	12–18	Lower symptom report by patients
Cooper et al,[50] 2013	7–11	Decrease in psychological distress measures
Cooper et al,[51] 2019	7–11	Improvement in parent measures
Individual Therapy		
Bickman et al,[52] 2011	11–18	Quicker symptom reduction
Douglas et al,[55] 2015	11–18	Therapists rated as more attuned to issues by patients
Bickman et al,[57] 2016	11–18	Dose-dependent improvement in both clinician-reported and patient-reported measures
Ogles et al,[65] 2006	M ± SD = 13.3 ± 3.0	No improvement in outcomes measured
Lester,[53] 2012	12–17	Higher therapeutic alliance
Nelson et al,[54] 2013	4–17	Dose-dependent improvement in outcomes
Timimi et al,[59] 2013	Children and adolescents	Improved therapeutic efficiency
Hansen et al,[56] 2015	9–17	Improvement in therapist-rated measures
Kodet et al,[58] 2019	6–17	Significantly reduced distress of patients
Group Therapy		
Shechtman & Sarig,[60] 2016	10–18	No improvement in outcomes
Shechtman & Tutian,[61] 2017	10–15	No improvement in outcomes

Abbreviations: M, mean; SD, standard deviation.

finding was particularly positive because a signal was found despite both low adherence rate (potentially reducing its overall effect) and small sample size.[51]

Nine implementation studies focus on MBC's impact on individual psychotherapy (see **Table 1**). Bickman and colleagues[52] conducted a randomized controlled trial (RCT) in 2011 showing that patients of therapists who were provided with patient-reported measures improved more quickly than patients of therapists who did not receive this information. In addition, patient response improved in a dose-dependent manner; the more their clinicians viewed results, the more they improved. This finding was despite the data being provided, on average, 9 days after each session.[52] In a secondary analysis in 2015, Douglas and colleagues[55] showed that MBC implementation led to therapists being significantly more attuned to issues rated as important by patients. In a second RCT in 2016, Bickman and colleagues[57] evaluated MBC at 2 clinic sites. Only 1 clinic showed significant benefits: at that site, MBC had a significant impact on both clinician-reported and patient-reported measures in a dose-dependent manner. The other clinic did not show benefit, which was particularly notable because it was likely caused by the underperforming clinic having a low implementation index, less day-to-day involvement from the senior administrator (because of distance), and using a noncomputerized measurement feedback system.[57] Although there was no difference in most mental health and demographic characteristics between sites, it is important that the underperforming clinic was in an urban (vs rural) setting and had a higher percentage of Medicaid patients (82% vs 30%).[64]

The remaining 6 studies of MBC in individual psychotherapy are positive overall, although they are of lower quality. In 2006, Ogles and colleagues[65] implemented MBC in an already intensive wraparound approach and found that MBC did not improve any outcomes measures. That study was limited because MBC was poorly implemented (measures were faxed to providers 4 times over 3 months and not reviewed with patients). In 2012, Lester[53] implemented MBC in a study with 120 hospitalized patients. The experimental group completed measures before and after each individual therapy session; all patients completed measures at admission and discharge. Although they found no significant differences in youth report of symptoms or length of hospitalization, they did find significantly higher therapeutic alliance in the experimental group. The study was limited because each participant only had 2 therapy sessions on average, likely affecting the primary outcome.[53]

In 2013, Nelson and colleagues[54] conducted a retrospective review of a youth early warning system (a system that attempts to identify those who are at risk of deterioration) that used standardized measures in 16,091 outpatients aged 4 to 17 years. Patients who completed more measures per month improved more quickly, even after controlling for the number of sessions.[54] In 2013, Timimi and colleagues[59] presented preliminary findings of their outcomes system implementation in a community mental health agency serving children and adolescents in the United Kingdom. This system led to improved therapeutic efficiency through multiple possible factors, including activation of resources for patients not progressing as expected and the creation of more curiosity in therapists, leading to changes in treatment.[59] In 2015, Hansen and colleagues[56] conducted a study in the Australian public health system with 73 outpatients aged 9 to 17 years with moderate to severe mental health issues. They implemented MBC by use of the ORS/SRS in the experimental group and found significant positive effects, but only on the therapist-rated measure and not on patient-rated measures. The study was limited because there was poor adoption by therapists, with only 3 therapists providing most of the data, potentially limiting the impact of MBC.[56]

In 2019, Kodet and colleagues[58] found that psychotherapy with MBC was effective in reducing distress among depressed youth in poverty. Unlike many effectiveness trials, where results are less robust than the original efficacy trial, the strength of effect was similar to that reported in clinical trials, suggesting MBC might be the tool needed to bridge the gap between research and clinical outcomes. The primary limitation of this study was the lack of a control group.[58] Overall, these 6 studies in individual psychotherapy provide support for the use of MBC in individual therapy.

Two studies have evaluated MBC in group therapy (see **Table 1**). The data in this setting are not supportive of MBC. In 2016, Shechtman and Sarig[60] conducted an

RCT of 220 children and adolescents with behavior problems and found no effect of MBC on outcomes or therapist alliance. In 2017, Shechtman and Tutian[61] conducted a quasiexperimental study of 230 children and adolescents with behaviors problems and did not find MBC to have an impact on outcomes. Both studies were limited by their use of unique populations and use of only 1 feedback measure. Although MBC implementation in group settings has been shown to be beneficial in adults,[66] there remains a lack of evidence for its benefit in the child and adolescent population. This lack of evidence may be caused by inherent increased dynamics (particularly in the children and adolescent populations studied) and limited individual contact in a group therapy setting.

In summary, the evidence base for MBC in child and adolescent mental health seems to support its use, at least in the individual care setting. The literature shows effectiveness in both school and outpatient settings despite less than ideal implementations of MBC itself, with respect to consistency of use and time frame of feedback. MBC has not shown benefits in group therapy for youth, although the literature base is limited.

EVIDENCE OF SYSTEM-LEVEL BENEFITS

A growing literature base shows system-level benefits for the consistent use of MBC. MBC is beneficial for clinicians to track treatment results for self-evaluation and for service-level quality improvement.[6,67] The analysis of aggregate data may allow more personalized care through the ability to find new treatment algorithms and patterns among patients.[68,69] Such data are important in determining payments and justification of service, and could eventually lead to improvements in reimbursement rates.[6,14,38]

BARRIERS

The literature exploring barriers to the implementation of MBC and strategies to mitigate them is expanding rapidly. Barriers identified to date include a lack of clinical time to review measures, financial implications (ie, providers with low response/remission rates having reduced reimbursement), concern that data would be used to punish providers, administrator turnover leading to a lack of champions who are committed to its implementation, a lack of consensus on which measures to use, a significant variation in the strength of psychometric properties of measures used, a lack of awareness of MBC, concern regarding patients' illnesses reducing validity of self-report measures, and patient complexity.[6,14,70]

SUMMARY

The original use of the term MBC in behavioral health care was with regard to providing more effective pharmacotherapy.[3] Available evidence from the adult literature clearly supports the benefits of MBC. The literature on MBC in children and adolescents, although less robust, is positive in supporting the use of MBC in youth. By routinely collecting data using standardized and validated measures to guide treatment, clinicians can improve patient outcomes and satisfaction. The literature supports that, to be effective, MBC must be administered immediately before or during every encounter, results must be available to and reviewed by providers immediately, results must be shared with the patient, and results must be used to guide treatment. Beyond the individual patients, MBC can move forward by providing data that lead to more personalized health care and proving value to payers. With the rapid evolution of the EHR and development of MFSs, it has become feasible to implement these practices into busy clinical workflows.

The authors believe a more rigorous definition of MBC, as defined in this article, should be adopted. Additional research is needed to understand the nuances of implementing MBC specifically in the child and adolescent population. In particular, attention should be paid to increasing the use of MBC in clinical practice by identifying, then mitigating, barriers. Further research is also needed to assess benefits specific to medication management settings. Despite specific literature supporting this, it is possible to extrapolate from the current research in children and adolescents and the medication management-specific research in adults to support its implementation in medication management in children and adolescents. Future educational initiatives should aim to incorporate MBC into the clinical curriculum of all health care professionals to enhance its use.

DISCLOSURE

Dr. Fristad had received Royalties from American Psychiatric Press, Child & Family Psychological Services, Guilford Press and Research support from Janssen. Rest of the authors have nothing to disclose.

REFERENCES

1. Whitney DG, Peterson MD. US national and state-level prevalence of mental health disorders and disparities of mental health care use in children. JAMA Pediatr 2019;173(4):389–91.
2. de Girolamo G, Dagani J, Purcell R, et al. Age of onset of mental disorders and use of mental health services: needs, opportunities and obstacles. Epidemiol Psychiatr Sci 2012;21(1):47–57. Available at: https://doi.org.proxy. lib.ohio-state.edu/10.1017/S2045796011000746.
3. Trivedi MH, Rush AJ, Wisniewski SR, et al. Evaluation of outcomes with citalopram for depression using measurement-based care in STAR*D: implications for clinical practice. Am J Psychiatry 2006;163(1):28–40.
4. Complying with Standard CTS.03.01.09: Behavioral Health Care Accreditation Program. In: The Joint Commission. Government Publication.
5. Aboraya A, Nasrallah HA, Elswick DE, et al. Measurement-based care in psychiatry—past, present, and future. Innov Clin Neurosci 2018;15(11-12):13–26.
6. Lewis CC, Boyd M, Puspitasari A, et al. Implementing measurement-based care in behavioral health: a review. JAMA Psychiatry 2019;76(3):324–35.
7. Krägeloh CU, Czuba KJ, Billington DR, et al. Using feedback from patient-reported outcome measures in mental health services: a scoping study and typology. Psychiatr Serv 2014;66(3):224–41.
8. Trivedi MH, Jha MK, Kahalnik F, et al. VitalSign6: a primary care first (PCP-first) model for universal screening and measurement-based care for depression. Pharmaceuticals 2019;12(2):71.
9. Zimmerman M, Young D, Chelminski I, et al. Overcoming the problem of diagnostic heterogeneity in applying measurement-based care in clinical practice: the concept of psychiatric vital signs. Compr Psychiatry 2012;53(2):117–24.
10. Kroenke K, Spitzer RL, Williams JBW. The PHQ-9: validity of a brief depression severity measure. J Gen Intern Med 2001;16(9):606–13.
11. Kroenke K, Spitzer RL, Williams JBW, et al. Anxiety disorders in primary care: prevalence, impairment, comorbidity, and detection. Ann Intern Med 2007; 146(5):317.

12. Gaynes BN, Rush AJ, Trivedi MH, et al. The STAR*D study: treating depression in the real world. Cleve Clin J Med 2008;75(1):57–66.

13. March JS, Silva S, Petrycki S, et al. The Treatment for Adolescents with Depression Study (TADS): long-term effectiveness and safety outcomes. Arch Gen Psychiatry 2007;64(10):1132–43.

14. Fortney JC, Unützer J, Wrenn G, et al. A tipping point for measurement-based care. Psychiatr Serv 2016;68(2):179–88.

15. Jensen-Doss A, Haimes EMB, Smith AM, et al. Monitoring treatment progress and providing feedback is viewed favorably but rarely used in practice. Adm Policy Ment Health 2018;45(1):48–61.

16. Scott K, Lewis CC. Using measurement-based care to enhance any treatment. Cogn Behav Pract 2015;22(1):49–59.

17. Hatfield DR, Ogles BM. Why some clinicians use outcome measures and others do not. Adm Policy Ment Health 2007;34(3):283–91.

18. Elmquist JM, Melton TK, Croarkin P, et al. A systematic overview of measurement-based care in the treatment of childhood and adolescent depression. J Psychiatr Pract 2010;16(4):217–34.

19. Cerimele JM, Goldberg SB, Miller CJ, et al. Systematic review of symptom assessment measures for use in measurement-based care of bipolar disorders. Psychiatr Serv 2019;70(5):396–408.

20. Kwan B, Rickwood DJ. A systematic review of mental health outcome measures for young people aged 12 to 25 years. BMC Psychiatry 2015;15(1):279.

21. Brooks SJ, Kutcher S. Diagnosis and measurement of adolescent depression: a review of commonly utilized instruments. J Child Adolesc Psychopharmacol 2001;11(4):341–76.

22. Pavuluri M, Birmaher B. A practical guide to using ratings of depression and anxiety in child psychiatric practice. Curr Psychiatry Rep 2004;6(2):108–16.

23. Lyon AR, Ludwig KA, Stoep AV, et al. Patterns and predictors of mental healthcare utilization in schools and other service sectors among adolescents at risk for depression. School Ment Health 2013;5(3). https://doi.org/10.1007/s12310-012-9097-6.

24. Tam HE, Ronan K. The application of a feedback-informed approach in psychological service with youth: systematic review and meta-analysis. Clin Psychol Rev 2017;55:41–55.

25. Elliott J, Nembhard M, Giannone V, et al. Clinical uses of an adolescent intake questionnaire. Soc Work Ment Health 2005;3(1-2):83–102.

26. Karver MS, Handelsman JB, Fields S, et al. Meta-analysis of therapeutic relationship variables in youth and family therapy: the evidence for different relationship variables in the child and adolescent treatment outcome literature. Clin Psychol Rev 2006;26(1):50–65.

27. McLeod BD. Relation of the alliance with outcomes in youth psychotherapy: a meta-analysis. Clin Psychol Rev 2011;31(4):603–16.

28. Owen J, Miller SD, Seidel J, et al. The working alliance in treatment of military adolescents. J Consult Clin Psychol 2016;84(3):200–10.

29. Lyon AR, Lewis CC, Boyd MR, et al. Capabilities and characteristics of digital measurement feedback systems: results from a comprehensive review. Adm Policy Ment Health 2016;43(3):441–66.

30. Black WE, Nagarkatti-Gude DR, Jetmalani A, et al. Harnessing technology to implement measurement-based care. Acad Psychiatry 2018;42(5):711–6.

31. Egeter J, Hüfner K, Sztankay M, et al. Implementation of an electronic routine outcome monitoring at an inpatient unit for psychosomatic medicine. J Psychosom Res 2018;105:64–71.

32. Walfish S, McAlister B, O'Donnell P, et al. An investigation of self-assessment bias in mental health providers. Psychol Rep 2012;110(2):639–44.

33. Jewell J, Handwerk M, Almquist J, et al. Comparing the validity of clinician-generated diagnosis of conduct disorder to the diagnostic interview schedule for children. J Clin Child Adolesc Psychol 2004;33(3):536–46.

34. Hatfield D, McCullough L, Frantz SHB, et al. Do we know when our clients get worse? an investigation of therapists' ability to detect negative client change. Clin Psychol Psychother 2010;17(1):25–32.

35. Lambert MJ, Whipple JL, Hawkins EJ, et al. Is it time for clinicians to routinely track patient outcome? a meta-analysis. Clin Psychol Sci Pract 2003;10(3): 288–301.

36. Hannan C, Lambert MJ, Harmon C, et al. A lab test and algorithms for identifying clients at risk for treatment failure. J Clin Psychol 2005;61(2):155–63.

37. Phillips LS, Branch WT, Cook CB, et al. Clinical inertia. Ann Intern Med 2001; 135(9):825–34.

38. Harding KJK, Rush AJ, Arbuckle M, et al. Measurement-based care in psychiatric practice: a policy framework for implementation. J Clin Psychiatry 2011;72(8): 1136–43.

39. Knaup C, Koesters M, Schoefer D, et al. Effect of feedback of treatment outcome in specialist mental healthcare: meta-analysis. Br J Psychiatry 2009;195(1): 15–22.

40. Carlier IVE, Meuldijk D, Van Vliet IM, et al. Routine outcome monitoring and feedback on physical or mental health status: evidence and theory: feedback on physical or mental health status. J Eval Clin Pract 2012;18(1):104–10.

41. Gondek D, Edbrooke-Childs J, Fink E, et al. Feedback from outcome measures and treatment effectiveness, treatment efficiency, and collaborative practice: a systematic review. Adm Policy Ment Health 2016;43(3):325–43.

42. Goodman JD, McKay JR, DePhilippis D. Progress monitoring in mental health and addiction treatment: a means of improving care. Prof Psychol Res Pract 2013;44(4):231–46.

43. Kendrick T, El-Gohary M, Stuart B, et al. Routine use of patient reported outcome measures (PROMs) for improving treatment of common mental health disorders in adults. Cochrane Database Syst Rev 2016;(7). https://doi.org/10.1002/14651858.CD011119.pub2.

44. Waldrop J, McGuinness TM. Measurement-based care in psychiatry. J Psychosoc Nurs Ment Health Serv 2017;55(11):30–5.

45. Shimokawa K, Lambert MJ, Smart DW. Enhancing treatment outcome of patients at risk of treatment failure: meta-analytic and mega-analytic review of a psychotherapy quality assurance system. J Consult Clin Psychol 2010;78(3):298–311.

46. Østergård OK, Randa H, Hougaard E. The effect of using the Partners for Change Outcome Management System as feedback tool in psychotherapy—a systematic review and meta-analysis. Psychother Res 2018;1–18. https://doi.org/10.1080/10503307.2018.1517949.

47. Duncan BL, Sparks JA. When meta-analysis misleads: a critical case study of a meta-analysis of client feedback. Psychol Serv 2019. https://doi.org/10.1037/ser0000398.

48. Bergman H, Kornør H, Nikolakopoulou A, et al. Client feedback in psychological therapy for children and adolescents with mental health problems. Cochrane Database Syst Rev 2018;(8):CD011729.

49. Melendez G. Effects of feedback to the therapist on child clinical outcomes: a patient -oriented approach to demonstrating effective practice 2002. Available at: http://search.proquest.com/docview/305552110/abstract/7083167461BE4EA8PQ/1. Accessed November 19, 2019.

50. Cooper M, Stewart D, Sparks J, et al. School-based counseling using systematic feedback: a cohort study evaluating outcomes and predictors of change. Psychother Res 2013;23(4):474–88.

51. Cooper M, Duncan B, Golden S, et al. Systematic client feedback in therapy for children with psychological difficulties: pilot cluster randomised controlled trial. Couns Psychol Q 2019;1–16. https://doi.org/10.1080/09515070.2019.1647142.

52. Bickman L, Kelley SD, Breda C, et al. Effects of routine feedback to clinicians on mental health outcomes of youths: results of a randomized trial. Psychiatr Serv 2011;62(12):1423–9.

53. Lester MC. The effectiveness of client feedback measures with adolescents in an acute psychiatric inpatient setting 2012. Available at: http://search.proquest.com/docview/1039541820/abstract/58FBE76F98C843A1PQ/1. Accessed November 19, 2019.

54. Nelson PL, Warren JS, Gleave RL, et al. Youth psychotherapy change trajectories and early warning system accuracy in a managed care setting. J Clin Psychol 2013;69(9):880–95.

55. Douglas SR, Jonghyuk B, de Andrade ARV, et al. Feedback mechanisms of change: how problem alerts reported by youth clients and their caregivers impact clinician-reported session content. Psychother Res 2015;25(6):678–93.

56. Hansen B, Howe A, Sutton P, et al. Impact of client feedback on clinical outcomes for young people using public mental health services: a pilot study. Psychiatry Res 2015;229(1):617–9.

57. Bickman L, Douglas SR, De Andrade ARV, et al. Implementing a measurement feedback system: a tale of two sites. Adm Policy Ment Health 2016;43(3):410–25.

58. Kodet J, Reese RJ, Duncan BL, et al. Psychotherapy for depressed youth in poverty: Benchmarking outcomes in a public behavioral health setting. Psychotherapy 2019;56(2):254–9.

59. Timimi S, Tetley D, Burgoine W, et al. Outcome orientated child and adolescent mental health services (OO-CAMHS): a whole service model. Clin Child Psychol Psychiatry 2013;18(2):169–84.

60. Shechtman Z, Sarig O. The effect of client progress feedback on child/adolescent's group-counseling outcomes. J Spec Group Work 2016;41(4):334–49.

61. Shechtman Z, Tutian R. Feedback to semi-professional counselors in treating child aggression. Psychother Res 2017;27(3):338–49.

62. Hofferth SL, Sandberg JF. How American children spend their time. Journal of Marriage and Family 2001;63(2):295–308.

63. Farmer EMZ, Burns BJ, Phillips SD, et al. Pathways into and through mental health services for children and adolescents. Psychiatr Serv 2003;54(1):60–6.

64. Gleacher AA, Olin SS, Nadeem E, et al. Implementing a measurement feedback system in community mental health clinics: a case study of multilevel barriers and facilitators. Adm Policy Ment Health 2016;43(3):426–40.

65. Ogles BM, Carlston D, Hatfield D, et al. The role of fidelity and feedback in the wraparound approach. J Child Fam Stud 2006;15(1):114–28.

66. Schuman DL, Slone NC, Reese RJ, et al. Efficacy of client feedback in group psychotherapy with soldiers referred for substance abuse treatment. Psychother Res 2015;25(4):396–407.
67. Lyon AR, Stirman SW, Kerns SEU, et al. Developing the mental health workforce: review and application of training approaches from multiple disciplines. Adm Policy Ment Health 2011;38(4):238–53.
68. Zwaanswijk M, Klip H, Laurenssen A, et al. Towards personalized child and adolescent psychiatry care by using routinely registered data from everyday clinical practice. Tijdschr Psychiatr 2018;60(11):750–5 [in Dutch].
69. Hickie IB, Scott EM, Cross SP, et al. Right care, first time: a highly personalised and measurement-based care model to manage youth mental health. Med J Aust 2019;211(S9):S3–46.
70. Fortney J, Sladek R, Unützer J. Fixing Behavioral Health Care in America A National Call for Measurement-Based Care in the Delivery of Behavioral Health Services.

Self-Report Rating Scales to Guide Measurement-Based Care in Child and Adolescent Psychiatry

Jessica Jeffrey, MD, MPH, MBA[a],*, Alexandra Klomhaus, MS[a,b],
Michael Enenbach, MD[a,c], Patricia Lester, MD[a],
Rajeev Krishna, MD, PhD[d]

KEYWORDS

• Measurement-based care • Rating scales • Self-report • Depression • Anxiety

KEY POINTS

• Measurement-based care in psychiatry is the consistent, repeated use of validated rating scales to enhance clinical evaluation, monitor treatment progress, and directly inform decisions relating to each patient's treatment.

• Rating scales should not be thought of as a replacement for, but instead used to enhance, the clinical interview, diagnostic formulation, and treatment plan.

• When using self-report rating scales in clinical practice, it is important for the clinician to select measures that are psychometrically validated. There are many brief, psychometrically validated rating scales within the public domain.

• Rating scales may be skillfully used to provide patients and their parents with psychoeducation, engage them in care, and enhance their overall experience with care.

INTRODUCTION

Measurement-based care (MBC) involves the practice of systematically administrating rating scales to patients in order to use the collected information to enhance clinical evaluation, monitor treatment progress, and directly inform decisions relating

Funding: The authors received no funding.
[a] Department of Psychiatry and Biobehavioral Sciences, Division of Population Behavioral Health, Nathanson Family Resilience Center, Jane and Terry Semel Institute for Neuroscience and Human Behavior at UCLA, 760 Westwood Plaza, A8-153, Los Angeles, CA 90095, USA; [b] Department of Biostatistics, UCLA Fielding School of Public Health, 650 Charles E. Young Dr. South, Los Angeles, CA 90095, USA; [c] Department of Psychiatry & Biobehavioral Sciences, Division of Child and Adolescent Psychiatry, Jane and Terry Semel Institute of Neuroscience and Human Behavior at UCLA, 760 Westwood Plaza, 48-270, Los Angeles, CA 90095, USA; [d] Psychiatry and Behavioral Health, Nationwide Children's Hospital, Psychiatry T5, 700 Children's Drive, Columbus, OH 43205, USA
* Corresponding author.
E-mail address: JJeffrey@mednet.ucla.edu

to the patients' treatment. Analogous to use the of physiologic and laboratory measurement in medical conditions, such as blood pressure readings to monitor hypertension and hemoglobin A1c tests to monitor diabetes, self-report behavioral health symptom rating scales are a key component to MBC in psychiatry. In child and adolescent psychiatric practice, obtaining youth and parent (defined within this report as primary caregiver) reports of the youth's symptoms are optimal to guide treatment.

Rating scale use is not a substitute for clinical judgment[1] but should be used to augment a provider's clinical interview. When used in isolation, rating scale scores are not sufficient to establish a diagnosis or create a treatment plan. Systematic use of rating scales in MBC helps providers to optimize the accuracy and consistency of their clinical assessment.[2] By allowing patients to provide responses to identical questions over the course of treatment, rating scale score monitoring provides opportunity for providers to assess nuanced changes in symptoms.[3] The concept of treatment to target involves treating patients to a level of outcome rather than to a specific medication dose or number of psychotherapy sessions.[4] Rating scales provide the data for providers to achieve this type of specificity in care.

Research has shown that, when used to guide clinical practice, the systematic use of rating scales improves clinical outcomes[2,5] and enhances patient experience.[6] The use of rating scales as a component of care enhances providers' attunement to patients' symptoms. Rating scales can be used as a tool to provide personalized psychoeducation to youth and their families, which allows them to become knowledgeable about behavioral health and more aware of the warning signs of relapse or recurrence.[7] Taking these benefits into consideration, MBC is considered an evidence-based practice by the Substance Abuse and Mental Health Services Administration.

This article provides a discussion of factors to consider when selecting and implementing self-report rating scales to conduct MBC within clinical practice. In addition, the article provides an overview of a selection of psychometrically validated, self-report rating scales applicable to the practice of child psychiatry that are available within the public domain. A case example shows the use of MBC to enhance clinical practice.

SUMMARY/DISCUSSION
Self-Report Rating Scales for Measurement-Based Care

Selection of rating scales
Several factors must be considered when selecting and implementing self-report rating scales for clinical practice. These factors relate to scales' functioning and the ease of administration within the practice setting. First, rating scales must be standardized and psychometrically sound to be useful within a clinical practice. Standardization is achieved by administering a rating scale to a specific population, thus allowing providers to compare patients' scores with their sociodemographic peers.[8] Standardized rating scales use uniform administration procedures, questions, and scoring.[9] The psychometric characteristics of a rating scale may vary by demographic and clinical factors of the population. Psychometrically, rating scales should be reliable (ie, items are consistent over time, across items, and across observers) and valid (ie, the scale should measure the true underlying condition). Criterion validity, the extent to which a score is related to the clinical outcome, is fundamental to MBC.[10,11] Of particular importance within a clinical setting is the concept of face validity, because patients, clinicians, and administrative staff are more likely to use ratings scales when perceived

as relevant to clinical care.[12,13] In addition, in order to achieve MBC, rating scales need to be sensitive to change, or reflect response to treatment over time.[11] Conceptually, there are 2 types of change clinicians must be aware of: reliable change and significant change. Reliable change concerns when changes in rating scale scores are unlikely to be caused by simple measurement unreliability.[14] Significant change relates to the clinical significance of a treatment effect.

However, many rating scales lack sufficient psychometric information to allow optimal application within clinical practice. Notably, no scale is completely reliable and valid; thus, clinicians must be aware there will be some error in measurement when interpreting and applying rating scale scores during clinical practice.[9]

When using rating scales within the clinical setting, consideration must be given to assessing the target symptoms that will best inform clinical decision making for a patient. Rating scales are most useful when they include questions that ask about both broad and specific aspects of a problem, which allows for capture of a range of symptoms.[9] For instance, anxiety rating scales may ask about feeling nervous and being scared to go to school. These questions allow providers to assess general endorsement of anxiety, as well as specific anxiety-provoking situations. Another issue to consider when choosing a rating scale is the availability of youth-report and parent-report versions of the scale. In general, youth are better reporters of internalizing symptoms and parents are more accurate reporters of externalizing behaviors.[15,16] As children become more developmentally mature, there tends to be greater correlation between youth and adult symptom report.[9]

Clinical workflows may be optimized when rating scales are brief and, thus, may be completed in a short time period. Brief rating scales also prevent response fatigue, and thus may lead to more accurate data being incorporated into the assessment and treatment plan. Administration may also be optimized when rating scales are available within the public domain, which not only eliminates additional workflows required to purchase rating scales but minimizes financial barriers to the incorporation of rating scales into clinical practice. Many health systems have invested in Web-based platforms to assist with capture of rating scale data; such systems may integrate these platforms into the electronic health record to allow ease of scoring and documentation, as well as customized clinical guidance.[17] However, these platforms may be financially prohibitive for smaller practices.[18]

Selection of publicly available self-report pediatric behavioral health rating scales
There are many brief, psychometrically validated rating scales available within the public domain. **Table 1** describes the properties of several such commonly used rating scales. To be used within an MBC framework, a rating scale needs to be responsive to change in symptoms. Although outside a strict MBC framework, select rating scales not meeting the criteria of responsiveness to change (Child PTSD [posttraumatic stress disorder] Symptom Scale for DSM-5 [Diagnostic and Statistical Manual of Mental Disorders, Fifth Edition], SNAP-IV [Swanson, Nolan, and Pelham-IV Questionnaire], CRAFFT [car, relax, alone, forget, friends, trouble]) have also been included in the table, because these scales may be used to optimize screening for patients and families.

Depression

Patient Health Questionnaire
The Patient Health Questionnaire-9 (PHQ-9),[19] originally validated by Kroenke and colleagues,[64] has been used to assess symptoms of depression in adolescents aged

Table 1
Properties of rating scales

Rating Scale	Reporter	Age Group (y)	# Items	Cutoff Score	Screening	Monitoring	Internal Consistency	Sensitivity (%)	Specificity (%)
Depression									
PHQ-9[4,19-21]	Youth	≥13	9	≥11	X	X[a]	α = .86-.89[b]	90	78
MFQ[22-26]	Youth	≥7	13-item and 34-item versions	13 items: ≥4; 34 items: ≥29	X	X	$\alpha_{13\text{-items}}$ = .84 $\alpha_{34\text{-items}}$ = .95	66 and 68	61 and 88
MFQ	Caregiver	≥7	13-item and 34-item versions	13 items: ≥4; 34 items: ≥27	X	X	$\alpha_{13\text{-items}}$ = .84; $\alpha_{34\text{-items}}$ = .96	66 and 61	66 and 85
Mania									
CMRS-p[27-29]	Caregiver	5-17	21	≥20	X	X	α = 0.96	82-84	94-98
CMRS-P	Caregiver	5-17	10	≥10	X	X	α = 0.91	84	83
YMRS–Parent Version[30,31]	Caregiver	5-17	11	≥17	X	X	α = 0.72	79	78
YMRS[32]	Youth, parent report Note, 1 study (Yee and colleagues[32]), both youth and parent interviewed with YMRS; clinical judgment used to resolve discrepancies	6-12	11	≥22.5	X	X	Cronbach alpha 0.76	68	86

Trauma

Scale	Respondent	Age	Items	Cutoff			α		
Child PTSD Symptom Scale for DSM-5[33]	Youth	8–18	27	≥31	X	NA	$\alpha = 0.63\text{–}.92$	93	82

Anxiety

SCARED[34,35]	Youth	≥9	38-item and 41-item versions	38 items: ≥15; 41 items: ≥25	X	X	$\alpha_{38\text{-items}} = 0.74\text{–}0.93$; $\alpha_{41\text{-items}} = 0.78\text{–}0.90$	67–80 and 71	50–84 and 61–71
SCARED	Caregiver	≥9	38-item and 41-item versions	38 items: ≥15; 41 items: ≥25	X	X	$\alpha_{38\text{-items}} = 0.74\text{–}0.93$; $\alpha_{41\text{-items}} = 0.78\text{–}0.90$	67–80	50–84
Spence Children's Anxiety Scale[36-40]	Youth	8–18	44	Screening, ≥22; Diagnostic, ≥33	X	X	$\alpha = 0.60\text{–}.92$	91 and 64	73 and 94
Spence Children's Anxiety Scale	Caregiver	6–18	38	Screening, ≥15; Diagnostic, ≥27	X	X	$\alpha = 0.62\text{–}.90$	91 and 62	53 and 94
C-YBOCS[41-44]	Youth and caregiver	6–17	10	≥14[c]	X	X	$\alpha_{child} = .78\text{–}.87$ and $\alpha_{parent} = .70\text{–}.86$	91	90

Family Functioning and Parenting

McMaster FAD[45,46]	Youth and caregiver	≥12	53-item and 60-item versions	1.9–2.3	X	X	$\alpha = 0.72\text{–}.92$	57–83	60–79

(continued on next page)

Table 1
(continued)

Rating Scale	Reporter	Age Group (y)	# Items	Cutoff Score	Screening	Monitoring	Internal Consistency	Sensitivity (%)	Specificity (%)
Substance Use									
CRAFFT[47]	Youth	12–18	Part A 3 and part B 6	2	X	NA	$\alpha = 0.68$	76–92	80–94
ADHD and Behavioral Symptoms									
SNAP-IV[48–50]	Caregiver	5–17	18-item, 26-item, and 90-item versions	1.44–1.88 per item	X	NA	$\alpha = 0.79$–.94	82	82
SNAP-IV	Teacher	5–17	18-item, 26-item, and 90-item versions	1.38–2.56 per item	X	NA	$\alpha = 0.92$–.97	91–97	26–31
VADTRS[51–53]	Teacher	6–12	43	2 or 3 on specific number of items based on subscale, and any score 4 or 5 in performance section	X	NA	$\alpha = 0.91$–.94	69	84
VADPRS	Parent	6–12	55	2 or 3 on specific number of items based on subscale, and any score 4 or 5 in performance section	X	NA	$\alpha = 0.93$–.95	80	75

Vanderbilt Teacher Follow-up	Teacher	6–12	26	Total score on ADHD symptoms should be added and performance scores averaged to track progress over time	No	X	NA	NA	NA
Vanderbilt Parent Follow-up	Parent	6–12	26	Total score on ADHD symptoms should be added and performance scores averaged to track progress over time	No	X	NA	NA	NA
Broad Rating Scales									
PSC[54-59]	Caregiver	4–16	35	4–5 y old, ≥24; 6–16 y old, ≥28	X	X	$\alpha_{4-5} = .78$ and $\alpha_{6+} = .91–.92$	64 and 95	93 and 68
PSC-Y	Youth	11–16 Bright Futures[60]	35	≥30	X	NA	$\alpha = 0.90–.91$	94	88

(continued on next page)

Table 1
(continued)

Rating Scale	Reporter	Age Group (y)	# Items	Screening	Monitoring	Cutoff Score	Internal Consistency	Sensitivity (%)	Specificity (%)
PSC-17[61-63]	Caregiver	4–16 Mental health screening	17	X	X	Total score: ≥15 Internalizing: ≥5 Externalizing: ≥7 Attention: ≥7	α = 0.78–87	77–87	68–81
PSC-17	Youth	11–16 Bright Futures[60]	17	X	NA	≥15	α = 0.68–81	NA	NA

Abbreviations: ADHD, Attention-Deficit/Hyperactivity Disorder; CMRS-P, Child Mania Rating Scale-Parent; CRAFFT, car, relax, alone, forget, friends, trouble; C-YBOCS, Children Yale-Brown Obsessive-Compulsive Scale; DSM-5, Diagnostic and Statistical Manual of Mental Disorders, Fifth Edition; FAD, Family Assessment Device; MFQ, Mood and Feelings Questionnaire; NA, not available; PHQ-9, Patient Health Questionnaire-9; PSC, Pediatric Symptom Checklist; PSC-Y, Pediatric Symptom Checklist- Youth Report; PTSD, post-traumatic stress disorder; SCARED, Screen for Child Anxiety-Related Disorders Scale; SNAP, Swanson, Nolan, and Pelham Questionnaire; VADPRS, Vanderbilt Attention-deficit/Hyperactivity Disorder Diagnostic Parent Rating Scale; VADTRS, Vanderbilt Attention-deficit/Hyperactivity Disorder Diagnostic Teacher Rating Scale; YMRS, Young Mania Rating Scale.

[a] Data from an adult population.
[b] Data from an adult population.
[c] Cutoff is based on most efficient prediction of clinical remission.

13 years and older.[20] This self-report questionnaire asks about symptoms present within the past 2 weeks. The PHQ-9 is composed of 9 questions, each scored on a Likert scale between 0 and 3 (0, not at all; 1, several days; 2, more than half the days; 3, nearly every day) that maps onto the DSM-IV diagnostic criteria for major depressive disorder. A tenth question, not included in the total score, asks about the extent to which symptoms have affected functioning. A total PHQ-9 score of 0 to 4 indicates minimal depression, 5 to 9 mild depression, 10 to 14 moderate depression, 15 to 19 moderately severe depression, and 20 to 27 severe depression.[19] Richardson and colleagues[20] investigated symptoms of depression in 442 youth, aged 13 to 17 years, recruited from patients who attended primary care appointments within a large health system. The study reported that, in adolescents, total PHQ-9 scores greater than or equal to 11 have a sensitivity of 89.5% and a specificity of 77.5% for detecting a major depressive episode (validated against DSM-IV criteria for major depression on the Diagnostic Interview Schedule for Children Version IV (DISC-IV)).

The PHQ-9 may be used as a screening tool to augment clinical interview during an initial psychiatric evaluation.[21] Data in adults suggest the PHQ-9 is sensitive to change and, thus, able to be used to track progress in treatment.[21] For example, when using the PHQ-9, a 3-point to 5-point change in score is considered clinically significant.[4] A greater than 50% decrease in score and/or a total score less than 10 is classified as treatment response, and a total score less than 5 is classified as remission.[4]

The Patient Health Questionnaire–Adolescent (PHQ-A) is a modified version of the PHQ-9. The rating scale includes characteristics of depression in adolescents and more age-appropriate language. Specifically, the PHQ-A asks about irritability in the question assessing depressed mood (item 1) and includes weight loss in the question assessing appetite (item 5). The PHQ-A also includes 3 additional questions, answered as either yes or no, querying symptoms of dysthymia ("In the past year have you felt depressed or sad most days, even if you felt okay sometimes?") and suicide ("Has there been a time in the past month when you have had serious thoughts about ending your life?" and "Have you ever, in your whole life, tried to kill yourself or made a suicide attempt?"). Although psychometric data are not available for the PHQ-A, the PHQ-A is almost identical to the PHQ-9 so the rating scale's developers have indicated that the use of PHQ-9 cutoffs is appropriate.[65]

Mood and Feelings Questionnaire

The Mood and Feelings Questionnaire (MFQ) has been validated to investigate symptoms of depression in youth aged 6 years and older.[22] The questionnaire is based on DSM-III-R criteria for depression. MFQ versions are available for youth self-report (MFQ-Y) and parent report (MFQ-P).[22,23] The MFQ-Y and MFQ-P questionnaires are available in long (34 questions) and short (13 questions) versions. MFQ items query whether cognitive and neurovegetative symptoms of depression have been present within the past 2 weeks. The items are scored on a Likert scale between 0 and 2 (0, not true; 1, sometimes; 2, true). The MFQ is reported to measure depression equivalently across sexes and ethnicities.[24] Both the long and short versions of the MFQ-Y have been reported to be sensitive to change.[24]

Long-version Mood and Feelings Questionnaire

Several studies have been conducted with the goal of validating the MFQ. Studies most comparable with youth commonly evaluated by child psychiatrists include those described here. Burleson Daviss and colleagues[25] investigated the performance of the long versions of the MFQ-Y and MFQ-P in a heterogeneous sample of 470 youth, including those with bipolar spectrum disorders and attention-deficit/hyperactivity disorder (ADHD), from clinic and community sources. A score greater than or equal to 29 on the MFQ-Y had a 68% sensitivity and 88% specificity for detecting a major depressive episode, and a score of 27 on the MFQ-P had a 61% sensitivity and 85% specificity for detecting a major depressive episode (validated against DSM-IV criteria for major depression using the Schedule for Mood Disorders and Schizophrenia for School-age Children–Present and Lifetime Version [K-SADS]).[25] The investigators of this study noted that combining youth and parent ratings was more discriminate than either measure used alone. Earlier studies, with similar findings to those of Burleson Daviss and colleagues,[25] include Wood and colleagues[66] and Kent.[67] Wood and colleagues[66] reported an optimal cutoff score greater than or equal to 27 for the diagnosis of major depressive episode while studying the validity of the MFQ-Y (assessed against standardized interview) in 104 adolescent outpatients, aged 10 to 19 years, attending a psychiatric clinic. Similarly, Kent[67] evaluated the performance of the MFQ-Y in 113 youth aged 7 to 17 years attending a psychiatric clinic (assessed against the K-SADS) and determined an optimal cutoff score greater than or equal to 29. Importantly, researchers noted the MFQ did not significantly differentiate between children with depressive and those with anxiety disorders.[67]

The most recent validation study of the MFQ-Y was conducted by Thabrew and colleagues.[24] Using a sample of 183 help-seeking adolescents aged 12 to 19 years recruited in primary care and school settings in New Zealand, they reported a cutoff score greater than or equal to 28 on the long-version MFQ-Y, and 84% sensitivity and 70.5% specificity for detecting a major depressive episode (validated against DSM-IV criteria for major depression on the Children's Depression Rating Scale–revised and the Reynolds Adolescent Depression Rating Scale 2 as the criterion standard).

Short-version Mood and Feelings Questionnaire
Several studies have been conducted with the goal of validating the short-version MFQ. Rhew and colleagues[26] examined a community sample of 521 sixth grade students, aged 11 to 13 years. For the short versions of the MFQ, a score greater than or equal to 4 on the MFQ-Y has a 66% sensitivity and 61% specificity for detecting a depressive disorder, and a score greater than or equal to 4 on the MFQ-P has a 66% sensitivity and 66% specificity for detecting a depressive disorder.[26] When youth and parent short-version reports are combined, a cut point greater than or equal to 10 has a 76% sensitivity and 78% specificity for detecting a depressive disorder.[26] In contrast, Thabrew and colleagues[24] and Turner and colleagues[68] reported higher cutoff scores. Thabrew and colleagues[24] noted that a cutoff score greater than or equal to 12 on the short-version MFQ-Y had an 84% sensitivity and 68% specificity for detecting a major depressive episode. Turner and colleagues[68] reported a short-version MFQ cutoff of greater than or equal to 11 in a community sample of adolescents aged 17 to 18 years (validated in relation to an adult depression measure administered in late adolescence).

The parallel structure and content of the MFQ-Y and MFQ-P allows clinicians to directly compare youth and parent ratings in order to examine potentially divergent ratings. Clinicians should weigh youth reports more strongly than parent reports, especially for youth in clinical settings and those with an anxiety or mood disorder.[25] Given strong correlations between long and short versions,[24] clinicians may consider using the short version in practice given time considerations.

Mania

Child Mania Rating Scale–Parent

The Child Mania Rating Scale–Parent (CMRS-P) has been validated to investigate symptoms of mania in youth aged 5 years and older.[27] The questionnaire is completed by parents only, consists of 21 items, and is based on DSM-IV criteria for mania. The items are scored on a Likert scale between 0 and 3 (0, never/rare; 1, sometimes; 2, often; 3, very often). Pavuluri and colleagues[27] examined 150 youth, aged 5 to 17 years, recruited from specialty psychiatry settings and community organizations. Youth were recruited with diagnoses of bipolar disorder (n = 50), ADHD (n = 50), or healthy controls (n = 50). A score greater than or equal to 20 on the CMRS-P has an 82% sensitivity, 94% specificity, and a positive likelihood ratio of 13.67 for differentiating bipolar disorder from ADHD. Furthermore, a score greater than or equal to 20 on the CMRS-P has an 84% sensitivity, 98% specificity, and positive likelihood ratio of 42 for differentiating bipolar disorder from healthy controls.[27]

The Brief Child Mania Rating Scale-Parent (B-CMRS-P) comprises 10 of the 21 questions on the B-CMRS-P. The measure also has strong sensitivity and specificity for differentiating youth with bipolar disorder from youth with ADHD and youth with bipolar disorder from healthy controls. A score greater than or equal to 10 has an 84% sensitivity and 83% specificity of differentiating bipolar disorder from ADHD.[28] Both the CMRS-P and B-CMRS-P have been shown to be sensitive to change.[29]

Young Mania Rating Scale

The Parent Version–Young Mania Rating Scale (P-YMRS) asks parents to identify potential symptoms of mania present in their children or adolescents. The rating scale is validated for ages 5 to 17 years.[21] The P-YMRS consists of 11 questions, scored from either 0 to 4 points or 0 to 8 points, with total score ranging from 0 to 60 points. Gracious and colleagues[30] validated the P-YMRS against the K-SADS, and clinical evaluation for approximately 75% of patients, using a sample of 117 children and adolescents, aged 5 to 17 years, recruited from an outpatient research center. Average scores on the P-YMRS were 25.4 in youth diagnosed with bipolar disorder type I; 20.2 in children with other bipolar disorders; 13.4 in children with disruptive disorders, such as ADHD; and 11.1 in youth with unipolar depression. Youth with a bipolar disorder diagnosis scored higher on the P-YMRS; however, classification rates were approximately 80% accurate.[30] Furthermore, the scale showed a 67% accuracy at differentiating bipolar disorder type I from other bipolar disorders. A high score on the P-YMRS may lend evidence for a bipolar disorder, but it does not determine a diagnosis. Gracious and colleagues[30] also reported that greater than or equal to 12-point changes in the P-YMRS were 95% likely to reflect a statistically reliable change in manic symptoms. In 2003, Youngstrom and colleagues,[31] following up on the work of Gracious and colleagues[30] and using the same study sample, reported that a score greater than or equal to 17 as reported by parents had a 79% sensitivity and 78% specificity for detecting any manic symptom disorder versus all other disorders (depressive, disruptive, no diagnosis). Given the P-YMRS was adapted from an adult mania rating scale, it has been noted that the item content in the measure is not as developmentally appropriate for children.[69]

In 2015, Yee and colleagues[32] validated the YMRS against the K-SADS in a clinical sample of 707 children and adolescents (162 youth with bipolar spectrum disorder and 545 without), aged 6 to 12 years, administered in an unfiltered manner, in which current symptoms are captured regardless of whether they occurred within the context of a mood episode. Separate interviews were conducted with youth and their parents. Interviewers used clinical judgment to resolve discrepant results. Yee and colleagues[32] determined that the YMRS has good discriminative validity for predicting bipolar disorder, with a cut point of 22.5. Furthermore, the YMRS was best able to discriminate bipolar disorder from ADHD and from anxiety. The investigators reported unfiltered administration of the YMRS as less discriminating than filtered administration.[32]

Trauma

Child posttraumatic Stress Disorder Symptom Scale for Diagnostic and Statistical Manual of Mental Disorders, Fifth Edition

The Child PTSD Symptom Scale (CPSS-5) is validated for youth aged 8 to 18 years and is used to assess for symptoms of PTSD. The questionnaire asks youth questions based on DSM-5 criteria for PTSD.[33] The CPSS-5 consists of 20 questions that ask about trauma symptoms over the past 1 month, scored on a 0 to 4 Likert scale (0, not at all; 4, 6 or more times weekly/severe), and 7 questions that ask about functioning (yes/no). Foa and colleagues[33] validated the CPSS-5 against the CPSS interview for DSM-5, using a sample of 64 children and adolescents, aged 8 to 18 years, who experienced a DSM-5 criterion A trauma. A cutoff score of 31 has a 93% sensitivity and 82% specificity for a probable PTSD diagnosis.[33]

Anxiety

Screen for Child Anxiety-related Disorders Scale

The Screen for Child Anxiety-related Disorders Scale (SCARED) was designed to assess anxiety and differentiate between depression, anxiety, and anxiety-related disorders in children and adolescents based on the DSM-IV criteria for childhood anxiety disorders.[34] The SCARED may be administered as a child report as well as a parent report. The original SCARED contained 38 items, with item responses scored on a Likert scale ranging from 0 to 2 (0, not true or hardly ever true; 1, somewhat true or sometimes true; 2, very true or often true). The SCARED was updated to a 41-item version with the addition of 3 questions on social phobia and contains information on 5 anxiety-related factors: panic/somatic, generalized anxiety, separation anxiety, social phobia, and school phobia.[35]

The development of the original 38-item SCARED among 341 outpatient children/adolescents aged 9 to 18 years and 300 parents showed good internal consistency for both the child- and parent reports, with coefficient alphas ranging from 0.74 to 0.93.[34] They also determined an optimal total score cutoff of 15, with a sensitivity of 70% and specificity of 50%, and recommend factor-specific cutoff scores with associated sensitivities and specificities ranging from 67% to 80% and 58% to 84%, respectively. In an outpatient sample of 190 children/adolescents and 166 parents, the 41-item SCARED showed good internal consistency, with the coefficient alpha for both the child-report and parent-report total score approximately 0.90, with factor-specific alpha values ranging from 0.78 to 0.87.[35] A cutoff score of 25 on the child-report total score yielded optimal sensitivity of 71%, whereas specificity varied for discriminating between anxiety and no anxiety (67%), anxiety and depression (61%), and anxiety and descriptive disorders (71%). A recent study addressed the use of the SCARED in predicting treatment response and remission, and included 438 youth and their parents.[70] The investigators found reductions of greater than or equal to 50% on the child report and greater than or equal to 55% on the parent report optimal for predicting treatment response, and greater than or equal to 60% on both reports optimal for predicting remission. A posttreatment total score of 12 on the child report and 10 on the parent report showed strong associations with remission in the overall sample, although the parent report showed increased efficiency when they used separate cutoffs for children and adolescents.

Spence Children's Anxiety Scale

The Spence Children's Anxiety Scale (SCAS)[63] assesses and evaluates symptoms related to 6 anxiety-related constructs in youth/adolescents: separation anxiety, social phobia, obsessive-compulsive disorder, panic-agoraphobia, generalized anxiety, and fears of physical injury.[36] There exists both a child self-report (SCAS) and a parent report (SCAS-P), both of which are designed to be brief and take around 10 minutes to complete. The child version comprises 44 items, 38 related to anxiety symptoms and 6 positively worded filler items,[37] whereas the parent version includes only the 38 anxiety-related items.[38] Item responses are scored on a Likert scale with a range from 0 to 3 (0, never; 1, sometimes; 2, often; 3, always), with the 6 filler items of the child version excluded in scoring. Separate subscale scores are calculated for each of the constructs listed earlier in addition to an overall total score. The Spence Children's Anxiety Scale may be used free of charge by individual clinicians.

An early validation study of the child version using a community sample of 2052 children aged 8 to 12 years found the following coefficient alphas: overall measure (0.92) and for the subscales, separation anxiety (0.70), social phobia (0.70), obsessive-compulsive disorder (0.73), panic-agoraphobia (0.82), generalized anxiety (0.73), and fears of physical injury (0.60).[37] The 6-month test-retest reliability among a subsample of children was acceptable, with a correlation coefficient of 0.60 on the SCAS total score. Another study examining the utility of the SCAS found similar internal consistencies in both the child and parent versions, with SCAS coefficient alphas ranging from 0.47 to 0.87 and SCAS-P coefficient alphas ranging from 0.62 to 0.90.[39] The same article explored the clinical utility of both the child and parent reports in predicting clinician diagnoses, and based on subscales and cut scores 1.5 standard deviations from community norms found SCAS sensitivity ranged from 33% to 78% and specificity from 42% to 84%, whereas SCAS-P sensitivity ranged from 32% to 100% and specificity from 32% to 82%. Recently, Olofsdotter and colleagues[40] conducted a validation study of both the child and parent versions of the SCAS among 104 Swedish youth from general outpatient psychiatric care, and their parents, and evaluated the SCAS against the K-SADS. For use as a screening tool, an SCAS total score greater than or equal to 22 had a sensitivity of 90.91% and specificity of 73.47%, and an SCAS-P total score greater than or equal to 15 had a sensitivity of 90.91% and specificity of 53.06%. For use as a diagnostic tool, an SCAS total score greater than or equal to 33 had a sensitivity of 63.64% and specificity of 93.88%, and an SCAS-P total score greater than or equal to 27 had a sensitivity of 61.82% and specificity of 93.75%. They also suggest screening and diagnostic cutoffs for the 6 subscales, with similar sensitivities and specificities.

Children Yale-Brown Obsessive-Compulsive Scale

The Children Yale-Brown Obsessive-Compulsive Scale (CY-BOCS) assesses symptom severity of obsessive-compulsive disorder (OCD) in children and adolescents,[41] and is a modified version of the original Y-BOCS developed for use among adults with OCD.[71] Clinicians can administer the measure as a child self-report and/or a parent report at their own discretion.[42] The CY-BOCS includes an obsessions symptoms checklist, a compulsions symptoms checklist, and a 10-item severity rating assessing the severity of both obsessions and compulsions over the past week. Only the 10 items relating to symptom severity are scored, with 5-item subscale scores for both obsessions and compulsions obtained from summing responses to the first 5 and last 5 items, respectively, and an overall total score obtained from summing all 10 items. Response options are scored on a Likert scale and range from 0 to 4 (items 1–4, 6–9: 0, none; 1, mild; 2, moderate; 3, severe; 4, extreme. Items 5–10: 0, complete control; 1, much control; 2, moderate control; 3, little control; 4, no control). Total CY-BOCS scores of 0 to 7, 8 to 15, 16 to 23, 24 to 31, and 32 to 40 are associated with subclinical, mild, moderate, severe, and extreme symptom severity, respectively.

Among a sample of 53 children and adolescents with OCD, the child and parent reports of the CY-BOCS total score were found to be internally consistent, with $\alpha = 0.87$ for the child-report and $\alpha = 0.86$ for the parent report.[43] The same sample showed acceptable internal consistency among the obsession ($\alpha = 0.78$) and compulsion ($\alpha = 0.81$) subscales of the child report, as well as the obsession ($\alpha = 0.83$) and compulsion ($\alpha = 0.70$) subscales of the parent report. Storch and colleagues[44] conducted a study comprising 109 youth with OCD, and reported percentage-reduction cutoffs for both treatment response and clinical remission and total score cutoffs for clinical remission. Receiver operating characteristic analyses suggested greater than or equal to 25% reduction in CY-BOCS as optimal for prediction of treatment response, with associated sensitivity of 0.98 and specificity of 0.75, and greater than or equal to 50% reduction in CY-BOCS as optimal for prediction of clinical remission, with associated sensitivity of 0.88 and specificity of 0.90. They additionally found the most efficient prediction of clinical remission based on a CY-BOCS total score cutoff to be 14, with sensitivity and specificity of 0.91 and 0.90, respectively.

Family Functioning and Parenting

McMaster Family Assessment Device
The Family Assessment Device (FAD) is a measure designed to assess characteristics of families and family functioning.[45] It includes 6 subscales that address specific family-related constructs: affective involvement, affective responsiveness, behavioral control, communication, problem solving, and roles, in addition to general functioning. Item responses are scored on a Likert scale and range from 1 to 4 (1, strongly agree; 2, agree; 3, disagree; 4, strongly disagree). The FAD was originally 53 items and was developed based on the McMaster Model of Family Functioning, although an updated version of the FAD includes 60 items. Epstein and colleagues[45] developed the FAD using a sample of 503 individuals, and found that Chronbach alphas suggested satisfactory internal reliability for all scales: problem solving (0.74), communication (0.75), roles (0.72), affective responsiveness (0.83), affective involvement (0.78), behavior control (0.72), and general functioning (0.92). A follow-up study evaluated cutoff scores for use in discriminating between healthy and unhealthy families.[46] A score of 2.0 for general functioning was associated with a sensitivity of 67% and specificity of 64%, whereas cutoff scores for the remaining subscales resulted in sensitivity between 57% to 83% and specificity between 60% to 79%. A recent study examined use of the FAD among both a community sample and help-seeking sample.[72] Using the cutoffs provided by Miller and colleagues,[46] they found scores from the help-seeking families were within the dissatisfied range, whereas scores from the community sample were within the satisfied range. In addition, intraclass correlation coefficients (ICCs) suggested moderate agreement between parents on all subscales except behavior control, whereas agreement between parents and adolescent children was similarly moderate, with low ICCs on problem solving in addition to behavior control.

Substance Use

CRAFFT
The CRAFFT is a well-validated screening tool for substance use disorders in adolescents aged 12 to 21 years. Its name is a mnemonic of the first letters of the key words in the 6 screening questions (car, relax, alone, forget, friends/family, and trouble). The test consists of 3 yes or no questions asking about use of alcohol, marijuana, or other

substances used to get high in the past 12 months. If the answer to any of those questions is yes, 6 follow-up yes or no questions are administered based on the mnemonic. Two or more yes answers to those 6 questions suggest a serious problem and need for further assessment. The percentage of patients with a DSM-5 substance use disorder is shown by CRAFFT score: 1 (32%), 2 (64%), 3 (79%), 4 (92%), and 5 to 6 (100%). Knight and colleagues[47] studied 538 patients in a large hospital-based general adolescent clinic (ages 14–18 years). A CRAFFT score of 2 or higher was optimal for identifying any problem (76% sensitivity, 94% specificity), any disorder (80% sensitivity, 86% specificity), and dependence (92% sensitivity, 80% specificity). Approximately one-fourth of patients scored 2 or higher. Validity was not significantly affected by age, sex, or race. The CRAFFT 2.0 was released in 2016 and changed the first 3 questions from yes/no to how many days used in the past 12 months.[73] More recently, CRAFFT 2.1 added edibles and vaping as methods of marijuana use.[74]

Attention-Deficit/Hyperactivity Disorder and Behavioral Symptoms

Swanson, Nolan, and Pelham–IV Questionnaire

The SNAP-IV[75] is a parent and teacher rating scale for ADHD in youth 5 to 17 years old. It consists of 90 items extracted from DSM-IV-based criteria for ADHD, oppositional defiant disorder (ODD), and other internalizing and externalizing disorders that may masquerade as ADHD, each scored on a Likert scale between 0 and 3 (0, not at all; 1, just a little; 2, quite a bit; 3, very much). Note that the SNAP-IV was not designed to be used in the formal process of diagnosing these non-ADHD disorders; scores of 2 or 3 warrant an assessment of these implicated disorders.

When screening for ADHD alone, the 18-item SNAP-IV is generally viewed as a brief, effective tool. It consists of 9 symptoms of inattention and 9 symptoms of hyperactivity. SNAP-IV subscales are calculated by summing the scores of the items in the specific subset (ie, inattention) and dividing by the number of items in the subset (9). There is also a 26-item SNAP-IV, which includes symptoms of ODD and is scored the same. This score is expressed as the average rating per item. Scores greater than the 95th percentile are considered clinically significant for ADHD and ODD subtypes, and corresponding cutoff scores are provided for parent and teacher ratings: ADHD-IT (inattentive type) (teacher 2.56, parent 1.78), ADHD-H/I (hyperactivity/impulsivity) (teacher 1.78, parent 1.44), ADHD-CT (combination type) (teacher 2.00, parent 1.67), and ODD (teacher 1.38, parent 1.88). Criticism has been leveled about the ability to generalize from the sample used to define these cutoffs,[48] because the subjects were a group of low-income Hispanic secondary school students.[76] There is also a dearth of evidence with regard to the predictive validity of the SNAP-IV. Following its use in the Multimodal Treatment Study for ADHD (MTA), Bussing and colleagues[48] evaluated the psychometric properties of the SNAP-IV and found acceptable internal consistency and item selection, and suggested that parent and teacher ratings satisfactorily distinguish children with varying levels of ADHD concerns. However, they cautioned the SNAP-IV's use for diagnostic purposes. Alda and Serrano-Troncoso[49] investigated the predictive validity of the parent-rated SNAP-IV in clinic-referred Spanish children, showing 82.3% sensitivity and 82.45% specificity with the clinicians' impression of ADHD. Nobel and colleagues[77] concluded that parent-report questionnaires may be acceptable to rate the overall severity of ADHD symptoms in treatment effect studies but not to detect the presence of ADHD in epidemiologic studies. Another study showed that parent ratings of inattention and hyperactivity/impulsivity on the SNAP-IV were good predictors of research but not clinician diagnosis. For teacher ratings, only hyperactivity/impulsivity scores were associated with research and clinician diagnosis. SNAP-IV scores showed high sensitivity but low specificity to clinician diagnosis, suggesting it is a valid outcome measure for use in randomized-controlled trials and clinical settings and is best used as a screening rather than a diagnostic tool for ADHD.[50]

Vanderbilt Attention-deficit/Hyperactivity Disorder Diagnostic Rating Scale

The Vanderbilt Attention-deficit/Hyperactivity Disorder Diagnostic Rating Scale (VADRS)[51] is an assessment tool for ADHD symptoms and their effects on behavior and academic performance in children aged 6 to 12 years. It elicits symptoms in domains of inattention, disruptive behavior, anxiety, and depression. Separate scales also assess school performance. There are both parent (VADPRS) and teacher (VADTRS) rating scales. The parent scale consists of 55 items and the teacher scale 43 items. There is also a parent/teacher follow-up scale with 26 items. The symptom questions are scored on a Likert scale between 0 and 3 (0, never; 1, occasionally; 2, often; 3, very often). The school performance questions are scored on a Likert scale between 1 and 5 (1, excellent; 2, above average; 3, average; 4, somewhat of a problem; 5, problematic).

The VADPRS contains 6 subscales, and behaviors are included in the total for each subscale if they are scored as a 2 or a 3. The VADTRS contains 5 subscales, and behaviors are included in the total for each subscale if they are scored as a 2 or a 3. A score of 1 or 2 on at least 1 question in the performance section indicates impairment. The parent and teacher follow-up scales have 18 questions limited to symptoms of ADHD and 9 performance questions, with 12 questions monitoring potential side effects of treatment. Scoring of these scales (total symptoms score items [18 items] and average performance score [9 items]) can be tracked over time with treatment.[78]

Wolraich and colleagues[52] examined the psychometric properties of the VADTRS and showed strong internal consistency and consistent latent dimension structure consistent with DSM-IV and other accepted measures of ADHD. The performance measures were correlated with the presence of problems in academic or behavioral performance. The performance measures are an important measure of the extent of impairment, although not sufficient alone to establish impairment. Wolraich and colleagues[53] also examined the psychometric properties of the VADPRS. Regarding reliability, factor structure, and concurrent validity to the VADTRS, it showed comparable internal consistency and factor structure. There was a high correlation with the performance questions of the Strengths and Difficulties Questionnaire (0.97). However, given that this was a study of a referred sample, sensitivity and specificity were not able to be established.

Broad Rating Scales

Pediatric Symptom Checklist

The Pediatric Symptom Checklist[60] (PSC) is a general psychosocial screening and functional assessment tool in the domains of attention, externalizing, and internalizing symptoms in children aged 6 to 12 years.[54] Developed from a revised version of the Washington Symptom Checklist,[79] the original PSC was intended for use among parents of school-aged children (6–12 years old) and was meant to take 3 to 5 minutes to complete. Subsequent applications of the PSC include responses on children aged 4 to 16 years, with certain school-specific questions excluded for the youngest children. In addition to the parent-report PSC, there is a 35-item youth self-report (PSC-Y) version, as well as abbreviated 17-item parent-report (PSC-17) and youth self-report (PSC-17-Y) versions. It is self-administered to youth (≥11 years old), and it is easy and quick to administer and score.

Pediatric Symptom Checklist (35 items)

The PSC is a 35-item measure designed to screen for difficulties in emotional and behavioral functioning in school-aged children.[54] Item responses are scored on a Likert scale and range from 0 to 2 (0, never; 1, sometimes; 2, often) and a total score is obtained by summing over responses to all items where higher scores suggest greater difficulties. Factor analysis of the original 35 items not only yielded the briefer PSC-17 but also further identified 3 subscales for internalizing, attention, and externalizing problems.[61]

In an early validation study of the 35-item PSC, Jellinek and colleagues[55] studied the validity of the PSC by screening 300 children in both a middle-class group practice and an urban health maintenance organization. Based on 48 children with in-depth interview assessments and pediatricians' ratings, a PSC cutoff score of 28 was associated with a sensitivity of 95% and specificity of 68%.

The PSC is also internally consistent across multiple formats, with high Cronbach alphas ($\alpha = 0.91$–0.92) in a clinic-based sample using English, Spanish, written, and oral versions of the PSC.[56] For children aged 4 to 5 years, a PSC cutoff score of 24 or more is associated with acceptable sensitivity (64%) and high specificity (93%), and yields a positive prevalence rate similar to the rate found among school-aged children.[57] For this age group, scores on 4 elementary school–related items are not included in the final score.[58] A following study assessing use of the PSC-Y as a self-report measure found using a cutoff score of 30 to be associated with optimal sensitivity (94%) and specificity (88%), with case/noncase agreement between the PSC and the PSC-Y of 79%.[80] Another study examined screening for psychosocial dysfunction in inner-city children and found the PSC to be a valid and reliable screening tool for economically disadvantaged and minority backgrounds, as it is for middle-class and upper-middle-class populations.[59] Using reliable and clinically significant change (Reliable Change Index) metrics, a change in the total PSC score of 6 or more was found to represent reliable change, whereas a change of 6 or more that included a shift across the measure's risk threshold suggested a clinically meaningful change in psychometric symptoms.[81] Similar analyses found that a change in score of 2 accompanied by crossing the risk threshold denoted clinically significant change on both the attention subscale[82] and the internalizing subscale.[83]

Pediatric Symptom Checklist-17

The PSC-17 is a brief checklist of 17 questions scored on a Likert scale (0, never; 1, sometimes; 2, often). The validity and reliability of the shortened PSC-17 is similar to that of the 35-item version. An early validation study using a large sample of primary care patients found that a cutoff score of 15 on the PSC-17 yielded a sensitivity of 82% and specificity of 81%.[61] Gardner and colleagues[61] also suggested cutoff scores for the 3 subscales: 5 for internalizing with sensitivity of 79% and specificity of 68%, 7 for externalizing with sensitivity of 77% and specificity of 80%, and 7 for attention with sensitivity of 87% and specificity of 79%. Higher scores indicate an increased likelihood of a behavioral health disorder being present. More recently, a large national study of 80,680 individuals from 325 pediatric offices found the PSC-17 continued to be internally reliable, with an overall Cronbach $\alpha = 0.87$, and $\alpha = 0.78$, $\alpha = 0.82$, and $\alpha = 0.80$ for the internalizing, attention, and externalizing subscales, respectively.[62] The PSC-17-Y yields similar, albeit slightly smaller, internal consistency statistics, with Cronbach $\alpha = 0.68$ to 0.81 for the overall and subscale scores.[63]

Parker and colleagues[84] examined the screening validity of the youth-report version of the PSC-17 in a child welfare population using multitrait multimethod matrices. Youth with any lifetime mental health diagnosis scored significantly higher on the total

PSC attention and internalizing subscales. Attention, internalizing, and total subscale scores were significantly correlated with psychosis, depression, and anxiety disorders, but not with externalizing scores. ADHD was associated with attention, externalizing, and total scores. Bipolar disorder was only weakly associated with externalizing and total subscale scores. Comparison between youth and foster parent scores showed the highest agreement on externalizing scores and lowest for internalizing scores. Jacobson and colleagues[85] similarly tested the reliability and validity of the PSC-17 in child welfare–involved youth in Washington State. The PSC-17 showed good convergent and divergent validity. Test-retest reliability was moderate over 6 months.

Case Example: Using Rating Scales to Care for an Adolescent Patient Within the Measurement-Based Care Framework

The following case example shows the use of self-report and parent-report behavioral health rating scales by a child psychiatrist working within an office-based practice. The case was created for the purposes of demonstrating the principles reviewed in this article.

Dr Williams is a child and adolescent psychiatrist working within a community outpatient clinic. The clinic staff use an electronic health record and Web-based platform to facilitate the collection of youth self-report and parent-report rating scales. This platform administers publicly available, standardized rating scales covering multiple symptom domains and administered by age range, with results and related clinical guidance transmitted directly into the electronic health record.

Intake appointment

Lily, a 16-year-old girl, is brought to see Dr Williams by her mother, at the suggestion of her primary care physician, after performing poorly in school. Lily's primary care provider told the family she believes Lily may be depressed. Before the appointment with Dr Williams, Lily and her mother are asked to complete the rating scales through the Web-based platform. An administrative assistant in the office describes the importance of obtaining Lily's "behavioral health vital signs," just as it is important to obtain height, weight, and blood pressure when attending a primary care appointment.[17] Lily completes the PSC-17-Y (broad measure), SCARED (anxiety), PHQ-9 (mood), CRAFFT (substance use), and the CPSS (trauma). The PSC, SCARED, and PHQ-9 are increased. Lily's mother completes the PSC-17, SCARED, SNAP-IV (ADHD symptoms), MFQ–Short Form (mood), and FAD (family functioning). The PSC-17, SCARED, MFQ–Short Form, and the FAD are increased. Lily's mother does not endorse observations consistent with ADHD. Abnormal results are shown in **Table 2**.

Dr Williams thanks Lily and her mother for completing the rating scales on the Web-based platform. She reinforces the concept of behavioral health vital signs and proceeds with a thorough interview. Dr Williams interviews Lily and her mother separately.

During the interview with Dr Williams, Lily says she has always been a perfectionist. She is a straight-A student and excels in theater and dance. Lily reports she has "always" experienced muscle tension and challenges "letting go" with friends, because she worries about various topics. Lily is frequently irritable; however, her irritability increased over the past 2 months following a breakup with her boyfriend. Lily's mood significantly decreased following this event. Lily has a passion for acting and she has a supporting role in the upcoming school play; however, has not been enjoying this activity as much as she used to. Lily has also been having difficulty remembering her lines, which is unlike her. Lily has trouble falling asleep at night, which she attributes to feeling responsible for the breakup. She has been tired during the

Table 2						
Abnormal results from the intake appointment						
Lily's Scores		**Intake**	**Mother's Scores**		**Intake**	
PSC	Total	20	PSC-17	Total	18
	Inattention	7		Inattention	6
	Internalizing	9		Internalizing	8
	Externalizing	4		Externalizing	4
SCARED	Total	26	SCARED	Total	25
(child)	Panic	5	(parent)	Panic	4
	Generalized Anxiety Disorder	16		Generalized Anxiety Disorder	15
	Separation	0		Separation	1
	Social	2		Social	2
	School	3		School	4
PHQ-9	Total	21	MFQ	Total	8
—	Question 9	1	FAD	Total	4

day and it has been hard to focus on her school work. Lily still wants to do well in her classes, but shares that, "I just can't seem to get my work done." Lily feels "bad" about herself. She shares that her parents have been worried about her and sometimes she thinks, "It would have been easier if I were not born," because she does not want to burden her parents. She denies having ever having had a plan or intent to end her life.

During interview, Lily's mother reports her daughter has been more irritable over the past 2 months. She has noticed Lily has been sad, observing she is still tearful about the breakup. Lily has been declining invitations to spend time with her friends. The patient's mother shares that she and Lily's father do not place pressure on Lily; however, Lily is driven to excel academically and in extracurricular activities. She is worried about her daughter. Lily's mother shares that she has struggled with depression, which has been successfully treated with Lexapro and psychotherapy. Dr Williams asks Lily's mother about her answers in the FAD (endorsed misunderstandings; challenges with feelings, expression, and communication) and she responds that there has been marital discord at home over the past 8 to 10 months, and she was thinking of this while answering the questions. Lily's mother reflects her belief that the home environment is also contributing to Lily's mood. Lily's mother asks Dr Williams whether she may be able to provide a referral for a couples therapist.

Dr Williams meets with Lily and her mother. She shares her belief that Lily is experiencing major depression and generalized anxiety disorder, because Lily's symptoms of anxiety have been long-standing, pervasive, and have affected her functioning. After a thorough interview, Lily is assessed to be low risk for suicide. Using the results of the PHQ-9 and SCARED, Dr Williams reviews symptoms of depression and anxiety with Lily and her mother. Specific attention is paid to the symptoms endorsed by Lily and her mother, noting where Lily and her mother were similar and where their reports differed. Lily states that it can be hard to describe her feelings and she was not sure what to expect from a psychiatry visit. She shares that the rating scales helped to guide her as to what sorts of symptom to discuss during the appointment.

Dr Williams provides Lily and her mother with a handout containing instructions on behavioral activation and challenging anxious thoughts. Dr Williams reviews treatment options with Lily and her mother. Lily agrees to participate in cognitive behavior therapy (CBT) for depression and anxiety. The patient and her mother are amenable to a trial of Lexapro, starting at 5 mg daily, to target low mood and anxiety, because this medication has been effective for Lily's mother. Lily's mother is also provided with referrals for couples therapy. Using the handout, Lily is encouraged to engage in behavioral activation and to challenge anxious thoughts. Dr Williams encourages Lily and her mother to monitor Lily's symptoms through the rating scales. The discussion of rating scale scores with Lily and her mother helps to facilitate psychoeducation, engage them in treatment, and promote shared decision making. Lily and her mother plan to follow up in 1 week by telephone, at which time the medication will be increased to 10 mg if Lily has been tolerating it well.

Two weeks later (2 weeks from intake)

Before the appointment with Dr Williams, Lily is asked to complete the rating scales that were increased during the intake visit, specifically the PSC-17-Y, SCARED, and PHQ-9. In the same vein, Lily's mother completes the PSC-17, SCARED, MFQ-SF, and FAD. They are again reminded of the value of these behavioral health vital signs. Abnormal results are shown in **Table 3**.

On interview, Lily reports she continues to feel down and anxious. Lily's mother reports her daughter has been slightly more engaged in school work and family activities. She endorses ongoing challenges with communication at home. Dr Williams reviews Lily's rating scales scores with her, noting specifically that Lily's PHQ-9 score reveals she has had mild improvements in sleep, energy, and appetite. She also remarks on the resolution of Lily's suicidal ideation since the last appointment. Lily states that she had not been aware of the slight improvements in sleep, energy, and appetite, but, now that she compares her scores on these items with her scores 2 weeks ago, she realizes she has already made some improvements. The SCARED reveals continued general anxiety symptoms, along with some school avoidance symptoms. Given the at-risk score on FAD, Dr Williams discusses the technique of active listening with Lily and her mother. Lily and her mother report that Lily has yet to start therapy; however, an intake appointment is scheduled for later in the week. Lily has been tolerating Lexapro without issue and the medication is continued at 10 mg daily. The patient's mother shares that she and her husband have had 1 appointment with the couples therapist. Lily and her mother are advised to follow up in 4 weeks.

Table 3
Abnormal results 2 weeks after intake

	Lily's Scores	Intake	2 wk		Mother's Scores	Intake	2 wk
PSC	Total	20	20	PSC-17	Total	18	14
	Inattention	7	7		Inattention	6	4
	Internalizing	9	9		Internalizing	8	6
	Externalizing	4	4		Externalizing	4	4
SCARED	Total	26	25	SCARED	Total	25	25
(child)	Panic	5	4	(parent)	Panic	4	4
	GAD	16	15		GAD	15	15
	Separation	0	0		Separation	1	0
	Social	2	2		Social	2	2
	School	3	4		School	4	4
PHQ-9	Total	21	14	MFQ	Total	8	7
—	Question 9	1	0	FAD	Total	4	4

Four weeks later (1.5 months from intake)

Lily is asked to complete the rating scales that were increased during the previous visit, specifically the PSC-17-Y, SCARED, and PHQ-9. Lily's mother completes the SCARED and FAD. They are again encouraged and reminded of the value of these assessments. Results are shown in **Table 4**.

During interview, Lily reports improvements in mood, supported by the decrease in PHQ-9 score. Using the PHQ-9, Lily and Dr Williams note particular challenges with self-esteem and concentration. Lily's SCARED reveals significant symptoms of generalized anxiety. Dr Williams and Lily discuss that poor ability to concentrate may be related to both depression and anxiety. Lily and her mother are provided with a handout of Lily's mother's scores, which again focus on effective communication skills such as active listening. Lily has begun weekly therapy and she reports that she enjoys working with her new therapist, Mr Lynn. Lexapro is continued at 10 mg daily. The patient's mother reports that she and Lily's father have been attending couples therapy, where they are working on effective communication. Dr Williams speaks with Mr Lynn and they discuss using CBT techniques to focus on negative evaluative thoughts. They also discuss focusing on mindfulness techniques in therapy to calm Lily's mind with hopes this will help to increase her ability to attend to assignments.

Dr Williams shares that she will monitor Lily's PHQ-9 score, with specific attention to the items that continue to remain most increased (self-esteem, concentration) because they are working toward a 50% reduction in score, with total score less than 5. However, Dr Williams notes that a 3-point to 5-point change in score is considered clinically significant. Lily reports that she believes she has made improvement in her symptoms (PHQ-9 score reduction of 10 since intake) and she says it is reassuring to see that her score has been decreasing. Dr Williams explains they will also continue to monitor the SCARED, working toward a 50% decrease in symptoms, as reported by Lily, and a total score of 12 or less. She also states they will continue to monitor family functioning. The patient and her mother are advised to follow up in 3 months.

Three months later (4.5 months from intake)

Lily is asked to complete the rating scales that were increased during the previous visit, specifically the SCARED and PHQ-9. Lily's mother completes FAD. Results are shown in **Table 5**.

During the interview, Lily reports improvements in mood and anxiety level. She notes that this is particularly remarkable because she has had more reasons to feel stressed lately, because she recently took her Scholastic Assessment Test (SAT). Dr Williams and Lily review her SCARED and PHQ-9 scores together. They note that Lily has made improvements in her ability to concentrate and to her self-esteem, which she attributes to therapy and to recently winning an essay contest she entered at school. Dr Williams tells Lily they will continue to work on residual symptoms of anxiety and low mood; however, also shares that Lily has made significant improvements in rating scale scores (achieved greater than 50% improvements on both SCARED and PHQ-9, with total SCARED <12). Lily's mother reports a more harmonious environment at home. Lily notes that this has also positively affected her mental state. Lily and her mother are provided with a handout of Lily's mother's FAD score. Dr Williams comments that the FAD is no longer increased in the at-risk range. The patient and her mother thank Dr Williams for being thorough in and attentive to Lily's care, citing systematic use of rating scales and discussion of the results, in addition to the clinical interview. They both report confidently knowing which symptoms they should monitor for continued improvement or worsening. Lily plans to continue weekly therapy and Lexapro. The patient's mother reports that she and Lily's

Table 4
Results 6 weeks after intake

		Lily's Scores					Mother's Scores		
		Intake	2 wk	6 wk			Intake	2 wk	6 wk
PSC	Total	20	20	14	PSC-17	Total	18	14	Within normal limits
	Inattention	7	7	5		Inattention	6	4	—
	Internal	9	9	6		Internal	8	6	—
	External	4	4	3		External	4	4	—
SCARED (child)	Total	26	25	25	SCARED (parent)	Total	25	25	20
	Panic	5	4	3		Panic	4	4	1
	GAD	16	15	18		GAD	15	15	15
	Separation	0	0	0		Separation	1	0	0
	Social	2	2	2		Social	2	2	2
	School	3	4	2		School	4	4	2
PHQ-9	Total	21	14	11	MFQ	Total	8	7	WNL
—	Question 9	1	0	0	FAD	Total	4	4	3

Table 5
Results 4 months after intake

Lily's Scores		Intake	2 wk	6 wk	4 mo	Mother's Scores		Intake	2 wk	6 wk	4 mo
PSC	Total	20	20	14	—	PSC-17	Total	18	14	WNL	—
	Inattention	7	7	5	—		Inattention	6	4	—	—
	Internal	9	9	6	—		Internal	8	6	—	—
	External	4	4	3	—		External	4	4	—	—
SCARED (child)	Total	26	25	25	11	SCARED (parent)	Total	25	25	20	WNL
	Panic	5	4	3	1		Panic	4	4	1	—
	GAD	16	15	18	7		GAD	15	15	15	—
	Separation	0	0	0	0		Separation	1	0	0	—
	Social	2	2	2	2		Social	2	2	2	—
	School	3	4	2	1		School	4	4	2	—
PHQ-9	Total	21	14	11	8	MFQ	Total	8	7	WNL	—
—	Question 9	1	0	0	0	FAD	Total	4	4	3	0

father will continue couples therapy. Dr Williams recommends Lily return for an appointment in 3 months.

Case Discussion

Dr William's treatment of Lily and her mother exemplifies skillful use of rating scales in patient treatment. According to MBC principles, rating scales were assessed frequently and concurrent with the clinical encounter. They were not used as a replacement for clinical interview, but enhanced the interview. Dr Williams used rating scale scores to inform her treatment plan and provide psychoeducation to Lily and her mother. During Lily's first follow-up appointment, she was pleasantly surprised to learn she had made improvement in several neurovegetative symptoms of depression even though she continued to feel down. This recognition of improvement may have given Lily and her mother increased hope that Lily could and would get better. Lily and her mother also noted that, even after Lily made treatment gains, they would continue to monitor symptoms.

Lily and her mother expressed increased confidence in Dr William's ability as a provider, because she consistently used rating scales to supplement her clinical interview. Lily and her mother thought themselves fortunate to have a provider that was so thorough and focused on outcomes. Lily reported increased ability to express herself through prompting with rating scale questions, especially during the intake appointment. The patient and her mother reported increased understanding of Lily's challenges and increased sense of agency. In this case, a benefit to using a rating scale such as the SCARED and PHQ-9 in a systematic way is that it afforded the opportunity for Lily and her mother to monitor particular symptoms (noted by specific questions) over time (such as self-esteem, concentration). In addition, the increased FAD score prompted Lily's mother to accept referrals for services to address the challenges in the relationship with her husband.

SUMMARY

MBC in psychiatry can be described as the consistent, repeated use of validated self-reported measures to track patient symptoms and impairment over the course of treatment. These measures are used to anchor the treatment process, establish treatment targets, and augment clinical decision making. In this way, they can be thought of as the psychiatric equivalent of monitoring laboratory tests or vital sign measures.

When using self-reported measures for this purpose, it is important that clinicians select measures that are psychometrically validated and address the symptoms or diagnosis of greatest concern. It is also important that clinicians have a sufficient understanding of the underlying psychometric properties of these measures to properly interpret changes in scored value over time and use these results to increase patient understanding and appropriately direct care.

An array of validated self-reported measures are available in the public domain, covering a wide range of potential mental disorders. This article offers a review of select public domain measures, and provides a summary of relevant psychometric properties that clinicians can put to immediate use to deploy MBC principles in clinical practice. A case example is offered to put the framework into context and describe the practical use of MBC to efficiently set and achieve target treatment goals.

DISCLOSURE

The authors have nothing to disclose.

REFERENCES

1. Harding KJ, Rush AJ, Arbuckle M, et al. Measurement-based care in psychiatric practice: a policy framework for implementation. J Clin Psychiatry 2011;72:1136–43.
2. Fortney JC, Unützer J, Wrenn G, et al. A tipping point for measurement-based care. Psychiatr Serv 2017;68(2):179–88.
3. Scott K, Lewis C. Using measurement-based care to enhance any treatment. Cogn Behav Pract 2015;2(1):49–59.
4. Kroenke K, Unutzer J. Closing the false divide: sustainable approaches to integrating mental health services into primary care. J Gen Intern Med 2016;32(4):404–10.
5. Bickman L, Kelley SD, Breda C, et al. Effects of routine feedback to clinicians on mental health outcomes of youths: results of a randomized trial. Psychiatr Serv 2011;62:1423–9.
6. Dowrick C, Leydon GM, McBride A, et al. Patients' and doctors' views on depression severity questionnaires incentivized in UK quality and outcomes framework: qualitative study. BMJ 2009;338:b66.
7. Valenstein M, Adler DA, Berlant J, et al. Implementing standardized assessments in clinical care: now's the time. Psychiatr Serv 2009;60:1372–5.
8. Sattler JM. Assessment of children: cognitive foundations. 5th edition. San Diego (CA): Jerome M. Sattler, Publisher, Inc; 2008.
9. Meyers K, Winters NC. Ten-year review of rating scales. I: overview of scale functioning, psychometric properties, and selection. J Am Acad Child Adolesc Psychiatry 2002;41:114–22.
10. Price PC, Jhangiani RS, Chiang IC. Reliability and validity of measurement. In: Research Methods in Psychology. Victoria, British Columbia, Canada: B.C. Open Textbook Project; 2015 Chapter 5. Available at: https://opentextbc.ca/researchmethods/chapter/reliability-and-validity-of-measurement/. Accessed July 14, 2020.
11. Löwe B, Kroenke K, Herzog W, et al. Measuring depression outcome with a brief self-report instrument: sensitivity to change of the Patient Health Questionnaire (PHQ-9). J Affect Disord 2004;1:61–6.
12. Priebe S, Mccabe R, Bullenkamp J, et al. The impact of routine outcome measurement on treatment processes in community mental health care: approach and methods of the MECCA study. Epidemiol Psichiatr Soc 2002;11:198–205.
13. Connell J, Carlton J, Grundy A, et al. The importance of content and face validity in instrument development: lessons learnt from service users when developing the Recovering Quality of Life measure (ReQoL). Qual Life Res 2018;27:1893–902.
14. Jacobson NS, Follette WC, Revenstorf D. Psychotherapy outcome research: methods for reporting variability and evaluating clinical significance. Behav Ther 1984;15:336–52.
15. Welner Z, Reich W, Herjanic B, et al. Reliability, validity, and parent child agreement studies of the Diagnostic Interview for Children and Adolescents (DICA). J Am Acad Child Adolesc Psychiatry 1987;26:649–53.
16. Yule W. Developmental considerations in child assessment. In: Ollendick TH, Hersen M, editors. Handbook of child and adolescent assessment. 167. Boston: Allyn & Bacon; 1993. p. 15–25.
17. Jefffrey J, Hajal NJ, Klomhaus A, et al. The use of behavioral health rating scales for primary care providers. Ment Health Fam Med 2019;15:884–92.

18. Ajami S, Bagheri-Tadi T. Barriers for adopting electronic health records (EHRs) by physicians. Acta Inform Med 2013;21(2):129–34.
19. Kroenke K, Spitzer RL, Williams JBW. The PHQ-9. J Gen Intern Med 2001;16: 606–13.
20. Richardson LP, McCauley E, Grossman DC, et al. Evaluation of the Patient Health Questionnaire (PHQ-9) for detecting major depression among adolescents. Pediatrics 2010;126(6):1117–23.
21. Beidas RS, Stewart RE, Walsh L, et al. Free, brief, and validated: standardized instruments for low-resource mental health settings. Cogn Behav Pract 2015; 22:5–19.
22. Angold A, Costello EJ, Messer SC, et al. The development of a short questionnaire for use in epidemiological studies of depression in children and adolescents. Int J Methods Psychiatr Res 1995;5:237–49.
23. Costello EJ, Angold A. Scales to assess child and adolescent depression: checklist, screens, and nets. J Am Acad Child Adolesc Psychiatry 1988;27(6):726–37.
24. Thabrew H, Stasiak K, Bavin LM, et al. Validation of the mood and feelings questionnaire (MFQ) and short mood and feelings questionnaire (SMFQ) in New Zealand help-seeking adolescents. Int J Methods Psychiatr Res 2018;7:e1610.
25. Burleson Daviss W, Birmaher B, Melhem NA, et al. Criterion validity of the Mood and Feelings Questionnaire for depressive episodes in clinic and non-clinic subjects. J Child Psychol Psychiatry 2006;47(9):927–34.
26. Rhew IC, Simpson K, Tracy M, et al. Criterion validity of the short mood and feelings questionnaire and one- and two-item depression screens in young adolescents. Child Adolesc Psychiatry Ment Health 2010;4:8.
27. Pavuluri MN, Henry DB, Devineni B, et al. Child mania rating scale: development, reliability, and validity. J Am Acad Child Adolesc Psychiatry 2006;45(5):55–560.
28. Henry DB, Pavuluri MN, Youngstrom E, et al. Accuracy of brief and full forms of the child mania rating scale. J Clin Psychol 2008;64(4):368–81.
29. West AE, Celio CI, Henry DB, et al. Child mania rating scale-parent version: a valid measure of symptom change due to pharmacotherapy. J Affect Disord 2011;128(1-2):112–9.
30. Gracious BL, Youngstrom EA, Findling RL, et al. Discriminative validity of a parent version of the young mania rating scale. J Am Acad Child Adolesc Psychiatry 2002;41(11):1350–9.
31. Youngstrom EA, Gracious BL, Danielson CK, et al. Toward an integration of parent and clinician report on the young mania rating scale. J Affect Disord 2003;77: 179–90.
32. Yee AM, Algorta GP, Youngstrom EA, et al, Lams Group. Unfiltered administration of the YMRS and CDRS-R in a clinical sample of children. J Clin Child Adolesc Psychol 2015;44(6):992–1007.
33. Foa EB, Asnaani A, Zang Y, et al. Psychometrics of the child PTSD symptom scale for DSM-5 for trauma exposed children and adolescents. J Clin Child Adolesc Psychol 2018;47(1):38–46.
34. Birmaher B, Khetarpal S, Brent D, et al. The screen for child anxiety related emotional disorders (SCARED): scale construction and psychometric characteristics. J Am Acad Child Adolesc Psychiatry 1997;36(4):545–53.
35. Birmaher B, Brent DA, Chiappetta L, et al. Psychometric properties of the screen for child anxiety related emotional disorders (SCARED): a replication study. J Am Acad Child Adolesc Psychiatry 1999;38(10):1230–6.
36. Spence SH. Structure of anxiety symptoms among children: a confirmatory factor-analytic study. J Abnorm Psychol 1997;106(2):280–97.

37. Spence SH. A measure of anxiety symptoms among children. Behav Res Ther 1998;36:545–66.

38. Spence SH. Spence children's anxiety scale (parent version). Brisbane (Australia): University of Queensland; 1999.

39. Brown-Jacobsen AM, Wallace DP, Whiteside SPH. Multimethod, multi-informant agreement and positive predictive value in the identification of child anxiety disorders using the SCAS and ADIS-C. Assessment 2011;18(3):382–92.

40. Olofsdotter S, Sonnby K, Vadlin S, et al. Assessing adolescent anxiety in general psychiatric care: diagnostic accuracy of the Swedish self-report and parent versions of the spence children's anxiety scale. Assessment 2016;23(6):744–57.

41. Scahill L, Riddle MA, McSwiggin-Hardin M, et al. Children's yale-brown obsessive compulsive scale: reliability and validity. J Am Acad Child Adolesc Psychiatry 1997;36(6):844–52.

42. Storch EA, Murphy TK, Geffken GR, et al. Psychometric evaluation of the children's yale-brown obsessive-compulsive scale. Psychiatry Res 2004; 129(1):91–8.

43. Storch EA, Murphy TK, Adkins JW, et al. The children's yale-brown obsessive-compulsive scale: psychometric properties of child- and parent-report formats. J Anxiety Disord 2006;20:1055–70.

44. Storch EA, Lewin AB, De Nadai AS, et al. Defining treatment response and remission in obsessive-compulsive disorder: a signal detection analysis of the children's yale-brown obsessive compulsive scale. J Am Acad Child Adolesc Psychiatry 2010;49(7):708–17.

45. Epstein NB, Baldwin LM, Bishop DS. The McMaster family assessment device. J Marital Fam Ther 1983;9(2):171–80.

46. Miller IW, Epstein NB, Bishop DS, et al. The Mcmaster family assessment device: reliability and validity. J Marital Fam Ther 1985;11(4):345–56.

47. Knight JR, Sherritt L, Shrier LA, et al. Validity of the CRAFFT substance abuse screening test among adolescent clinic patients. Arch Pediatr Adolesc Med 2002;156(6):607–14.

48. Bussing R, Fernandez M, Harwood M, et al. Parent and teacher SNAP-IV ratings of attention deficit hyperactivity disorder symptoms: psychometric properties and normative ratings from a school district sample. Assessment 2008;15(3):317–28.

49. Alda JA, Serrano-Troncoso E. Attention-deficit hyperactivity disorder: agreement between clinical impression and the SNAP-IV screening tool. Actas Esp Psiquiatr 2013;41(2):76–83.

50. Hall CL, Guo B, Valentine AZ, et al. The validity of the SNAP-IV in children displaying ADHD symptoms. Assessment 2019;16. 1073191119842255.

51. Wolraich ML, Bard DE, Deas B, et al. The psychometric properties of the vanderbilt attention-deficit hyperactivity disorder diagnostic teacher rating scale in a community population. J Dev Behav Pediatr 2013;34(2):83–93.

52. Wolraich ML1, Feurer ID, Hannah JN, et al. Obtaining systematic teacher reports of disruptive behavior disorders utilizing DSM-IV. J Abnorm Child Psychol 1998; 26(2):141–52.

53. Wolraich ML1, Lambert W, Doffing MA, et al. Psychometric properties of the Vanderbilt ADHD diagnostic parent rating scale in a referred population. J Pediatr Psychol 2003;28(8):559–67.

54. Jellinek MS, Murphy M, Burns BJ. Brief psychosocial screening in outpatient pediatric practice. J Pediatr 1986;109(2):371–8.

55. Jellinek MS, Murphy JM, Robinson J, et al. Pediatric symptom checklist: screening school-age children for psychosocial dysfunction. J Pediatr 1988; 11(2):201–9.
56. Murphy JM, Ichinose C, Hicks RC, et al. Utility of the pediatric symptom checklist as a psychosocial screen to meet the federal Early and Periodic Screening, Diagnosis, and Treatment (EPSDT) standards: a pilot study. J Pediatr 1996;129(6): 864–9.
57. Little M, Murphy JM, Jellinek MS, et al. Screening 4- and 5-year-old children for psychosocial dysfunction: a preliminary study with the Pediatric Symptom Checklist. J Dev Behav Pediatr 1994;15(3):191–7.
58. Pagano M, Murphy JM, Pedersen M, et al. Screening for psychosocial problems in 4-5-year-olds during routine EPSDT examinations: validity and reliability in a Mexican-America Sample. Clin Pediatr 1996;35(3):139–46.
59. Murphy JM, Reerde J, Jellinek MS, et al. Screening for psychosocial dysfunction in inner-city children: further validation of the pediatric symptom checklist. J Am Acad Child Adolesc Psychiatry 1992;31:6.
60. Pediatric symptom checklist. Available at: http://www.brightfutures.org. Accessed December 27, 2019.
61. Gardner W, Murphy M, Childs G, et al. The PSC-17: a brief pediatric symptom checklist with psychosocial problem subscales. A report from PROS and ASPN. Ambul Child Health 1999;5(3):225–36.
62. Murphy JM, Bergmann P, Chiang C, et al. The PSC-17: subscale scores, reliability, and factor structure in a new national sample. Pediatrics 2016;138(3): e20160038.
63. Bergmann P, Lucke C, Nguyen T, et al. Identification and utility of a short form of the Pediatric Symptom Checklist-Youth self-report (PSC-17-Y). Eur J Psychol Assess 2018;1–9. https://doi.org/10.1027/1015-5759/a000486.
64. Kroenke K, Spitzer RL, Williams JB. The PHQ-9: validity of a brief depression severity measure. J Gen Intern Med 2001;6:606–13.
65. Lewandowski RE, O'Connor B, Bertagnolli A, et al. Screening and diagnosis of depression in adolescents in a large HMO. Psychiatr Serv 2016;67(6):636–41.
66. Wood A, Kroll L, Moore A, et al. Properties of the mood and feelings questionnaire in psychiatric outpatients: a research note. J Child Psychol Psychiatry 1995;36(2): 327–34.
67. Kent L. Detection of major and minor depression in children and adolescents: evaluation of the mood and feelings questionnaire. J Child Psychol Psychiatry 1997;38:565–73.
68. Turner N, Joinson C, Peters TJ, et al. Validity of the short mood and feelings questionnaire in late adolescence. Psychol Assess 2014;26(3):752–62.
69. Axelson D, Birmaher BJ, Brent D, et al. A preliminary study of the kiddie schedule for affective disorders and schizophrenia for school-age children mania rating scale for children and adolescents. J Child Adolesc Psychopharmacol 2004; 13(4):463–70.
70. Caporino NE, Sakolsky D, Brodman DM, et al. Establishing clinical cutoffs for response and remission on the screen for child anxiety related emotional disorders. J Am Acad Child Adolesc Psychiatry 2017;56(8):696–702.
71. Goodman WK, Price LH, Rasmussen SA, et al. The yale-brown obsessive compulsive scale I. Development, use, and reliability. Arch Gen Psychiatry 1989;46(11):1006–11.
72. Mansfield AK, Keitner GI, Dealy J. The family assessment device: an update. Fam Process 2015;54(1):82–93.

73. Harris SK, Knight JR Jr, Van Hook S, et al. Adolescent substance use screening in primary care: validity of computer self-administered vs. clinician-administered screening. Subst Abus 2015;37(1):197–203.
74. Knight J. The CRAFFT Interview (Version 2.1). Center for Adolescent Substance Abuse Research (CeASAR), Boston Children's Hospital, 2018. Available at http://crafft.org/wp-content/uploads/2018/08/FINAL-CRAFFT-2.1_provider_manual_with-CRAFFTN_2018-04-23.pdf. Accessed July 14, 2020
75. Swanson JM. The Swanson, Nolan, and Pelham Teacher and Parent Rating Scale (SNAP-IV). Irvine (CA): Child Development Center, University of California; 1995.
76. Gaub M, Carlson CL. Behavioral characteristics of DSM-IV ADHD subtypes in a school-based population. J Abnorm Child Psychol 1997;25(2):103–11.
77. Nobel E, Brunnekreef RJ, Van den Hoofdakker BJ, et al. Parent–clinician agreement in rating the presence and severity of attention-deficit/hyperactivity disorder symptoms. Atten Defic Hyperact Disord 2019;11(1):21–9.
78. American Academy of Pediatrics. National Initiative for Children Healthcare Quality (NICHQ) [Internet]. 2002. Available from: http//www.nichq.org/toolkits_publications/.../07Scoring%20Instructions.pdf. Accessed July 14, 2020.
79. Wimberger RC, Gregory RJ. A behavior checklist for use in child psychiatry clinics. J Am Acad Child Psychiatry 1968;7:677–81.
80. Pagano ME, Cassidy LJ, Little M, et al. Identifying psychosocial dysfunction in school-age children: the pediatric symptom checklist as a self-report measure. Psychol Sch 2000;37(2):91–106.
81. Murphy JM, Blais M, Baer L, et al. Measuring outcomes in outpatient child psychiatry: reliable improvement, deterioration, and clinically significant improvement. Clin Child Psychol Psychiatry 2015;20(1):39–52.
82. McCarthy A, Asghar S, Wilens T, et al. Using a brief parent-report measure to track outcomes for children and teens with ADHD. Child Psychiatry Hum Dev 2016;47:407–16.
83. Kamin HS, McCarthy AE, Abel MR, et al. Using a brief parent-report measure to track outcomes for children and teens with internalizing disorders. Child Psychiatry Hum Dev 2015;46:851–62.
84. Parker EM, Jacobson J, Pullmann MD, et al. Identifying psychosocial problems among children and youth in the child welfare system using the PSC-17: exploring convergent and discriminant validity with multiple informants. Child Psychiatry Hum Dev 2019;50:108–20.
85. Jacobson JH, Pullmann MD, Parker EM, et al. Measurement based care in child welfare-involved children and youth: reliability and validity of the PSC-17. Child Psychiatry Hum Dev 2019;50:332–45.

Section II: Clinical Applications

Measurement-Based Care in the Treatment of Adolescent Depression

Arthur Reese Abright, MD[a],*, Eugene Grudnikoff, MD[a,b]

KEYWORDS

- Measurement-based care • Adolescents • Depression • Suicide prevention

KEY POINTS

- Measurement-based care is a helpful adjunct to clinical assessment in monitoring and improving outcomes in treatment of adolescent depression and prevention of suicide.
- Clinicians can implement measurement-based care through the use of validated rating scales and other instruments for screening, assessment and treatment planning.
- Obstacles to implementation include concerns about costs and time involved in administration of rating scales and acceptability to patients and clinicians.
- Clinicians can facilitate implementation and acceptability by selecting measures and other instruments that are brief, easy to administer and score, available in the public domain, and compatible with electronic health record systems.

Abbreviations	
ASQ	Ask suicide-screening questions
C-SSRS	Columbia Suicide Severity Rating Scale
MBC	Measurement-based care
PHQ-9	Patient Health Questionnaire-9
SAFE-T	Suicide Assessment Five-step Evaluation and Triage
TJC	The Joint Commission
USPSTF	US Preventive Services Task Force

INTRODUCTION

The use of baseline and outcome measures is a cornerstone of psychiatric research and the evidence base for psychiatric treatments but has been slow to gain

[a] New York City Health + Hospitals/Elmhurst, Icahn School of Medicine at Mount Sinai, 79-01 Broadway, Elmhurst, NY 11373, USA; [b] South Oaks Hospital, 400 Sunrise Highway, Amityville, NY 11701, USA
* Corresponding author.
E-mail addresses: abrighta@nychhc.org; arabright@gmail.com

Child Adolesc Psychiatric Clin N Am 29 (2020) 631–643
https://doi.org/10.1016/j.chc.2020.06.003
childpsych.theclinics.com

acceptance in clinical practice. The term measurement-based care (MBC) refers to the use of standardized measures for screening, assessment, and outcome monitoring to assist in treatment planning and prevention of treatment failures in clinical settings.[1] MBC concepts are incorporated in the Joint Commission (TJC) requirements for behavioral health care organizations for use of standardized instruments or tools to monitor outcomes and inform care, treatment and services[2] and for hospitals and behavioral health care organizations accredited by TJC to use validated screening tools to screen for suicide risk, an evidence based process or tool in determination of suicide risk, and guidelines for monitoring, reassessment and safety planning.[3] The goals intrinsic to these requirements—improving outcomes and preventing suicide—are applicable across clinical and practice settings, including those not under TJC regulations.

The term adolescent depression as used in the present article refers to symptoms and impairments associated with diagnoses of depressive disorders ranging from subclinical presentations to dysthymic disorder and major depressive disorder in adolescence. Depressive disorders in this age group are common, disabling, enduring, recurring, and associated with comorbid medical and psychiatric disorders and increased risk for suicide, which is now the second leading cause of death in individuals ages 15 to 24 years old.[4] Effective treatments include depression-focused psychotherapies (cognitive–behavioral therapy and interpersonal therapy) and antidepressant medications, but there remains substantial room for improvement in rates of treatment response and remission[4] and adherence to evidence-based guidelines.[5]

Clinical guidelines developed by professional and national organizations in the United States and other countries[6–9] vary in strategies for literature searches, reliance on expert consensus, participation of stakeholders, adherence to current standards for guideline development,[10,11] and specifics regarding the timing and types of treatment interventions, but share common themes. These themes include the role of screening; the importance of engaging and educating patients and families about depression and treatments; the need for comprehensive psychiatric, medical, and psychosocial assessments; evaluation and safe management of suicide risk; reduction of stressors; a stepped approach to treatment based on severity beginning with supportive interventions and proceeding to psychotherapy and antidepressant medication alone or in combination; and recommendations for clinicians to use standardized measures for baseline and outcome assessments. The US Preventive Services Task Force (USPSTF) recommends screening for depression in adolescents age 12 to 18 years, but concluded that current evidence is insufficient to recommend such screening in children age 11 years and younger.[12]

In recognition of the need for increased awareness regarding depression in children and adolescents, associated impairments and available treatments, the American Academy of Child and Adolescent Psychiatry has established a Depression Resource Center (aacap.org) for clinicians and families with links to related resources.[13–15] In contrast with the age range in the USPSTF recommendation, the American Academy of Child and Adolescent Psychiatry recommends screening for depression in children and adolescents age 8 and older across health care settings and assessment for depressive symptoms in children ages 3 years and older referred for emotional and behavioral problems.[16]

MBC has been associated with increased adherence to treatment algorithms and improvement in outcomes in depression in adults[16] and adolescents.[17,18] Challenges for child and adolescent psychiatrists and other clinicians in implementing MBC and complying with current regulatory requirements for the use of standardized instruments in screening, assessment and management of depression and suicide risk include concerns about time and expense involved in the selection, administration, and interpretation of rating scales and other instruments and integration of results with clinical assessments and decision making.[19,20] The purpose of the present article is to provide a framework for addressing these challenges. Topics covered include MBC in adolescent depression, relevant regulatory requirements, and a practical approach to implementation of MBC across a range of clinical settings. The article does not cover MBC in children, a topic that merits a separate discussion.

MEASUREMENT-BASED CARE IN ADOLESCENT DEPRESSION

In a systematic review of MBC for treatment of depression in children and adolescents, Elmquist and colleagues[21] discuss the established benefits of rating scales in tracking symptom severity and treatment efficacy in research studies of depression in children and adolescents, note limited implementation in clinical practice and barriers including time constraints and need for training, review psychometric properties, advantages and limitations of available scales; and conclude by advocating for studies regarding use of such scales in practice. Evidence in support of the effectiveness of quality improvement interventions comparing the use of standardized measures together with flexible application of clinical guidelines to usual practice includes findings by Wells and colleagues[17] and Asarnow and colleagues[18] of improved outcomes for depressed adolescents receiving quality improvement interventions.

Recent reports have described examples of innovative approaches to use of health information technology in implementation of MBC and quality improvement efforts in children and adolescents. Liu and colleagues[22] describe a cloud-based digital measurement feedback system that provides baseline and repeated measures completion rates for a library of behavioral health measures. Corathers and colleagues[23] report on the use of electronic tablets with automated score reports together with a software platform that facilitates integration into the electronic health record of screening and follow-up scores over time for depression and suicidal ideation in adolescents with diabetes. The authors note accommodations in implementation in response to patient preference for shorter surveys and less frequent screening. Efforts to achieve compliance with the current regulatory requirements described in the next sections are likely to present further opportunities for clinical and quality improvement studies of the use of MBC in depression and other disorders.

THE JOINT COMMISSION STANDARD FOR MONITORING OUTCOME OF CARE, TREATMENT, OR SERVICES (CTS 03.01.09)

This standard was modified in January 2018 to require that behavioral health organizations use a standardized tool or instrument to monitor outcomes and inform and improve care for individuals and populations served.[2]

Requirements for this standard are summarized in **Fig. 1** and specify that ideally the tool or instrument monitors progress from the individual's perspective and may have

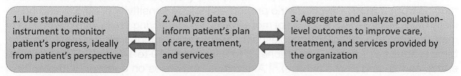

Fig. 1. Summary of the 3 elements of performance for outcomes measures standard, as outlined in TJC CTS.03.01.09 for behavioral health organizations.

either a global (distress, quality of life) or more targeted focus (depression or anxiety). TJC guidance for this standard[2] notes the growing role of MBC in behavioral health, cites evidence for the value of MBC in improving outcomes and preventing failure of care, lists criteria for outcome measures (including reliability, validity, sensitivity to change), and provides references to measurement-based tools[24] but leaves the choice of instruments or tools to the organization. The guidance emphasizes that the use of a standardized tool or instrument is in and of itself insufficient to meet the standard and that data gathered from the instrument must be used to track the progress of individuals or lack thereof; inform care, treatment, or services for individuals; and be aggregated to inform quality improvement efforts for the organization. In practice, this requirement imposes on clinicians and organizations a responsibility to select and implement appropriate measures and demonstrate use of results of such measures in treatment planning and quality improvement efforts. These elements of performance as applied to adolescent depression are discussed elsewhere in this article.

RATING SCALES FOR DEPRESSION IN ADOLESCENTS

Zimmerman[25] summarizes desirable features in depression rating scales, including brevity, acceptability to patients and clinicians, sensitivity to change, ability to assess suicidal thoughts, ease of scoring, and low expense. D'Angelo and Augenstein[26] provide a cogent discussion of the distinctions between structured and unstructured clinical evaluations, the high prevalence of anxiety and other comorbid symptoms in depression, and integration of evidence-based measures with clinical practice and suggest a format in which findings on broad band screening of mood-related symptoms are followed by depression-specific measures and focused clinical assessments.

Options available to child and adolescent psychiatrists and other providers in selection of rating scales for depression in children and adolescents include broad based instruments that cover a range of symptoms and disorders such as the Pediatric Symptom Checklist[27] and instruments specific to depression, including the Children's Depression Inventory, Beck's Depression Inventory, Center for Epidemiologic Studies – Depression Scale, Reynolds Adolescent Depression Scale, Mood and Feelings Questionnaire, and Quick Inventory of Depressive Symptoms. These instruments and their psychometric properties, as well as those of other scales for internalizing disorders in children and adolescents, are well-described and referenced in reviews by Elmquist and colleagues,[21] Myers and Winters,[28] D'Angelo and Augenstein,[26] and Stockings and colleagues.[29]

The focus of the present discussion is on the Patient Health Questionnaire-9 (PHQ-9) because of its current widespread use as a screening and outcome measure, ease of administration and scoring, availability in the public domain and in multiple languages and compatibility with electronic health record systems. The PHQ-9 is a 9-item self-report questionnaire covering *Diagnostic and Statistical Manual of Mental Disorders*-IV criteria for major depressive disorder rated over the previous 2 weeks.[30] Items are rated on a scale from 0 (not at all) to 3 (nearly every day) with total scores ranging from 0 to 27. Psychometric properties include sensitivity of 89.5% and specificity of 77.5% for PHQ-9 scores of more than 10 in identifying youth with diagnoses of major depressive disorder in adolescents and severity ranges for depressive symptoms in adults as follows: 0 to 4 (none), 5 to 9 (minimal), 10 to 14 (mild), 15 to 19 (moderate), and 20 and above (severe).[31] Affirmative responses on question 9 (thoughts of self-harm and suicide) require concurrent further assessment for suicide risk as discussed elsewhere in this article with the National Patient Safety Goal for Suicide

Prevention. The PHQ-2 is a 2-item self-report questionnaire that may be used for brief screening for depression in adults and has been shown to have a sensitivity of 74% and a specificity of 75% for identifying major depressive disorder in youth ages 13 to 17.[32] Sensitivity in detection of change in outcomes over time has been established in adults[33] but evidence for sensitivity to change with the PHQ-9 is more limited in adolescents.[34]

Table 1 summarizes the likelihood ratios of PHQ-9 score ranges in adults with diagnoses of depressive disorders in adults and includes suggestions regarding use of PHQ-9 to inform decisions regarding referral, evaluation and treatment.

Issues in use of the PHQ-2, PHQ-9, and other scales in screening and assessment for depression in adolescents are comprehensively discussed by Zuckerbrot and colleagues,[7] who conclude that self-report scales can improve detection of depression but emphasize the importance of follow-up clinical assessment in confirming diagnoses and developing treatment plans. The PHQ-9 has been modified for use in adolescents (PHQ-9M)[34] with minor changes in scored questions and addition of nonscored questions regarding depressed mood in the past year, impairments in functioning, suicidal thoughts in the past month, and lifetime history of suicide attempts.

NATIONAL PATIENT SAFETY GOAL FOR THE PREVENTION OF SUICIDE

TJC new and revised National Patient Safety Goal for Prevention of Suicide (goal 15.01.01) became effective July 1, 2019.[2] Discussion of this National Patient Safety Goal is included in the present article because of the increased risk of suicide in depressed adolescents, increased rates of suicide in persons ages 10 to 24 years in the period from 2007 to 2017,[35] and the requirement for the use of validated tools in screening, assessment, monitoring, and reduction of suicide risk.

The elements of performance for this National Patient Safety Goal are summarized in Fig. 2 and include environmental assessment for ligature points and other suicide

Table 1
Interpretation of PHQ-9 severity scores based on study in adult population and treatment considerations for corresponding scores in adolescents

PHQ-9 Score	Likely Diagnostic Correlates	Positive Likelihood Ratio	Referral, Evaluation and Treatment Considerations for Adolescents
0–4	Almost always signifies absence of a depressive disorder	0.04	Psychoeducation and regular screening
5–9	Patients with either no depression or subthreshold depression	0.5	
10–14	A spectrum of depressive disorders, including dysthymia and MDD, mild or moderate	2.6	Consultation with collaborative care and/or referral for diagnostic evaluation and treatment; safety/suicidality screening and risk assessment
15–19	Indicates MDD, moderate or severe	8.4	
20–27	Indicates MDD, severe	36.8	

The interpretation of positive likelihood ratio: a PHQ-9 score in the range 10 to 14 is 2.6 times as likely in a patient with actual major depressive disorder, compared with a patient without major depression.
Abbreviation: MDD, major depressive disorder.
Data from Kroenke K, Spitzer RL, Williams JBW. The PHQ-9: validity of a brief depression severity measure. J Gen Intern Med. 2001;16(9):606–13.

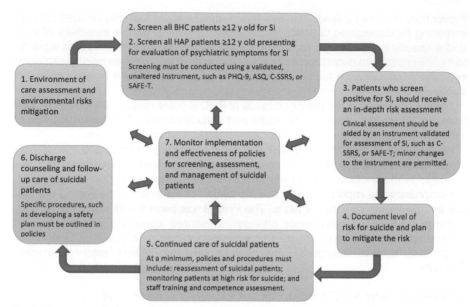

Fig. 2. Summary of the 7 elements of performance as outlined in TJC's National Patient Safety Goal 15.01.01. BHC, behavioral health care; HAP, hospital accreditation program.

risks and actions to minimize such risk, use of a validated suicide risk screening tool for all individuals served in behavioral health care settings and individuals identified with behavioral health problems in nonbehavioral care settings, use of an evidence-based process for assessment of all individuals who have screened positive for suicide risk, documentation of overall level of risk for suicide in such individuals (high, medium, or low) and plan to mitigate such risk, guidelines for reassessment, and training for staff who care for individuals at risk for suicide. TJC specifies that screening for suicidal ideation with a validated screening tool is required for all individuals age 12 and older in behavioral health settings and all individuals age 12 and older being evaluated for behavioral health problems in nonbehavioral health settings.[2]

The focus in the requirement on individuals who may have an increased risk for suicide in association with mental health disorders rather than on the general population of patients across nonbehavioral care settings seems to be consistent with the conclusion by the USPSTF that there is insufficient evidence regarding benefits and risks to recommend screening for suicide risk in the general population of adolescents, adults, and older adults in primary care settings.[36] In a thoughtful commentary, Henderson and colleagues[37] discuss concerns raised by this regulatory mandate, including limitations in the evidence base for determination of risk levels, possible underestimation of risk in some cases, and possible over-referral to emergency and inpatient settings in accord with risk stratification protocols. These concerns highlight the importance of the role of clinical judgment in use of standardized tools such as those described elsewhere in this article.

TOOLS FOR SCREENING AND ASSESSMENT OF SUICIDE RISK

Examples provided by TJC of screening tools include the Ask Suicide-Screening Questions (ASQ),[38] the PHQ-9, which is described in the preceding section of the present article; and the Columbia Suicide Severity Rating Scale (C-SSRS),[39] which is cited as an example of a scale that can be used both for screening and assessment.

The ASQ, developed by the National Institute of Mental Health, is a 5-item scale for youth ages 10 to 24 years that can be administered for screening in emergency, inpatient, and primary care settings; is available in multiple languages; is in the public domain; and is reported to be effective in identifying individuals at risk for suicide and requiring further assessment or immediate interventions for safety. Information about the ASQ can be downloaded from the National Institute of Mental Health website.[40]

The C-SSRS is a 6-item scale that includes questions about passive and active suicidal ideation, method, intent, plan, and behaviors. Description of the C-SSRS is available through the Columbia Lighthouse project website,[41] which includes information about psychometric properties; use in health care, military, school, and other settings; versions based on intervals (screening, recent, lifetime) and age groups (children, adolescents, adults) covered; availability in multiple languages and at no cost for health care institutions; and compatibility with electronic health record systems.

The Suicide Assessment Five-step Evaluation and Triage (SAFE-T)[42] provides a structured approach to assessment that incorporates TJC requirements for the identification of risk and protective factors; inquiry about thoughts, plans, and behaviors; determination of risk level and interventions; and documentation of rationale for risk level and interventions and may be combined with the C-SSRS for screening and assessment as the SAFE-T Protocol with C-SSRS available through the Columbia Lighthouse Project website.[41] Determination of risk levels as low, moderate or high and decisions about interventions including need for hospitalization for safety are based on presence or absence of suicidal thoughts, intent, plan, and current or past behaviors; risk and protective factors; and clinical judgment.

Safety plans developed in collaboration with adolescent patients and their parents or other legal guardians to assist in identifying warning signs, coping strategies, distractions, personal and professional resources, and environmental safety concerns are important components in interventions designed to reduce suicide risk.[43]

IMPLEMENTATION

An awareness of the potential benefits of MBC in care of adolescents with depression and other disorders may be accompanied by understandable concerns by child and adolescent psychiatrists and other clinicians about practical issues in adding rating scales and other instruments to an already lengthy list of other requirements for clinical assessment and documentation during intake and follow-up visits in a range of programs and settings across the continuum of care. Such concerns may be tempered by the selection of instruments that are brief and easy to administer and score, as well as attention to the management of obstacles. Approaches developed in 1 program or institution consistent with MBC principles and regulatory requirements may vary in specifics from those in other programs and institutions, and there remains ample room for discussion and study as to which approaches may be most feasible, most consistent with current evidence, and most likely to be associated with improved outcomes.

Practical considerations in implementation include:

- Selection, type (self-report, parent-rated, clinician rated), and number of standardized instruments to be used.
- Advantages and limitations of instruments selected: For example, the PHQ-9M provides a brief survey of recent depressive symptoms from the patient's

perspective but does not cover manic or hypomanic symptoms, bipolar or other disorders, history, or stressors. The C-SSRS provides standardized questions about suicidal thoughts and behaviors, but additional inquiry is required to distinguish nonsuicidal self-injurious behaviors (ie, self-cutting) from those with suicidal intent. The SAFE-T provides a structured format for identification of risk and protective factors, but formulation of the level of suicidal risk and interventions for safety and risk mitigation requires careful clinical judgment regarding acuity, setting (ie, inpatient vs ambulatory), intent, and available supports.

- *Mode* (paper or electronic), *place* (waiting room, clinician's office), and *timing* (before or during visits) of administration.
- *Responsibility for administration* (eg, clerical staff for initial screening with PHQ-9M, clinician staff for C-SSRS, and SAFE-T) and for *data entry* into electronic health record systems.
- *Responsibility for alerting clinicians to positive findings* on screening, especially with regard to red flag items such as affirmative responses on PHQ-9M question 9 or C-SSRS regarding suicidal ideation, plan or intent.
- *Resources available* for concurrent clinical assessment and interventions for the safety of patients who screen positive for suicide risk and for referral for further assessment and treatment when indicated.
- *Diversity* (cultural, linguistic, cognitive, developmental, gender, and socioeconomic) in the populations screened and treated for depression and suicide risk and applicability of instruments used.
  - *Education* provided to minor patients, parents or other legal guardians, and program staff regarding depression and reasons for use of rating scales and other instruments, how results will be used, and the confidentiality of findings. Clinicians should be familiar with institutional policies and procedures, and state and federal regulations regarding disclosure of minor's health information to parents or other legal guardians, including information about findings indicating potential risk of harm to self or others.
  - *Engagement of patients* in the use of rating scales and other instruments as valuable tools in identifying and tracking symptoms, identification of treatment goals, and progress rather than as pro forma exercises necessary to meet requirements. An important step in this process is for the clinician to review with the patient the patient's responses to individual items rather than focusing only on total score.
- The use of findings from standardized instruments in conjunction with clinical assessment and clinical guidelines[7] to inform care of individual patients.
  - *Example*: A psychiatrist recommends addition of antidepressant medication when a 14-year-old patient's PHQ-9M scores remain in range of moderate severity of depressive symptoms after 4 to 6 weeks of monotherapy with cognitive–behavioral therapy.
- *Aggregation of data* from standardized instruments to improve care of population served.
  - *Example*: Findings of PHQ-9M scores of 10 or greater in 20% of adolescent patients screened in an outpatient clinic may be used in support of a recommendation for increased training and supervision for program staff in cognitive–behavioral therapy or other evidence-based therapy for depression.
  - References for *National Center for Quality Assurance*[44] and *Healthcare Effectiveness Data and Information Set*[45] recommendations for quality measurements of depression screening, follow-up and monitoring remission or response are included in the reference list at the end of this article.

MEASUREMENT-BASED CARE ACROSS THE CONTINUUM OF CARE

Studies of MBC in adolescent depression have usually focused on specific settings (for example, collaborative care programs). However, current regulatory standards require use of standardized instruments for assessment and monitoring outcome and suicide risk across a range of settings. The model in **Fig. 3** is based on the authors' experiences in a large urban teaching hospital and is intended to be illustrative rather than prescriptive. Key components include the following.

- *Screening with the PHQ-9M* for depression in all adolescents in pediatric, other medical, and psychiatric settings.
- *Referral for clinical assessment and treatment* for depressive symptoms in patients with a PHQ-9M of 10 or higher, or other indicators of significant emotional distress.
- *Screening and assessment for suicide risk with C-SSRS and SAFE-T and clinical assessment* for all adolescents in psychiatric settings and for adolescents in pediatric settings with a PHQ-9M of 10 of higher, or other red flags, including affirmative responses on question 9 regarding suicidal thoughts, or other indicators of significant emotional or behavioral problems.
- *Safety interventions and referral for emergency evaluation and inpatient hospitalization* for patients determined to be at high risk for suicide on SAFE-T and clinical assessment.
- *Feedback* based on results from repeat monitoring with PHQ-9M and C-SSRS together with clinical assessment to inform care and adjust treatment goals, methods and plans when indicated.

CLINICAL VIGNETTE

A 16-year-old girl is referred from an adolescent medicine clinic for emergency psychiatric evaluation after she completes a PHQ-9M with a score of 18 and positive responses on question 9 regarding suicidal thoughts in the past 2 weeks and a nonscored question regarding thoughts of ending her life in the past month, but

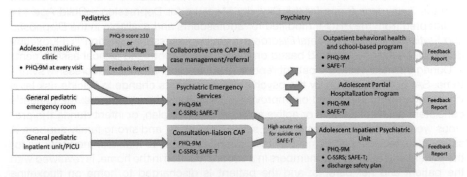

Fig. 3. Implementation of outcomes measures in assessment and treatment of depression and suicidality across services and levels of care. "Red Flags" that warrant involvement of collaborative care services include: patient reporting significant suicidal thoughts or behaviors; patient answering "yes" on PHQ-9M question 9; or patient presenting with significant emotional distress. "Feedback Report" refers to collection and analysis of outcomes data to monitor and inform patient's treatment and to improve facility's overall outcomes. CAP, child and adolescent psychiatrist; PHQ-9M, Patient Health Questionnaire, modified for Adolescents; PICU, pediatric intensive care unit; SSRS, Columbia Suicide Severity Rating Scale.

negative response on a nonscored question regarding lifetime history of suicidal attempts. A review of the medical record indicates that the patient's scores on the PHQ-9 at time points 6 months and 1 year previously were both below 5.

On clinical assessment in the emergency room, the patient confirms her responses on the PHQ-9M and states that she has been experiencing depressive symptoms with intermittent thoughts of "not wanting to be here anymore" and of taking an overdose of over-the-counter analgesics after a break up with a boyfriend about 2 weeks previously. Assessments in the emergency room include the C-SSRS with responses indicating passive and active suicidal ideation with method (overdose) but without plan or intent and SAFE-T with documentation of risk factors (including depressive symptoms and active suicidal ideation), protective factors (including family support), and formulation of acute suicide risk as moderate rather than high owing to the absence of current active suicidal intent. In view of the patient's report of continuing active suicidal ideation, significant depressive symptoms, and risk of exacerbation of suicidal ideation, the psychiatrist recommends inpatient hospitalization for safety and stabilization.

The patient and her parents agree and the patient is admitted to the hospital's adolescent psychiatric inpatient unit, where a diagnosis of major depressive episode, single, moderate severity, without psychotic features is confirmed.

The PHQ-9M is completed by the patient the day after admission with score of 18, indicating continued depressive symptoms of moderate severity. Suicide risk assessments based on mental status examination and C-SSRS since last visit assessments are positive for continued passive suicidal ideation and negative for current active suicidal ideation or intent during the first week of the admission and become negative for both passive and active ideation during week 2. The psychiatrist discusses treatment options with the patient and her parents, including psychotherapy and antidepressant medication. After a discussion of the potential benefits and risks, including a black box warning from the US Food and Drug Administration regarding suicidal risk, the patient's parents consent and the patient assents to a trial of fluoxetine, which is initiated at 10 mg/d. One week after admission, the patient's score on the PHQ-9M regarding symptoms in the past week is 16, indicating continued depressive symptoms of moderate severity. (Administration of PHQ-9M focused on past week instead of past 2 weeks provides an interim measure during brief hospitalizations and is consistent with the 7-day time frame for the Severity Measure for Depression – Child Age 11–17 adapted from the PHQ-9 modified for adolescents and available in the *Diagnostic and Statistical Manual of Mental Disorders*-5 Online Assessment section[46]). Fluoxetine dose is increased to 20 mg/d based on the PHQ-9M score and clinical assessment.

During the next week, the patient reports gradual improvement in depressive symptoms. SAFE-T formulation by the psychiatrist documents change in suicide risk level from moderate to low based on improvement in depressive symptoms; the patient's consistent denial of passive or active suicidal ideation, plan, or intent during the previous week; an absence of a history of suicide attempts; and strong family support. A safety plan, including agreement by the patient's parents to maintain medications for the patient and other family members in a secure location in the home, is reviewed with the patient and her parents; and the patient is discharged to home on fluoxetine 20 mg/d with plan for follow-up in the partial hospital program. Her PHQ-9 M on discharge is 8, with a negative response on question 9. Treatment in the partial hospital program and subsequently in the child and adolescent outpatient program includes repeat PHQ-9M's at 2-week intervals and suicide risk assessment with C-SSRS at each visit as adjuncts to clinical assessment and treatment planning to achieve goals of further remission of depressive symptoms, improvement in functioning, and prevention of recurrence of depressive episode and suicidal risk.

SUMMARY

MBC has been found to be a helpful adjunct to clinical assessment in improving outcomes in depression in adults and adolescents. MBC principles are incorporated in current regulatory requirements for use of standardized instruments in efforts to improve care and prevent suicide. Challenges for child and adolescent psychiatrists and other clinicians in implementing MBC include concerns about time and expense involved in administration and interpretation of results from rating scales and other instruments. Implementation can be facilitated by selection of instruments that are brief, easy to administer and score, compatible with electronic health record systems and available in the public domain.

DISCLOSURE

The authors have nothing to disclose.

REFERENCES

1. Aboraya A, Nasrallah HA, Elswick, et al. Measurement-based care in psychiatry – past, present and future. Innov Clin Neurosci 2018;15(11-12):13–26.
2. The Joint Commission. Revised outcome measures standard for behavioral health care. R 3 report: requirement, rationale, reference. Issue 13 2018. Available at: https://www.jointcomission.org/assets/1/18/R3_Outcome_measures_1_30_18_FINAL.pdf. Accessed December 19, 2019.
3. The Joint Commission. National patient safety goal for suicide prevention. R3 report: requirement, rationale, reference. Issue 18 2019. Available at: https://www.jointcommission.org/standards/r3-report/r3-report-issue-18-national-patient-safety-goal-for-suicide-prevention/. Accessed December 19, 2019.
4. Brent DA. Depressive disorders. In: Martin A, Bloch MH, Volkmar FR, editors. Lewis's child and adolescent psychiatry: a comprehensive textbook. 5th edition. Philadelphia: Wolters Kluwer Health; 2018. p. 473–82.
5. Soria-Saucedo R, Walter HJ, Cabral H, et al. Receipt of evidence-based pharmacotherapy and psychotherapy among children and adolescents with new diagnoses of depression. Psychiatr Serv 2016;67(3):316–23.
6. Birmaher B, Brent D, Bernet W, et al. Practice parameter for the assessment and treatment of children and adolescents with depressive disorders. J Am Acad Child Adolesc Psychiatry 2007;46(11):1503–26.
7. Zuckerbrot RA, Cheung A, Jensen PS, et al. GLAD-PC Steering Group. Guidelines for adolescent depression in primary care (GLAD-PC): part I. Practice preparation, identification, assessment, and initial management. Pediatrics 2018;141(3):e20174081.
8. Cheung AH, Zuckerbrot RA, Jensen PS, et al. GLAD-PC Steering Group. Guidelines for adolescent depression in primary care (GLAD-PC): part II. treatment and ongoing management. Pediatrics 2018;141(3):e20174082.
9. National Institute for Health and Care Excellence. NICE guideline. Depression in young people: identification and management 2019. Available at: www.nice.org.uk/guidance/ng134. Accessed December 21, 2019.
10. Walter HJ, Bukstein OG. Forward to the future: clinical updates and clinical practice guidelines. J Am Acad Child Adolesc Psychiatry 2017;56(10):811–2.
11. Lewandowski ER, Acri MC, Hoagwood KE, et al. Evidence for the management of adolescent depression. Pediatrics 2013;132:e996–1009.

12. Siu AL. On behalf of the US Preventive Services Task Force. Screening for depression in children and adolescents: US Preventive Services Task Force Recommendation statement. Pediatrics 2016;137(3):e20154467.
13. American Academy of child and adolescent psychiatry. Available at: https://www.aacap.org/AACAP/Families_and_Youth/Resource_Centers/Depression_Resource_Center/Depression_Resource_Center.aspx. Accessed December 21, 2019.
14. Wagner KD. Presidential address: depression awareness and screening in children and adolescents. J Am Acad Child Adolesc Psychiatry 2018;57(1):6–7.
15. American Academy of Child and Adolescent Psychiatry. Policy statement on depression screening. Available at: https://www.aacap.org/AACAP/Policy_Statements/2019/Policy_Statement_on_Depression_Screening.aspx. Accessed December 29, 2019.
16. Guo T, Yu-TaoX, Le X, et al. Measure-based care versus standard care for major depression: a randomized controlled trial with blind raters. Am J Psychiatr 2015; 172:1004–13.
17. Wells KB, Tang L, Carlson GA, et al. Treatment of youth depression in primary care under usual practice conditions: observational findings from Youth Partners in Care. J Child Adolesc Psychopharmacol 2012;22(1):80–90.
18. Asarnow JR, Jaycox LH, Duan N, et al. Effectiveness of a quality improvement intervention for adolescent depression in primary care clinics - a randomized controlled trial. JAMA 2005;293(3):311–9.
19. Boswell JF, Kraus DR, Miller SD, et al. Implementing routine outcome monitoring in clinical practice: benefits, challenges, and solutions. Psychother Res 2015;25(1):6–19.
20. Rush J. Isn't it about time to employ measurement-based care in practice? Am J Psychiatry 2015;172(10):934–6.
21. Elmquist JM, Melton TK, Croarkin P, et al. A systematic overview of measurement-based care in the treatment of childhood and adolescent depression. J Psychiatr Pract 2010;16(4):217–34.
22. Liu FF, Cruz RA, Rockhill CM, et al. Mind the gap: considering disparities in implementing measurement-based care. J Am Acad Child Adolesc Psychiatry 2019;58(4):459–61.
23. Corathers S, Mara CA, Chundi PK, et al. Depression screening of adolescents with diabetes: 5-years of implementation and outcomes. J Am Acad Child Adolesc Psychiatry 2019;58(6):628–31.
24. Wren G, Fortney J. Core set of outcome measures for behavioral health across service settings. Washington, DC: The Kennedy Forum, ca; 2015. Available at: http://thekennedyforum-dot-org.s#.amazonaws.com/documents/MBC supplement.pdf. Accessed December 18, 2019.
25. Zimmerman M. Using scales to monitor symptoms and treat depression (measurement based care). UpToDate. Available at: https://www.uptodate.com/contents/using-scales-to-monitor-symptoms-and-treat-depression-measurement-based-care. Accessed December 21, 2019.
26. D'Angelo EJ, Augenstein TM. Developmentally informed evaluation of depression: evidence-based instruments. Child Adolesc Psychiatr Clin N Am 2012;21(2):279–98.
27. Jellinek MS, Murphy JM, Little M, et al. Use of the pediatric symptom checklist (PSC) to screen for psychosocial problems in pediatric primary care: a national feasibility study. Arch Pediatr Adolesc Med 1999;153(3):254–60.
28. Myers K, Winters NC. Ten-year review of rating scales. II. scales for internalizing disorders. J Am Acad Child Adolesc Psychiatry 2002;41(6):634–59.
29. Stockings E, Degenhardt L, Lee YY, et al. Symptom screening scales for detecting major depressive disorder in children and adolescents: a systematic review

and meta-analysis of reliability, validity and diagnostic utility. J Affect Disord 2015; 174:447–63.

30. Kroenke K, Spitzer RL, Williams JBW. The PHQ-9: validity of a brief depression severity measure. J Gen Intern Med 2001;16:606–13.

31. Richardson LP, McCauley E, Grossman DC, et al. Evaluation of the patient health questionnaire-9 item for detecting major depression among adolescents. Pediatrics 2010;126(6):1117–23.

32. Richardson LP, Rockhill C, Russo JE, et al. Evaluation of the PHQ-2 as a brief screen for detecting major depression among adolescents. Pediatrics 2010; 125(5):e1097–103.

33. Lowe B, Kroenke K, Herzog W, et al. Measuring depression outcome with a brief self-report instrument: sensitivity to change of the patient health questionnaire (PHQ-9). J Affect Disord 2004;81:61–6.

34. Nandakumar AL, Vande Voort JL, Nakonezny PA, et al. Psychometric properties of the patient health questionnaire-9 modified for major depressive disorder in adolescents. J Child Adolesc Psychopharmacol 2019;29(1):34–40.

35. Curtin SC, Heron M. Death rates due to suicide and homicide among persons aged 10 -24: United States, 2000 – 2017. NCHS Data Brief. No. 352 2019. Available at: https://www.cdc.gov/nchs/data/databriefs/db352-h.pdf. Accessed December 26, 2019.

36. LeFevre ML. Screening for suicide risk in adolescents, adults, and older adults in primary care: U.S. Preventive Services Task Force Recommendation Statement. Ann Intern Med 2014;160(10):719.

37. Henderson SW, Gerson R, Phillips B. What is "high risk" and what are we actually supposed to do about it? J Am Acad Child Adolesc Psychiatry 2019;58(6):561–4.

38. Horowitz LM, Bridge JA, Teach SJ, et al. Ask suicide-screening questions (ASQ): a brief instrument for the pediatric emergency department. Arch Pediatr Adolesc Med 2012;166(12):1170–6.

39. Posner K, Brown GK, Stanley B, et al. The Columbia-suicide severity rating scale: internal validity and internal consistency findings from three multisite studies with adolescents and adults. Am J Psychiatry 2011;168:1266–77.

40. ASQ information Sheet. Available at: https://www.nimh.nih.gov/research/research-conducted-at-nimh/asq-toolkit-materials/inpatient/asq-information-sheet.shtml. Accessed December 26, 2019.

41. The Columbia Lighthouse project. Available at: http://www.cssrs.columbia.edu/. Accessed December 26, 2019.

42. SAFE-T. Suicide assessment five-step evaluation and triage for mental health professionals. Available at: www.sprc.org. Accessed December 26, 2019.

43. Stanley B, Brown GK. Safety planning intervention: a brief intervention to mitigate suicide risk. Cogn Behav Pract 2012;19:256–64.

44. Zima BT, Murphy JM, Scholle SH, et al. National quality measures for child mental health care: background, progress and next steps. Pediatrics 2013; 131:S38–49.

45. HEDIS depression measures for electronic clinical data. Available at: https://www.ncqa.org/hedis/the-future-of-hedis/hedis-depression-measures-for-electronic-clinical-data/. Accessed December 30, 2019.

46. American Psychiatric Association. Online assessment measures. In Diagnostic and statistical manual of mental disorders (5th ed.). 2013. https://www.psychiatry.org/psychiatrists/practice/dsm/educational-resources/assessment-measures. Accessed February13, 2020.

Measurement-Based Care in the Treatment of Anxiety

Courtney Romba, MD*, John Lavigne, PhD, John Walkup, MD, Rachel Ballard, MD

KEYWORDS

- Measurement-based care • Child and adolescent psychiatry • Pediatric anxiety
- Patient-reported outcome measures • Reliable change

KEY POINTS

- Measurement-based care is the administration of rating scales at the patient level to guide clinical decisions, track symptom improvement, and monitor response to treatment.
- The evidence base for measurement-based care in the clinical practice of child psychiatry is limited, but well-established in randomized controlled trials with growing interest in standardizing use.
- Parent and child agreement about a child's anxiety tends to be low, and measures from both parent and child should be obtained, if possible.
- Measures used to track pediatric anxiety should be brief, accessible, sensitive to change, and reliable.

Abbreviations	
GAD	Generalized anxiety disorder
PROMIS	Patient-Reported Outcomes Measurement Information System
RCI	Reliable change index
SCARED	Screen for Child Anxiety Related Disorders

INTRODUCTION TO MEASUREMENT-BASED CARE

Measurement-based care involves the systematic administration of rating scales and the application of the results to guide patient-specific clinical decisions.[1–4] Although randomized controlled trials have implemented measurement-based care for years, its use is not yet common in clinical practice. Measurement-based care builds on data collected from the clinical interview and improves awareness and engagement between the psychiatrist and patient about the target of treatment.[5] Close systematic

Pritzker Department of Psychiatry and Behavioral Health, Ann and Robert H. Lurie Children's Hospital of Chicago, 225 East Chicago Avenue, Box 10, Chicago, IL 60611, USA
* Corresponding author.
E-mail address: cromba@luriechildrens.org

Child Adolesc Psychiatric Clin N Am 29 (2020) 645–661
https://doi.org/10.1016/j.chc.2020.06.004
1056-4993/20/© 2020 Elsevier Inc. All rights reserved.
childpsych.theclinics.com

monitoring of symptoms also builds patient and family confidence and instills hope and optimism in the treatment process.[2] More specifically, measurement-based care guides treatment by identifying change in symptoms over time, monitoring adverse effects, in the long term promotes the goal of remission, and decreases the risk of recurrence.

By increasing information available to the psychiatrist, the psychiatrist is provided with additional information to be used in the decision-making process and, by assisting the patient to focus on patterns of change in specific symptoms rather than relying solely on the patients global impressions of improvement, that information can help the patient to be more actively engaged in treatment decisions.[1,2,5] Existing studies in the adult population suggest that use of measurement-based care decreases time to response and remission in the treatment of depression.[5] When measurement-based care is connected to algorithmic treatment in adult depression, patients achieve symptom remission more quickly and more completely compared with care as usual.[3,4]

There is less evidence for the use of measurement-based care in pediatric mental health disorders, but a growing interest in implementing outcome measurement more regularly into practice. Although many mental health providers often use clinical judgment alone to assess for symptom change, it has been suggested that the actual rates of provider identification of patient deterioration are quite low, with 1 study suggesting mental health clinicians detect deterioration for only 21% of their patients who experience increased symptom severity.[6]

Among child psychiatrists, there can be varying definitions of response and remission. It is generally understood that remission refers to the state of being symptom free, whereas response refers to a clinically meaningful change in symptoms compared with baseline.[7] In this article, we use this understanding of the terms response and remission to guide our discussion.

CHALLENGES IN MEASUREMENT-BASED TREATMENT OF PEDIATRIC ANXIETY

In contrast with adult depression, which has a fairly uniform presentation, pediatric anxiety is a group of disorders that has distinct presentations, ages of onset, and symptom sets. Any individual child or adolescent may manifest symptoms of 1 or several anxiety disorders at a time. That same child or adolescent may go on to develop symptoms of a different anxiety disorder at a later time. The ideal instrument to measure symptomatic change over time would parsimoniously capture the presence and severity of the major pediatric anxiety across the pediatric age range. The clinician treating a child for a particular anxiety disorder needs to be mindful of the importance of monitoring changes in all types of anxiety symptoms during the course of treatment.

Anxiety Subtypes

As described in the *Diagnostic and Statistical Manual of Mental Disorders,* 5th edition, pediatric anxiety consists of a group of disorders, including separation anxiety, generalized anxiety, social anxiety, and panic disorder. The symptoms associated with these disorders differ across diagnostic entities, there are differences in the age of onset for some of these conditions (eg, separation anxiety is more likely to emerge in preschool), and some children may show symptoms associated exclusively with 1 type of anxiety and not another. Comorbidity across different anxiety disorders, however, is very common; any individual child or adolescent may manifest symptoms of 1 or several anxiety disorders at a particular time, or a child or adolescent may present with symptoms with one particular type of anxiety, but then symptoms of a different anxiety disorder at a later time. The interrelation between types of anxiety symptoms is reflected in the moderate to high correlations on different dimensions of anxiety that are measured in the same anxiety questionnaires. The ideal instrument to measure symptomatic change over time would parsimoniously capture the presence and severity of the major pediatric anxiety across the pediatric age range, and the clinician treating a child for a particular anxiety disorder needs to be mindful of the importance of monitoring changes in all types of anxiety symptoms during the course of treatment.

Combining Parent and Child Reports of Anxiety Symptoms

Diagnosis and treatment in all pediatric fields involves some combination of parent-given history, patient-given history, examination of the patients, and supplementary assessments completed by a parent and/or the child. The younger the child, the greater the reliance on parent-given history and parent-completed assessments. Symptom criteria for internalizing disorders such as anxiety include a combination of internal experiences ("persistent and excessive worry about losing major attachment figures or about possible harm to them, such as illness, injury, disasters, or death") and observable behaviors ("persistent reluctance or refusal to sleep away from home or to go to sleep without being near a major attachment figure"). Child self-report scales are generally validated for children ages 8 and older, with third grade being the time at which reading and cognitive levels are adequate for the child to respond meaningfully to questions about symptoms.

Parent and child agreement about the child's behaviors and emotions tends to be low. Studies using the Screen for Child Anxiety Related Disorders (SCARED),[8] Multidimensional Anxiety Scale for Children,[9] and the Spence Children's Anxiety Scale,[10] have examined parent–child agreement on symptoms of anxiety and show that correlations between parent and child ratings of anxiety symptoms range from 0.18 to 0.69, with a mean of 0.46 for total symptom scales and similar results on subscales.[8,11–20] Two studies indicate that parent–child agreement is slightly higher for adolescents than younger children, but the difference is not clinically important because parent–adolescent agreement is still only moderate (Birmaher and colleagues[11]: children 0.08; adolescents 0.39; Wei and colleagues[18]: children 0.47; adolescents 0.57). Overall, these levels of correlation suggest that parent and child are providing ratings of a similar underlying construct of anxiety, but they are not high enough to suggest that the parent rating can serve as a proxy for the child's report, or vice versa, and negate the need to assess anxiety symptoms as reported by both raters. The clinician must then decide how to resolve discrepancies in parent and child reports. Clinical trials assessing treatment of anxiety in children and adolescents have used various approaches to reconciling parent–child disagreements. This process can include following the "and" rule (child meets criteria for anxiety disorder if both the child's and the parent's ratings are consistent with an anxiety diagnosis), the "or" rule (child meets criteria for an anxiety disorder if either the parent's or the child's report meets criteria for an anxiety disorder), or the use of an independent evaluator who weighs evidence from all sources and makes a composite decision. For measurement-based care, it is important that the clinician recognize that child and parent ratings are not interchangeable, and monitor changes in both parent and child report to assess treatment progress.

Because of the need to capture 3 or more types of anxiety, anxiety scales used as diagnostic aids are longer and more cumbersome than are depression scales. When considering instruments to track response to treatment in a child or adolescent with a single anxiety diagnosis, it may be preferable to use a briefer instrument that captures symptoms of only that diagnosis. Currently, this option is only available for generalized anxiety disorder (GAD). A potential risk in such an approach is that one may miss the emergence of new anxiety symptoms related to a different anxiety disorder. Anxiety disorders tend to emerge in predictable stages of pediatric and adolescent development, and a young person followed chronologically may, for example, develop symptoms of panic disorder after social phobia has partially resolved.

MEASUREMENT-BASED ASSESSMENT VERSUS MEASUREMENT-BASED CARE: PSYCHOMETRIC ISSUES

The psychometric properties of a particular measure of attitudes, emotions, or behavior refer to that measure's validity (measuring what it is intended to measure) and reliability (measuring a construct consistently across time, individuals, and situations). Reliability includes 3 concepts: (a) internal consistency measures the consistency of people's responses across the items on a multiple-item measure and often reported as Cronbach's alpha, α; (b) inter-rater reliability is the extent to which different observers are consistent in their judgments and is reported as a correlation when the measures are continuous or, when they are categorical, as Cohen's kappa, κ; and (c) test–retest reliability, which is discussed elsewhere in this article. In general, although there are exceptions, a score of 0.8 or greater for Cronbach's α indicates good reliability, as does a kappa of 0.80. There is no clear standard for the value of the Pearson correlation that is acceptable.

In tracking response to treatment in measurement-based care, the test–retest reliability of the instrument is particularly important. Because there is always some measurement error, it is possible that the change in test scores across 2 time points could be due to measurement error rather than to a change in the underlying construct (eg, anxiety) purportedly being measured. If the test–retest reliability is known, a statistical known as the standard error of a difference can be calculated. A reliable change index (RCI) can then be calculated. That value represents the 95% confidence interval for the difference score; if the magnitude of change is greater than or equal to the RCI, there is a 95% chance that the change is not due to measurement error. The more reliable the test is, the smaller the magnitude of change in scores must be to be confident the change is not due to measurement error. There is no absolute standard for acceptable test–retest reliability; if a test is chosen for which reliability is poor, the consequence is that the change on the test needed to be confident the change is unlikely to be due to measurement error increases, so it behooves the clinician to find a reliable test for measurement-based care. It is important to keep in mind that the magnitude of the test–retest reliability of a measure decreases with longer intervals between test administrations. For measures of emotional or behavior problems, one seeks an interval long enough to detect random variation in scores but shorter than that in which clinical change unrelated to treatment should be anticipated.

Although reliable change is change that is greater than would be attributable to measurement error, a change that is reliable may nonetheless be too small to be meaningful or clinically significant. Thus, although achieving a reliable change is 1 standard of improvement in treatment, a second standard is needed, a change to a level that is also clinically meaningful. Clinically significant change must meet 2 standards: it must be reliable change, and it must cross some threshold of significance.[21] Thresholds can be established in relation to (a) distance from the mean score in a population with the active diagnosis, (b) distance from the mean score in a healthy population, or (c) some point between (a) and (b). **Fig. 1** illustrates relationships between reliable change and clinically significant change.

We can illustrate some of the issues involved in determining whether a patient has achieved a clinically significant change for the widely used SCARED measure. The first step involves calculating the RCI by measuring test–retest reliability and its standard deviation. The RCI vary from sample to sample, and some clinical judgment must be exercised in determining whether the sample for which that information is available is a good match for the one of interest to you. For the SCARED, Birmaher and colleagues[8] calculated the test–retest reliability for a 38-item version. Subsequently, they refined

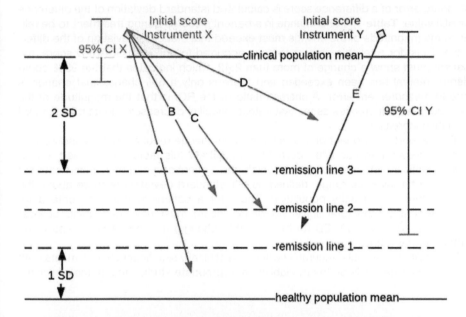

Reliable change and potential definitions of clinically significant change
Reliable change= >95% CI of the clinical population mean
Confidence interval (CI) X represents Instrument X with high test-retest validity
CI Y represents Instrument Y with low test-retest validity
Clinically significant change must be:
(1). Greater than the 95% CI for the test-retest validity of the instrument used
AND (2): one of the following:
Line A: improvment to less than 1 standard deviation (SD) above the healthy population mean
Line B: improvement to greater than 2 SD below the clinical population mean
Line C: improvement to or below the midpoint between 1 SD above the healty population mean and 2 SD below the clinical population mean
****
Line D represents reliable change using Instrument X but lack of clinically significant change
Line E represents lack of clinically significant change: while change in score is large, it is less than the 95% CI of test-retest reliability for Instrument Y

Fig. 1. Reliable change and potential definitions of clinically significant change.

the measure by adding items, creating the 41-item version now in use. The developers of the SCARED did not report a revised test–retest reliability for the refined measure, but 2 subsequent studies have done so. Boyd and colleagues[22] reported 6-month test–retest reliability for a small sample of African American adolescents. Typically, the longer the interval between test administrations, the lower the test–retest reliability will be. Haley and colleagues[23] examined the 3-month test–retest reliability in a sample of white adolescents ages 14 to 18 years. A clinician would have to decide which of these 2 samples best matches their patient population.

We illustrate the use of the RCI for the SCARED based on the Haley and colleagues study.[23] Although other approaches to calculating the RCI have been developed, we use the original approach described by Jacobson and Truax.[24] In that approach the standard error of a difference score is calculated (standard deviation of the difference or RCI value; **Table 1**). For a change in a patient's scores during treatment to be reliable, the magnitude of the change must exceed that standard deviation of the difference. Thus, for a reliable change to have occurred for the total SCARED score, the patient must show a change of more than 2.42, which indicates that the 95% confidence interval has been exceeded and there is only a 5% chance that change is due to measurement error. A characteristic of the RCI is that the magnitude of the needed change increases as the test–retest reliability decreases and as the standard deviation increases.

The second component of assessing clinical change requires that the individual's scores cross an appropriate threshold. To illustrate this factor, we defined a clinically significant change as one in which the patient's symptoms after treatment fall within the average range, defined as +1 standard deviation or more above the mean score in a healthy population. Thus, for a patient to meet the criteria for improvement on the total scale, his or her score must have decreased at least 2.42 points on the SCARED (to be a reliable change) and be 24.37 or less to be in the normal range.

The ability to calculate accurately whether a clinically significant change meets both these criteria depends on the availability of appropriate studies that fit the clinician's

Table 1
Mean, standard deviation, and reliable change value on the SCARED in a population of adolescent males

	Mean	SD	r	RCI Value (S-diff)	Normal Range Cutoff
Total	21.24	3.13	0.7	2.42	24.37
GAD	6.44	4.24	0.62	3.69	10.68
SAD	2.91	2.86	0.69	2.25	5.77
Social phobia	5.28	3.74	0.83	2.18	9.02
School phobia	1.93	1.8	0.46	1.87	3.73
Somatic/panic	4.77	4.52	0.58	4.14	9.29

Abbreviations: r, test–retest correlation; SAD, social anxiety disorder; SD, standard deviation; S-diff, standard deviation of difference.

Data from Haley T, Puskar K, Terhorst L. Psychometric properties of the Screen for Child Anxiety Related Emotional Disorders in a rural high school population. J Child Adolesc Psychiatr Nurs. 2011;24(1):23-32.)

sample of interest. For most groups and most measures, there are presently no useful studies. For others, as with white adolescents in the Haley and colleagues, sample, there is reasonably good information upon which to determine clinically significant change.

The absence of psychometric measures underpinning clinically significant change does not preclude the use of the instruments developed to screen for pediatric anxiety disorder in measurement-based care. Clearly, better scores are likely to be consistent with improvement and worse scores with a greater symptom burden. The benefits as described, including aiding in structuring and focusing the follow-up visit, clarifying language used for symptoms, and guiding the patient in monitoring their internal symptom scale, are not negated by a lack of psychometric precision. It is important to remember, however, that scales cannot be thought of as the definitive target of treatment in the way that a diastolic blood pressure of less than 120 mm Hg or a body mass index of less than 25 kg/m^2 can be a target.

ANXIETY SYMPTOM MEASURES

Selecting an outcome measure for your practice should include a measure that is established as reliable and valid, sensitive to change, brief, easily accessible, and preferably has versions for multiple raters (child, parent, and/or teacher). **Table 2** provides an overview of several measures that can be used in the assessment of anxiety in children and adolescents.

Many of the measures in **Table 2** are inclusive of multiple anxiety disorders, whereas GAD-7 only addresses symptoms of GAD. In an adolescent who is reporting only GAD symptoms, this scale may be practical to use, because it is brief and publicly available. In an adolescent with multiple anxiety disorders, the GAD-7 is not comprehensive enough to include these specific symptoms and a broader scale may be more appropriate. The measure includes a brief assessment of functional impairment, with an added item asking how anxiety impacts the ability "to do your work, take care of things at home, or get along with other people." The Pediatric Anxiety Rating Scale is unique in that it is a clinician-rated instrument that assesses level of impairment.[25] The Pediatric Anxiety Rating Scale was used as the dimensional outcome measure in Child/Adolescent Anxiety Multimodal Study.[26] In this measure, the clinician rates the severity of 7 dimensions: (1) number of symptoms (none to >10), (2) frequency (none to several hours per day), (3) severity of distress associated with anxiety symptoms (none to extreme), (4) severity of physical symptoms (none to extreme), (5) avoidance (none to extreme), (6) interference at home (no interference to totally or almost totally unable to function at home), and (7) interference out of home (no interference to totally or almost totally unable to function out of home such as with peers or at school). This scale does not provide for patient self-report and in an outpatient practice setting, is less likely to be utilized as the only outcome measure. The Patient-Reported Outcomes Measurement Information System (PROMIS) project was instituted by NIH to advance patient reported outcomes in chronic illness. Within pediatrics, the PROMIS Pediatric project developed patient reported outcome measures across several pediatric health domains, for ages 8 to 17 years; these domains include measures for depression, anxiety, anger, pain interference, peer relationships, fatigue, mobility, and asthma. The PROMIS anxiety items assess the following domains with subscales noted in parentheses over a 7-day period: fear (fearfulness, panic), anxious misery (worry, dread), hyperarousal (tension, nervousness, restlessness), and somatic symptoms related to arousal (racing heart, dizziness). The test–retest reliability has not been established for the PROMIS anxiety items.

Table 2
Selected instruments used in the evaluation and ongoing treatment of pediatric anxiety

Instrument	Age Range (y)		Subscales	Number of Items (Short Version)	Likert Scale Points	Rater	Cost	Test Reliability	Languages
	Child Version	Parent Version							
Multidimensional Anxiety Scale for Children (March et al, 2013)	8–19	8–19	SEP, GAD, SOC, harm avoidance, physical symptoms, obsessions/compulsions)	50	4	Patient/parent	–	(r = 0.79; March et al., 1997).	–
SCARED (Birmaher et al 1997, 1999)	8–18	8–18	SEP, GAD, SOC, PD, school refusal	41(5)	3	Patient/parent	Free	r = 0.7 (Haley et al, 2007)	English, Spanish
Spence Children's Anxiety Scale (Spence et al 1998)	8–12	2.5–6.5	Panic attacks and agoraphobia, SEP, physical injury fears, SOC, obsessive-compulsive, and GAD	34–45 (19)	4	Patient/parent	–	0.92	Several languages
GAD Scale (GAD-7) (Spitzer, Kroenke, Williams, & Lowe, 2006)	≥12	N/A	GAD only	7	4	Patient	Free	Not available	–
Preschool Anxiety Scale (PAS)	N/A	3–6	None	29–34		Parent		Not available	Several languages
PROMIS anxiety scale	8–17	5–17	None	8	5	Patient/parent	free	Not available	–
Pediatric Anxiety Rating Scale (Riddle et al, 2002)			SOC, SEP, GAD, specific phobia, physical signs and symptoms	50 + 7 severity items	6	Clinician		Not available	–

Abbreviations: PD, panic disorder; SEP, separation anxiety disorder; SOC, social anxiety disorder.

ANXIETY IMPAIRMENT MEASURES

An alternate approach to measuring response to treatment in pediatric anxiety disorders is to take a functional rather than symptomatic approach. The scales listed in **Table 2** primarily measure the child's internal experience of worries, or the parent's inference of those experiences in their child. A functional approach to assessing anxiety looks at the ways in which anxiety interferes with the child's daily activities, or in which the child's anxiety has created a system of accommodations that interferes with the daily activities of those around her. A functional approach may involve mapping out the ways in which anxiety is interfering with functioning and/or causing suffering in the individual child and her family, and tracking changes in those areas.

The Children's Global Assessment Scale is a clinician-rated, diagnosis-agnostic, single-item measure of symptom severity and functional interference on a scale from 1 to 100, indicated for ages 4 to 16 years.[27] The Children's Global Assessment Scale has been widely used as a supplemental measure in randomized controlled trials of both psychopharmacologic and psychotherapeutic interventions in pediatric mental health. Shaffer and colleagues[27] demonstrated both inter-rater and test–retest reliability of the Children's Global Assessment Scale to be excellent.

The Child Anxiety Impairment Scale is a 27-item measure of the impact of anxiety on a child's capacity to engage in developmentally appropriate activities in home, school, and social settings.[28] Langley and colleagues[28] originally developed a parent-report instrument, and later, a mirroring child/adolescent instrument was added and factor analysis of both the parent and child versions was conducted as part of the Child/Adolescent Anxiety Multimodal Study. The test–retest reliability of the Child Anxiety Impairment Scale has not been established.

The Top Problems method approaches measurement of functional change by helping the child and parent identify specific impairments attributable to a disorder that matter most to them.[29] Top Problems lends itself to a treatment-to-target strategy by helping remind clinicians, patients and families of treatment goals and documenting when they have been achieved, and what new goals may follow.

MEASUREMENT-BASED CARE IN PEDIATRIC ANXIETY: A CASE
Initial Evaluation

Leticia Salas is 10-year-old fourth grader referred to you by her pediatrician. At a recent well-child check, Leticia's mother, Ms Salas, expressed concern about anxiety and emotional regulation. Leticia seems to be anxious and tense often. She is stressed around new social situations at school and at playdates. She talks with her mother but has difficulty expressing her emotions. Leticia has never told her mother she is anxious.

Meeting with you for an initial visit, you find that these symptoms have been present for about 6 months. Before that, Leticia was less irritable but has always been a little shy, and tends to apprehensive about new place, people, or activities. She has 1 close friend, but difficulty making new friends. She makes average grades in school, where she is seen as a quiet child and does not get into any trouble. Leticia does not have a sustained depressed mood or thoughts of death or of self-harm. She does not have obsessions, compulsions, or psychotic symptoms. She sleeps well as long as she sleeps with her parents. She has been eating larger quantities and gaining weight, crossing body mass index curves from the 60th to the 85th percentile over the last year.

Leticia's father tends to be anxious, but has never been diagnosed with any mental health disorder. Leticia's maternal grandmother suffered from post partum depression.

After you conduct your clinical interview, you ask Ms Salas and Leticia to complete the parent and child versions of the SCARED. Leticia attempts the first question, but is unsure of what answer to put, and becomes so distraught at having to answer questions about anxiety that she is unable to continue. Her mother completes the SCARED parent form with the following scores.

Parent SCARED

Total SCARED	Panic Subscale	Generalized Anxiety Subscale	Separation Anxiety	Social Phobia	School Avoidance
34	3	18	8	4	1

You explain that Leticia has symptoms consistent with separation anxiety disorder and GAD, and that Leticia's irritability and difficulty regulating her emotions are related to her being anxious most of the time. You explain that GAD in children and adolescents can be treated with medication, psychotherapy, or a combination thereof. Ms Salas states a strong preference to avoid medication. You refer her to a colleague for cognitive–behavioral therapy and ask to see her back in 8 weeks.

Visit #2 (8 Weeks After Evaluation)

Ms Salas reports that Leticia continues to be anxious and irritable at times. Leticia is finding it difficult to engage in cognitive–behavioral therapy strategies targeting her GAD symptoms. She is unable to identifying coping strategies that help. Her parents have learned about their role in accommodating Leticia's separation anxiety, and, through graded exposures, gotten Leticia to sleep in her own bed and be more independent around the house. Now that she has gotten used to naming her anxiety symptoms in therapy, Leticia is able to complete the SCARED.

Parent SCARED

Total SCARED	Panic Subscale	Generalized Anxiety Subscale	Separation Anxiety	Social Phobia	School Avoidance
31	4	17	4	5	1

Child SCARED

Total SCARED	Panic Subscale	Generalized Anxiety Subscale	Separation Anxiety	Social Phobia	School Avoidance
31	5	16	5	4	1

You review the evidence for combined therapy for moderate to severe GAD, which is not responding to cognitive–behavioral therapy alone. After a discussion of risks, benefits, and side effects, Ms Salas consents to a trial of sertraline for Leticia.

Visit #3 (12 Weeks After Evaluation)

Leticia is tolerating sertraline 25 mg without side effects. She thinks she may be a little less anxious but cannot really tell. She continues in therapy. Ms Salas describes Leticia as a little more relaxed and less reactive to minor stresses.

Parent SCARED

Total SCARED	Panic Subscale	Generalized Anxiety Subscale	Separation Anxiety	Social Phobia	School Avoidance
27	4	14	4	4	1

Child SCARED

Total SCARED	Panic Subscale	Generalized Anxiety Subscale	Separation Anxiety	Social Phobia	School Avoidance
26	3	12	5	5	1

You recommend a dose increase to sertraline 50 mg, and Ms Salas agrees.

Visit #4 (16 Weeks After Evaluation)

Leticia returns today and announces that she is feeling better. She wants to join a dance group that her best friend has recently joined.

Parent SCARED

Total SCARED	Panic Subscale	Generalized Anxiety Subscale	Separation Anxiety	Social Phobia	School Avoidance
15	3	6	4	2	0

Child SCARED

Total SCARED	Panic Subscale	Generalized Anxiety Subscale	Separation Anxiety	Social Phobia	School Avoidance
13	2	5	2	3	1

You review Leticia's symptoms, level of functioning, and the trajectory of the SCARED scores. You tell Leticia that you think her anxiety is currently much better, and she and Ms Salas agree. You discuss with Leticia and her mother that you would like to see them back in 4 weeks to monitor the stability of her symptoms.

In this case example, the child's completion of the SCARED measure at the second visit helped to identify the elevated subscale score for GAD and further indicated that Leticia was considerably symptomatic despite 8 weeks of therapy. This additional information provided by the outcome measure prompted the psychiatrist to start medication management expediently. If the child did not complete the SCARED, it is probable that medication initiation could have been delayed.

ADDITIONAL CLINICAL ISSUES AND CONSIDERATIONS IN MEASUREMENT-BASED CARE

Beyond the discussed benefits and limitations of measurement-based care in pediatric anxiety, the use of measurement-based care prompts additional clinical considerations for the child psychiatrist.

LITERACY AND HEALTH LITERACY

At the patient level, younger children and children with cognitive/intellectual and physical/visual impairments may be unable to complete measures. Efforts must be made to accommodate the special needs of the child while also examining the appropriateness for the patient to engage in measurement-based care. The literacy level of the child and parent, as well as the family's understanding of mental health and language nuances, may impact understanding of items and reports provided on measures. It may be helpful, before administering a measure, for the psychiatrist to discuss the family's literacy framework and understanding of specific items. For instance, the use of clarification questions, such as, "What does this question mean to you?" and "Did you have any trouble understanding these questions?" can broaden the conversation to include not only symptom reporting, but the patient and family understanding of mental health. If a child or parent is unable to complete measures owing to literacy issues, consider using an alternate measure, reading the instrument to the respondent, or using a clinician-rated scale.

COMORBIDITIES

We commonly see patients who have a primary anxiety disorder and multiple other comorbid psychiatric diagnosis (depression, attention deficit hyperactivity disorder, oppositional defiant disorder), and there is no guideline on how to effectively and efficiently use multiple measurement-based care outcomes to monitor all diagnoses in a child with comorbidities. In such a case, multiple outcome measures may be necessary to monitor all active symptoms; however, the appropriateness and practicality of a child and her parent completing multiple measures should be further considered. Outcome measures are meant to be efficient and time sensitive, and excessive use may place additional burden on the patient by making visits laborious for child and parent. The psychiatrist must be able to review all measures obtained with the patient directly to ensure that there is appropriate discussion around elevated items, as well as to note improvement in items. The psychiatrist may need to develop an organized system to monitor and record multiple measures and incorporate them into the treatment in a meaningful, not overwhelming, way.[30]

USING MEASUREMENT TO EXPLORE LACK OF CLINICAL RESPONSE

Measurement-based care can add structure and provide support to clinical decision making, but it cannot replace clinical judgment. Particularly when measurement-based care indicates lack of response to evidence-based treatment, it is important to step back and identify possible reasons for a lack of improvement. It may be that the instrument chosen is not a valid measure for what the patient has, and diagnostic reevaluation is needed. In pediatric anxiety disorders, it may be that factors outside the child reinforce the anxiety disorder through accommodation of the child's symptoms or even through reinforcement of a parent's anxiety, as when a father quits a stressful job to stay home with an anxious child. In these cases, measurement of the child's symptoms may not actually measure "the problem" that must be resolved to reduce symptoms. An assessment of family functioning and accommodation can help to identify the extent to which the family is participating in the child's anxiety. Lebowitz and colleagues[31] modified Calvocoressi's Family Accommodation Scale for Obsessive–Compulsive Disorder to assess accommodation across all childhood anxiety disorders, with creation of the Family Accommodation Scale—Anxiety. The following are items the Family Accommodation Scale—Anxiety uses to assess level of parental distress and negative outcomes of accommodation: (1) Does helping your child in these ways cause you distress? (2) Has your child become distressed/anxious when you have not provided assistance? (3) Has your child become angry/abusive when you have not provided assistance? and (4) Has your child's anxiety been worse when you have not provided assistance?[31] The Family Accommodation Scale—Anxiety shows good internal consistency and convergent and divergent validity and can be used at the outset of treatment and during course of treatment to monitor level of accommodation.

Sometimes, before treatment even begins, one should measure readiness for change on the part of the patient and of key family members. Readiness for change is a component of motivational interviewing and at its most basic involves 2 questions: (1) How important is it for you to make this change? (2) How confident are you that you can make this change? Readiness to change and expectancy of treatment response are closely linked concepts. Expectancy is generally understood as the extent to which a child believes she will benefit from treatment. Strawn and colleagues[32] studied the influence of expectancy on treatment response in children receiving pill-placebo in Child/Adolescent Anxiety Multimodal Study.[28] In this analysis, child/parent expectations were assessed using a 5-point Likert rating for the following items: (1) "I expect to get control over my anxiety through this treatment"; (2) "I expect to get better or become less anxious through this treatment"; and (3) "I expect my life to get better in some ways through this treatment." Children with higher, more positive treatment expectancy were more likely to be placebo responders. Similarly, parents of placebo responders also had higher expectation that the treatment would be effective.[32] The psychiatrist can use knowledge of the patient and family's expectations to explore biases that may be influencing treatment and to increase the family's education about the treatment, as well as its evidence base and response rates. In patients with a negative expectancy, the psychiatrist may be able to work more closely with patient and family to identify small, positive changes on measurement outcomes to increase awareness of positive change when it occurs.

Knowledge of factors that impact a child's likelihood to reach response or ideally, remission, can also help the psychiatrist to monitor for risk factors that may portend to a poor response. Ginsburg and colleagues[33] analyzed patient-level predictors of remission in anxious children, and the most consistent predictors were younger age, lower anxiety at baseline and absence of social anxiety at baseline. At the family level, family functioning and caregiver strain can impair response to treatment. Compton and colleagues[34] demonstrated that a higher level of caregiver strain is known to be associated with poorer treatment response. Children with these risk factors may require longer or more intensive treatment and consideration of adjunctive treatment measures and may not demonstrate response to treatment as expected.

PRACTICE-LEVEL CONSIDERATIONS

As discussed elsewhere in this article, measurement-based care is not yet standardized in outpatient psychiatric practice, although interest in implementation continues to emerge. Although it is difficult to estimate the number of psychiatrists who are currently implementing measurement-based care regularly, smaller studies of psychiatrist (adult) engagement in measurement-based care have indicated that these numbers are quite small and most psychiatrists are not routinely using measures.[35,36] It is unclear how many child psychiatrists are regularly using measures. Many factors may affect the psychiatrist's readiness to implement measurement-based care into practice; among these factors are the provider's familiarity and previous training in the application of progress monitoring. To increase familiarity with measures, it may be necessary to start introducing measurement-based care into residency programs and embed this into the training process. An alternative approach would be brief training on the use of measures for practicing psychiatrists and this may require designation of a champion, if in a group or hospital practice, to disseminate the instruction.

Although we have discussed the importance of measurement-based care to the child's treatment course, the psychiatric clinician may also think about measurement-based care at a practice level to monitor prescribing trends (at what symptom threshold and severity are dose changes made), rates of patient remission and recurrence of symptoms, and time to length of remission. In this way, measurement-based care can be used as a platform for clinician growth and an understanding of personal practice trends.

On more structural and systematic levels, providers often note that time constraints influence their choice to implement measurement-based care.[37,38] The amount of time allotted for the physician to review and discuss measures and conduct treatment planning is largely related to the practice setting, whether private practice, group, community hospital, or academic. In a setting with increased resources, the physician may have ample time to have the child and parent complete the measure, and perhaps multiple measures as appropriate, before the visit. In such settings, staff members may be available to enter data from measures into an electronic system. More commonly, the psychiatrist will be in a private practice setting and may not have access to electronic charting or to additional staff to assist with data entry and tracking. Reviewing completed measures directly with the patient is essential to measurement-based care, and the resources of the particular practice setting as well as time allotted for visits may influence how the psychiatrist chooses to use outcome measures, if at all.

CONCLUDING THOUGHTS

In review, anxiety disorders are among the most prevalent conditions in pediatric mental health, and several outcome measures are available to monitor the child's progress toward remission. Child psychiatrists are using these measures in variable ways, though there are no formalized guidelines to use patient outcome measures. In the future, we recommend more formalized study of the use of outcome measures in a clinical population of anxious children and evidence base for use in pediatric anxiety will be strengthened.

DISCLOSURE

Dr R. Ballard receives royalties from American Psychiatric Publishing, Inc, for co-edited books on general child and adolescent psychiatry. Dr J. Walkup is on the advisory board for the Anxiety Disorders Association of America, Tourette Association, and Trichotillomania Learning Center. He receives royalties from Guilford Press, Oxford University Press, and Wolters Kluwer. Dr J. Lavigne and Dr C. Romba have nothing to disclose.

REFERENCES

1. Elmquist JM, Melton TK, Croarkin P, et al. A systematic overview of measurement-based care in the treatment of childhood and adolescent depression. J Psychiatr Pract 2010;16(4):217–34.
2. Jackson WC. The benefits of measurement-based care for primary care patients with depression. J Clin Psychiatry 2016;77(3):e318.
3. Ricken R, Wiethoff K, Reinhold T, et al. Algorithm-guided treatment of depression reduces treatment costs–results from the randomized controlled German Algorithm Project (GAPII). J Affect Disord 2011;134(1-3):249–56.
4. Bauer M, Pfennig A, Linden M, et al. Efficacy of an algorithm-guided treatment compared with treatment as usual: a randomized, controlled study of inpatients with depression. J Clin Psychopharmacol 2009;29(4):327–33.
5. Guo T, Xiang YT, Xiao L, et al. Measurement-based care versus standard care for major depression: a randomized controlled trial with blind raters. Am J Psychiatry 2015;172(10):1004–13.
6. Lambert MJ, Harmon C, Slade K, et al. Providing feedback to psychotherapists on their patients' progress: clinical results and practice suggestions. J Clin Psychol 2005;61(2):165–74.
7. Frank E, Prien RF, Jarrett RB, et al. Conceptualization and rationale for consensus definitions of terms in major depressive disorder. Remission, recovery, relapse, and recurrence. Arch Gen Psychiatry 1991;48(9):851–5.
8. Birmaher B, Khetarpal S, Brent D, et al. The screen for child anxiety related emotional disorders (SCARED): scale construction and psychometric characteristics. J Am Acad Child Adolesc Psychiatry 1997;36(4):545–53.
9. March JS, Parker JD, Sullivan K, et al. The Multidimensional Anxiety Scale for Children (MASC): factor structure, reliability, and validity. J Am Acad Child Adolesc Psychiatry 1997;36(4):554–65.
10. Spence SH. A measure of anxiety symptoms among children. Behav Res Ther 1998;36(5):545–66.
11. Birmaher B, Brent DA, Chiappetta L, et al. Psychometric properties of the screen for child anxiety related emotional disorders (SCARED): a replication study. J Am Acad Child Adolesc Psychiatry 1999;38(10):1230–6.
12. Rappaport BI, Pagliaccio D, Pine DS, et al. Discriminant validity, diagnostic utility, and parent-child agreement on the Screen for Child Anxiety Related Emotional Disorders (SCARED) in treatment- and non-treatment-seeking youth. J Anxiety Disord 2017;51:22–31.
13. Weems CF, Feaster DJ, Horigian VE, et al. Parent and child agreement on anxiety disorder symptoms using the DISC predictive scales. Assessment 2011;18(2):213–6.
14. Muris P, Merckelbach H, van Brakel A, et al. The revised version of the screen for child anxiety related emotional disorders (SCARED-R): further evidence for its reliability and validity. Anxiety Stress Coping 1999;12(4):411–25.
15. Muris P, Dreessen L, Bogels S, et al. A questionnaire for screening a broad range of DSM-defined anxiety disorder symptoms in clinically referred children and adolescents. J Child Psychol Psychiatry 2004;45(4):813–20.
16. Wren FJ, Bridge JA, Birmaher B. Screening for childhood anxiety symptoms in primary care: integrating child and parent reports. J Am Acad Child Adolesc Psychiatry 2004;43(11):1364–71.

17. Wren FJ, Berg EA, Heiden LA, et al. Childhood anxiety in a diverse primary care population: parent-child reports, ethnicity and SCARED factor structure. J Am Acad Child Adolesc Psychiatry 2007;46(3):332–40.
18. Wei C, Hoff A, Villabø MA, et al. Assessing anxiety in youth with the multidimensional anxiety scale for children. J Clin Child Adolesc Psychol 2014;43(4):566–78.
19. Su L, Wang K, Fan F, et al. Reliability and validity of the screen for child anxiety related emotional disorders (SCARED) in Chinese children. J Anxiety Disord 2008;22(4):612–21.
20. Hariz N, Bawab S, Atwi M, et al. Reliability and validity of the Arabic screen for child anxiety related emotional disorders (SCARED) in a clinical sample. Psychiatry Res 2013;209(2):222–8.
21. Saps M, Lavigne JV, van Tilburg MA, et al. Endpoints, reliability, and meaningful changes in clinical trials for children with irritable bowel syndrome. The Rome foundation pediatric subcommittee on clinical trials. Neurogastroenterol Motil 2018;30(5):e13308.
22. Boyd RC, Ginsburg GS, Lambert SF, et al. Screen for child anxiety related emotional disorders (SCARED): psychometric properties in an African-American parochial high school sample. J Am Acad Child Adolesc Psychiatry 2003;42(10):1188–96.
23. Haley T, Puskar K, Terhorst L. Psychometric properties of the screen for child anxiety related emotional disorders in a rural high school population. J Child Adolesc Psychiatr Nurs 2011;24(1):23–32.
24. Jacobson NS, Truax P. Clinical significance: a statistical approach to defining meaningful change in psychotherapy research. J Consult Clin Psychol 1991;59(1):12–9.
25. The pediatric anxiety rating scale (PARS): development and psychometric properties. J Am Acad Child Adolesc Psychiatry 2002;41(9):1061–9.
26. Walkup JT, Albano AM, Piacentini J, et al. Cognitive behavioral therapy, sertraline, or a combination in childhood anxiety. N Engl J Med 2008;359(26):2753–66.
27. Shaffer D, Gould MS, Brasic J, et al. A children's global assessment scale (CGAS). Arch Gen Psychiatry 1983;40(11):1228–31.
28. Langley AK, Falk A, Peris T, et al. The child anxiety impact scale: examining parent- and child-reported impairment in child anxiety disorders. J Clin Child Adolesc Psychol 2014;43(4):579–91.
29. Weisz JR, Chorpita BF, Frye A, et al. Youth Top Problems: using idiographic, consumer-guided assessment to identify treatment needs and to track change during psychotherapy. J Consult Clin Psychol 2011;79(3):369–80.
30. Scott K, Lewis CC. Using measurement-based care to enhance any treatment. Cogn Behav Pract 2015;22(1):49–59.
31. Lebowitz ER, Woolston J, Bar-Haim Y, et al. Family accommodation in pediatric anxiety disorders. Depress Anxiety 2013;30(1):47–54.
32. Strawn JR, Dobson ET, Mills JA, et al. Placebo response in pediatric anxiety disorders: results from the Child/Adolescent Anxiety Multimodal Study. J Child Adolesc Psychopharmacol 2017;27(6):501–8.
33. Ginsburg GS, Kendall PC, Sakolsky D, et al. Remission after acute treatment in children and adolescents with anxiety disorders: findings from the CAMS. J Consult Clin Psychol 2011;79(6):806–13.
34. Compton SN, Peris TS, Almirall D, et al. Predictors and moderators of treatment response in childhood anxiety disorders: results from the CAMS trial. J Consult Clin Psychol 2014;82(2):212–24.

35. Zimmerman M, McGlinchey JB. Why don't psychiatrists use scales to measure outcome when treating depressed patients? J Clin Psychiatry 2008;69(12): 1916–9.
36. Lewis CC, Boyd M, Puspitasari A, et al. Implementing measurement-based care in behavioral health: a review. JAMA Psychiatry 2019;76(3):324–35.
37. Hatfield DR, Ogles BM. Why some clinicians use outcome measures and others do not. Adm Policy Ment Health 2007;34(3):283–91.
38. Aboraya A, Nasrallah HA, Elswick DE, et al. Measurement-based care in psychiatry-past, present, and future. Innov Clin Neurosci 2018;15(11-12):13–26.

Measurement-Based Care in the Treatment of Attention-Deficit/Hyperactivity Disorder and Disruptive Behavior Disorders

Claudine Higdon, MD[a],*, Joseph Blader, PhD[b],
Vamsi K. Kalari, MD[a], Victor M. Fornari, MD, MS[a]

KEYWORDS

- Attention-deficit/hyperactivity disorder (ADHD) • Measurement based care
- Children and adolescents • Disruptive behavior disorders
- Evidence-based medicine

KEY POINTS

- ADHD entails impairments that have extensive and profound detrimental effects on many critical developmental areas.
- A quantitative measurement strategy to treat ADHD is a valuable component of care that helps to determine the need for treatment, specify treatment goals, monitor clinical progress and outcome, and thereby hasten relief from symptoms.
- Features of ADHD and its pharmacotherapy make measurement-based care especially useful.
- There are many well-validated rating scales used to assess ADHD symptom severity and according to several practice guidelines are considered minimum standard.
- A basic requirement of measurement-based care is that outcome data be available in a format that is intelligible and actionable.

INTRODUCTION

Rationale for Measurement-Based Care in Attention-Deficit/Hyperactivity Disorder

Attention-deficit/hyperactivity disorder (ADHD) is one of the most common mental health disorders of childhood with prevalence rates ranging from 5% to 12%.[1] The core symptoms of ADHD include inattention, impulsivity, and hyperactivity. Children with ADHD show impairments in multiple domains of functioning including family, social, and academic. ADHD entails impairments that have extensive and profound detrimental effects on many critical developmental areas. Children with ADHD exhibit poor

[a] Donald & Barbara Zucker School of Medicine at Hofstra/Northwell, 7559 263rd Street, Glen Oaks, NY 11004, USA; [b] University of Texas Health Science Center at San Antonio, 7703 Floyd Curl Drive, MS 7719, San Antonio, TX 78229, USA
* Corresponding author.
E-mail address: chigdon@northwell.edu

Child Adolesc Psychiatric Clin N Am 29 (2020) 663–674
https://doi.org/10.1016/j.chc.2020.06.005
1056-4993/20/© 2020 Elsevier Inc. All rights reserved.
childpsych.theclinics.com

organizational skills and noncompliance with adult requests leading to negative inter-actions with family members. Parents of children with ADHD report more frequent and severe interparental discord and child-rearing disagreements, more negative parenting practices, greater parenting stress, and caregiver strain and more psycho-pathology themselves.[2,3] Children with ADHD have poor boundaries with peers and siblings, being seen as intrusive, overbearing, silly and immature, boastful, and aggressive often causing unsuccessful involvement in socialization opportunities. Studies of children with ADHD in classroom settings have documented that they are more off-task, complete less assigned work and with less accuracy, are more disrup-tive and break more classroom rules.[3,4] They are less likely to follow directions compared with their peers. The behavioral problems at school often lead to lower levels of academic achievement and higher rates of disciplinary referrals, retention, and later dropout.[3,5] High impulsiveness also raises the risks for injury, and, among adolescents, substance use and other behaviors with severe consequences.[6] Longer persistence of these problems and risks worsens their cumulative impact, making it more likely they will adversely affect the child's life trajectory well beyond youth. Whereas core symptoms of ADHD may improve with age, the functional impairments often persist into adolescence and adulthood. In the management of ADHD, therefore, time is of the essence.

A quantitative measurement strategy to treat ADHD is a valuable component of care that helps determine the need for treatment, specify treatment goals, monitor clinical progress and outcome, and thereby hasten relief from its symptoms. Some features of ADHD and its pharmacotherapy make measurement-based care especially useful. The leading first-line treatments, chiefly stimulant medications, have large effect sizes up to 0.8, but for a given patient seemingly small changes in dose strongly affect outcome.[7,8] These dose-response relationships also show high individual variability. One consequence is that establishing an optimal regimen is a dose-finding exercise. Rating scales that quantify behavioral response make the comparison of various medi-cation and dose combinations much easier and accurate than reliance on narrative notes or memory.

Most medications for ADHD demonstrate their effects right away, unlike many other psychiatric treatments that take time to achieve a steady-state concentration and to impact symptoms. Their offset of action is also rapid, with little to no carryover from 1 day to the next. In outpatient settings, one can usually determine the effectiveness and tolerability of a regimen in 1 to 2 weeks. Most behavioral ratings scales to track ADHD symptoms are designed for just this type of serial administration, and ask infor-mants to use observations over the past week as the basis for their responses.

ADHD symptoms do not always improve in unison.[7,9] For instance, it is not uncom-mon for attention span to improve with a given regimen, whereas other problems, such as impulsivity or emotional lability, may only respond to a higher dose of the specific medication, if at all. Sometimes, a dose may worsen an area, as when treatment-emergent irritability, obsessiveness, or hyperacusis cause discomfort or impair func-tioning. It becomes important to differentiate and measure these responses as they occur, and several rating scales in common use provide separate scores for specific domains of ADHD-related symptoms.

Because ADHD often co-occurs with other disorders, it is important to determine how these other problems are affected by treatment. Half of children and adolescents with ADHD have oppositional-defiant disorder or conduct disorder.[10,11] Twenty-five percent to 30% of children with ADHD have anxiety disorder and 20% to 25% of chil-dren with ADHD have a learning disorder.[12–14] There is an increased risk of mood dis-orders with studies showing up to 33% of patients with ADHD meeting criteria for a depressive disorder.[14] Biederman and colleagues[12] found that 16% of a sample of ADHD patients met criteria for mania.

Several practice guidelines strongly endorse quantifying symptoms and treatment response with observer-completed or self-reported rating scales. They were crafted with an eye toward feasibility in routine care and before current technologies that enabled more diverse means to capture and score data than paper and pencil. One implication is that they should be taken as minimal standards for the acquisition and use of patient assessment and outcomes information.[15–17] ADHD rating scales are reliable and effective at discriminating between clinical and nonclinical groups.[18] ADHD rating scales are measures of treatment outcome and are sensitive to behavioral and pharmacologic treatment effects.[19]

Rating scales yield a measure of ADHD behaviors, but they can also help screen for other psychiatric disorders, such as depression or anxiety, which may be comorbid with ADHD. Mild mood lability, such as shouting out, crying, being quick to frustrate, or temper, is common in ADHD[15] and should be distinguished from a comorbid depressive disorder. When a major depressive disorder is present with ADHD, the affective disorder is often addressed first. Measurement instruments are sensitive to not just core symptoms of ADHD but also associated problems, more global functioning impairments, and comorbid diagnoses. Rating scale assessments may not show improvement when there are continued difficulties with academic performance, social interactions, low self-esteem, and dysphoria, all of which may stem directly from the ADHD. These associated problems often respond to stimulant optimization. Furthermore, aggressive children with ADHD with callous-unemotional traits or proactive aggression do not show worsened outcome with optimized stimulant pharmacotherapy.[20] Overall aggressive acts and antisocial behavior decline as evidence by improvement in ADHD rating scales and measures of aggression when patients with ADHD are treated with optimal stimulant pharmacotherapy.[15,21]

TACTICS AND IMPLEMENTATION
Informants

Parents/caregivers
There are many well-validated, standardized instruments used to assess family, social, and school functioning in children with ADHD. These include reports from parents/caregivers, teachers, and peers and assessment of IQ and academic achievement. The Vanderbilt rating scale[22] and the Swanson, Nolan, and Pelham Rating Scale and broadband rating scales, such as the Child Behavior Checklist and Teacher Report Form, include comorbid symptoms of other disorders.[23] Scales used to determine diagnosis and baseline symptoms are longer and more multidimensional, whereas scales for assessing response to ongoing treatment are often briefer and more focused. **Table 1** provides an overview of some common scales. Internal consistency and test-retest reliabilities are high for many of the rating scales, although interrater reliability for these scales (not shown in **Table 1**) is lower, around 0.3 to 0.4. One common complication of interpretation occurs when different people provide this information over the course of treatment. Unlike, say, a lipid profile that should yield essentially the same results from different laboratories using the same specimen, rating scales do reflect the rater at least to some extent and scores can vary between informants. Furthermore, some of the difference may stem from true variation in child behavior with different adults. A portion also results from differences in response biases of the informants themselves. Parental depression can bias rating scales

Table 1
Overview of common scales

Name of Scale	Description	Reliability
ADHD Rating Scale-5 (DuPaul et al, 2016)	Home and school version based on DSM-5 diagnostic criteria Consist of 2 symptom subscales, Inattention (9 items) and Hyperactivity–Impulsivity (9 items), and a Total Scale (18 items) Assesses 6 domains of impairment: 1. Relationships relationships with significant others (family members for the home version and teachers for the school version) 2. Peer relationships 3. Academic functioning 4. Behavioral functioning 5. Homework performance 6. Self-esteem https://www.guilford.com/books/ADHD-Rating-Scale-5-for-Children-and-Adolescents/DuPaul-Power-Anastopoulos-Reid/9781462524877/technical-information	Internal consistency $\alpha = 0.89$–0.96 Test-retest over 6 wks $r = 0.90$–0.93 school version, and 0.80–0.87 for home version https://www.guilford.com/books/ADHD-Rating-Scale-5-for-Children-and-Adolescents/DuPaul-Power-Anastopoulos-Reid/9781462524877/technical-information
Conners Parent Rating Scale – Revised; Conners Teacher Rating Scale – Revised (Conners, 1997)	Available in long (broad-band) or short versions for parent, teacher, and adolescent completion Parent and adolescent self-report versions (Conners, 1997)	Internal consistency α (parent) = 0.86–0.94 α (teacher) = 0.88–0.95 Test-retest r (parent over 6–8 week period) = 0.62–0.85 r (teacher) = 0.72–0.92
Swanson, Nolan, and Pelham (SNAP-IV) (SNAP; Atkins et al, 1985; Atkins et al, 1988; Gaub & Carlson, 1997; MTA Cooperative Group, 1999a; Pelham & Bender, 1982)	26-item scale that contains DSM-IV criteria for ADHD and screens for other DSM diagnoses (Swanson, 1992)	Internal consistency not reported Test-retest r (teacher) = 0.77–0.80

(continued on next page)

Table 1 (continued)		
Name of Scale	Description	Reliability
Vanderbilt ADHD Diagnostic Parent and Teacher Scales (Wolraich et al, 2003)	Teachers rate 35 symptoms, 8 performance items measuring ADHD and other common comorbid conditions Parent version contains all 18 ADHD symptoms with items assessing comorbid conditions and performance (Wolraich et al, 2003)	Internal consistency = α (parent) = 0.94–0.95 α (teacher) = 0.90–0.94 Test-retest not reported

Abbreviation: DSM, Diagnostic and Statistical Manual of Mental Disorders.

when active depressive symptoms are present making it seem that a child has ADHD when in fact they do not.[3,24] This underscores the importance of obtaining additional evaluations from teachers or other sources.

Children often have numerous caregivers (parents, legal guardians, adult siblings, grandparents) involved in their lives and, accordingly, one out of several adults may accompany a child to his or her outpatient appointments. As a condition whose symptomatology and treatment response are best assessed by repeated standardized measurements via clinical rating scales, the variability in reporters accompanying the child poses a challenge to tracking ADHD symptoms because interreporter variability is significant. Cross-informant reliabilities are low showing that raters differ in how they evaluate ADHD behaviors.[15] The utility of the clinical rating scales filled out by the accompanying adult is particularly diminished if the accompanying adult does not typically spend a significant amount of time with the child or if the adult has a strong bias regarding a child's illness (eg, denial regarding diagnosis or tendency to overpathologize).

Overall, more reliable information over time comes from the same person who has had enough involvement with the patient. If a different person than usual is bringing the child for a follow-up appointment, we recommend getting ratings from the regular informant. This could be accomplished by providing physical copies of scales to the designated rater ahead of time or obtaining the ratings electronically. It is usually too burdensome to obtain this information by telephone interview–type administration, but we do on occasion ask a parent who can call in to the appointment to do so. As telepsychiatry becomes more common and alternate care settings, such as school-based clinics, spread to improve access, hybrids like this (eg, child in person, main adult informant involved by telecommunication) may become more accepted. In light of the COVID-19 pandemic, telepsychiatry has become the care delivery model for much of the United States and having the consistent in-home informant as well as other in-home informants participate in the telehealth visit is recommended.

Teachers and other out-of-home informants

The high prevalence of ADHD-related impairments in the school setting often require information about functioning from school personnel directly for initial assessment and outcome monitoring. The fact that the diagnosis of ADHD requires symptoms and impairment in more than one setting has made the acquisition of this information routine and practically expected by teachers who are well aware of a student's difficulties and are often eager for his or her treatment to get underway.

Several rating scales have versions that parallel the parent-completed one whose content is adapted to school settings. A few also have normative data based on teacher ratings.[25–27] The traditional way to get this information has been to give the scale to the parent to bring or send along to the teacher, who can then return it via the parent or by fax. However, getting paper forms back in a timely manner is a challenge. Parents have difficulties getting the school to deliver and retrieve forms, the child may not reliably bring forms back and forth, and overworked teachers view rating scale completion a low priority. Directly sending requests via email is becoming more acceptable and efficient but needs parental consent and locating email addresses. In light of the COVID-19 pandemic and transformation of outpatient care delivery to telepsychiatry, email communication, scanning of rating scales and/or use of Research Electronic Data Capture (REDCap https://www.project-redcap.org) may become standard of practice in the future.

In addition, the age at which children begin having several teachers for core subject areas over the school day has been lowering. It is not uncommon in the United States for fifth graders to be in departmentalized programs of this type, and in middle schools housing the sixth grade it is standard practice. This means there are more teachers involved, but each probably has less familiarity with the patient than in elementary school settings. One practice is to solicit information and ratings from the two settings where the patient encounters the most difficulties. Except for highly impaired and disorganized patients, most adolescents can self-report about overall attention and concentration in relation to academic work.

For preschoolers with ADHD, parent training in behavioral management and/or behavioral classroom interventions are first-line treatment.[17] Pharmacologic interventions are considered when children with ADHD present with moderate to severe dysfunction. Children in daycare or preschool programs can display severe hyperactivity and impulsiveness that imperils the willingness of staff to keep them in these settings. That in turn can put parents' livelihoods at risk. Primary care clinicians are often uncertain about ADHD pharmacotherapy for those younger than 6, which, with a few exceptions, is off-label use that adds to their discomfort. Preschool versions of some behavioral rating scales, which focus more on overactivity and impulsiveness, are available and useful in helping clinicians determine the severity of the child's difficulties.[28] In some locations and for some payers, psychopharmacotherapy for preschoolers requires preauthorization, and quantification of symptoms by observers is good documentation for this purpose.

Global Assessments

Ratings of impairment and adaptive skills are included in many of the diagnostic-based rating scales, but there are also separate scales that measure impairment specifically. The Children's Global Assessment of Functioning[29] is clinician completed and the Columbia Impairment Rating Scale,[30,31] the Impairment Rating Scale,[3] and the Vanderbilt[22] ask parents to rate the child's level of impairment. All scales show adequate reliability and validity. The Impairment Rating Scale has shown sensitivity to behavioral and pharmacologic treatment effects.

The Individualized Target Behavior Evaluation (ITBE)[3] is a simple observational scheme that uses teacher- or parent-implemented frequency counts as proxies for more extensive observations by independent observers. The ITBE operationalizes the target behaviors and sets a criterion for each behavior evaluated. The parent and teacher rate whether the child met the behavioral goal in the time period specified (eg, interrupts three or fewer times during each class period). The ITBE can be used as part of the daily report card. Furthermore, the ITBE correlates well with standard measures of ADHD behavior and is sensitive to the effects of medication and behavior modification.[3,32,33]

Frequency of Assessments

The use of brief scales sensitive to treatment effects on ADHD symptoms at each office visit should be strongly considered. The lookback period for these is about 1 week, so data are most often a fair reflection of the impact of the current regimen, at least for stimulants. For α_2-agonists at least 2 to 4 weeks is needed to get more accurate reflection of the impact of medication changes. Obtaining information from teachers can be less frequent. Just like having laboratory studies ordered and received before a follow-up visit in medicine, when logistics permit, it is worthwhile to have school data on hand at the time of the visit.

Patient Self-Report

Many adolescents with ADHD can identify and discuss problems with attention, concentration, and not being fully in charge of their behavior, and furnish essential information for measurement-based treatment. Numerous patient-report versions of widely used parent behavioral rating systems are available. Nevertheless, some teenagers with ADHD tend to underestimate the severity of their impulsive behavior and restlessness, or they blame other and situational factors, with the net effect that rating scale data misrepresent the degree of their impairment. In general, patient self-report in the treatment of adolescents with ADHD should be accompanied by observations of a parent or other person. Children with ADHD often lack insight into their symptoms and the associated impairments, and therefore, there is a lack of support for child report measures in clinical assessments for ADHD.[34,35]

The comorbidity of ADHD with depression and anxiety is high, especially in adolescents.[19] Because these problems are often less evident to others, a measurement strategy that includes patient report for these areas is important.

CHALLENGES IN IMPLEMENTATION
Data Management and Electronic Medical Record Limitations

A basic requirement of measurement-based care is that outcome data be available in a format that is intelligible and actionable. Rating scales obtained during any one appointment are indicative of a single snapshot in time over the course of a child's illness. Although an isolated data point is useful in making an initial diagnosis, maximum use of these measurements is achieved through analysis of various longitudinal data points in conjunction with concurrent changes in treatment and social factors. To this end, the ability to efficiently store, retrieve, and compare data obtained from rating scales is paramount to make the data clinically actionable.

Today, it is possible to obtain data by direct entry by patients through a tablet, smartphone, or a computer workstation. However, in many settings, there is a lack of the necessary infrastructure to get rating scale data onto a computer system. Many clinical settings lack the digital interface needed for parents and teachers to input their rating data and then have it transferred and displayed to the physician in an actionable format. Without this level of data processing the steps involved in scoring and recording information in tables or graphs that reflect patient status are cumbersome and involve someone keying in responses from paper. In many settings paper forms filled out by parents at initial visits would be looked over rather than scored and then filed somewhere in the patient's chart or perhaps scanned into the electronic record. In settings where the burden of this data entry falls to physicians it results in less time being spent meaningfully interacting with patients and could predispose to even more burnout.

Some publishers of ADHD assessment tools provide digital data capture on a subscription basis, but if one needs several measures from different companies it is costly and unwieldy to have measures in separate formats rather than collected in one place. A few developers now provide suites for patient outcomes that combine the full path from patient/informant data entry to reports with tables and graphs, and some also include proprietary scales. However, these data are typically siloed in a separate computer system rather than the electronic medical record (EMR) that is home to most clinical documentation. Consequently, clinicians usually have to interface with at least two systems to review assessment and outcome data and to complete their documentation requirements.

Site-specific solutions can be developed, but require expertise to develop and maintain. An example of such a system is shown in **Fig. 1**. It was developed for a demonstration project for which some scale publishers had given permission to develop alternative administration and report formats. Parents completed rating scales on a tablet at each visit before seeing the clinician. On submission, data were scored, standard scores were computed, and displayed to the clinician's office computer through Microsoft Excel. Scores were colored as a heat map to draw attention to ratings of higher symptom severity. The result is that one can see current status and trajectories before the family enters the office, with a significant time saving at each visit. **Fig. 1** presents the "supervisor" view, in which a clinical director can view many patients at once.

Another hurdle is combining symptom outcome information with information about treatment. Ideally, systems will be able to amalgamate treatment data from a service setting's EMR with outcome data captured from patients or other raters. Unfortunately, no single EMR implementation that allows for this level of data management is currently widely used. Given the COVID-19 pandemic and increase in telepsychiatry service delivery, there is greater likelihood of having the EMR better integrate with

IDENTIFICATION					Visit Info	Conners Global Index		Child Behavior Checklist									
Clinician	Visit Date	Type	Patient	Age	Medication Summary	Restless & Inattentive	Emotional Lability	INT	EXT	A/D	W/D	SOM	SOC	THGT	ATT	RULES	AGGR
GarzaD	1/17/20	OV	John Martin	11.2	Concerta 54mg	59	56										
GarzaD	11/21/19	OV	John Martin	11.1	None	70	74										
GarzaD	10/19/19	OV	John Martin	11	Concerta 54mg	54	49										
GarzaD	3/13/19	OV	John Martin	10.4	Concerta 36mg	66	74										
GarzaD	2/12/19	3MO	John Martin	10.4	Concerta 36mg	63	75	69	70	68	77	59	62	66	70	70	66
GarzaD	1/15/19	OV	John Martin	10.3	Concerta 18mg	87	90										
GarzaD	1/4/19	OV	John Martin	10.2	Concerta 18mg	75	81										
GarzaD	11/9/18	INTK	John Martin	10	None	78	87	73	77	74	80	59	64	62	83	74	79

Fig. 1. Sample output from measurement-based care system. Display of partial data from a measurement-based care approach showing a patient whose parent completed the Conners Global Index at each visit and the Child Behavior Checklist at intake and 3 months later. Scores shown are standardized T scores (mean of 50, standard deviation of 10). Cells are color-coded to draw attention to more severe ratings. 3MO, 3-month review; A/D, anxiety/depression; AGGR, aggressive behavior; ATT, attention problems; EXT, externalizing behavior; INT, internalizing behavior; INTK, intake; OV, office visit; RULES, rule-breaking behavior; SOC, social problems; SOM, somatic problems; THGT, thought problems; W/D, withdrawal/depression.

intake forms, handwritten psychosocial assessments, rating scales, and other clinically useful outcome measures.

Practice Setting

Most children with ADHD are treated by their primary care physician rather than a subspecialist. Therefore, for the benefits of measurement-based care to reach as many children with ADHD as possible it needs to be easily deployable in a primary care setting.[36–39] Obstacles to this include the aforementioned general lack of EMR optimization to handle rating scale data and the time-crunch inherent in most primary care appointments. The logistical challenge of incorporating numerous disorder-specific approaches in the primary care setting is substantial. However, this disorder-specific approach to care must be the goal to enhance the adherence to and reliability of measurement-based care. If adeptly implemented this approach could even help with efficiency and possibly alleviate some of the time constraints experienced by patient and physician during these appointments.

Trial and Error Approach

Another challenge inherent with primary care physicians providing most of the pharmacologic treatment of ADHD is the paradigm shift needed to engage in the trial and error system of treating ADHD versus the more typically regimented approach to treating other medical conditions, such as infections. Measurement-based care can serve to add some more clarity and standardization to this process because it would at least provide reproducible data that can easily be interpreted to tailor pharmacologic treatment as needed. The trial and error process is akin to personalized trial designs also known as N-of-1 trials.[37] The most common form of N-of-1 trials uses a multiple crossover design, that is, multiple exposures to reversible treatment given in random order, and the patient's response to each treatment is compared with each of his or her other responses. N-of-1 trials are most applicable to chronic conditions, such as ADHD, which have measurable markers for treatment effectiveness, and the treatment assessed in N-of-1 trials should have rapid onset of action and a short washout period, such as stimulant treatment.[40] This form of precision medicine can alleviate some degree of primary care physicians' feelings of discomfort with regards to the hit and miss nature of treating ADHD. More generally, there is a need for continued education of primary care physicians regarding dose titrations and the role of interval measurements to guide this streamlined and more regimented process.

Financial and Cultural Factors

Some validated rating scales are too expensive for large practices. As of yet reimbursement is not linked to quality of care and/or clinical outcomes.

Many see psychiatry as one of the few remaining fields in medicine where physicians and patients and their families regularly have meaningful conversations. Therefore, for some, using rating scales to collect information rather than relying on discussion and clinical interview can seem to suggest that meaningful conversations are no longer useful. Rating scale data should supplement clinical interview and not be a stand-alone assessment tool. It is also important to educate providers, patients, and their families about the clinical utility of rating scales so they understand the rationale for their use.

Adherence

A full discussion of psychiatric adherence and non-adherence in ADHD is beyond the scope of this chapter. Although, a necessary component of measurement-based care is to assess patient and caregiver adherence to the recommended treatment plan and to assess barriers to full adherence to treatment recommendations.

Psychiatric nonadherence is common in ADHD and for a complete discussion of this topic please see Dr. Blader's chapter entitled "Nonadherence in Childhood Disorders: Attention-Deficit/Hyperactivity Disorder" in the text Psychiatric Nonadherence: A Solutions-Based Approach edited by Drs. Victor Fornari and Ida Dancyger.[41] Use of the recommended Psychiatric Treatment Adherence Checklist outlined by Drs. Fornari and Dancyger can be an important step in the implementation of measurement-based care.[42]

SUMMARY

Measurement-based care is a necessary component in the proper diagnosis and treatment of ADHD and other disruptive behavioral disorders. It aids clinical-decision making around effectiveness of behavioral and medication interventions and provides needed outcome data thereby improving the quality of care. Information technology infrastructure that allows rating scale data to become embedded in the EMR is paramount to ensuring widespread dissemination of measurement-based care.

DISCLOSURE

Drs. Higdon, Kalari, and Fornari have no commercial or financial conflicts of interest to disclose. Dr. Blader has received research support from Texas Health and Human Services and Abbott Laboratories (now AbbVie) and consultant's honoraria from Arbor Pharmaceuticals and Supernus Pharmaceuticals.

REFERENCES

1. Martin A, Volkmar FR, Lewis M. Lewis's child and adolescent psychiatry: a comprehensive textbook. Philadelphia: Lippincott Williams & Wilkins; 2007.
2. Johnston C, Mash EJ. Families of children with attention-deficit/hyperactivity disorder: review and recommendations for future research. Clin child Fam Psychol Rev 2001;4(3):183–207.
3. Pelham J, William E, Fabiano GA, et al. Evidence-based assessment of attention deficit hyperactivity disorder in children and adolescents. J Clin child Adolesc Psychol 2005;34(3):449–76.
4. Atkins MS, Pelham WE, Licht MH. A comparison of objective classroom measures and teacher ratings of attention deficit disorder. J Abnorm Child Psychol 1985; 13(1):155–67.
5. DuPaul G, Stoner G. ADHD in the schools: assessment and intervention strategies. 2nd edition. New York: Guilford; 2003.
6. Barkley RA, Fischer M, Smallish L, et al. Young adult follow-up of hyperactive children: antisocial activities and drug use. J Child Psychol Psychiatry 2004;45(2): 195–211.
7. Douglas VI, Barr RG, Amin K, et al. Dosage effects and individual responsivity to methylphenidate in attention deficit disorder. J Child Psychol Psychiatry 1988; 29(4):453–75.
8. Rapport MD, Stoner G, DuPaul GJ, et al. Attention deficit disorder and methylphenidate: a multilevel analysis of dose-response effects on children's impulsivity across settings. J Am Acad Child Adolesc Psychiatry 1988;27(1):60–9.

9. Rapport MD, Kelly KL. Psychostimulant effects on learning and cognitive function: findings and implications for children with attention deficit hyperactivity disorder. Clin Psychol Rev 1991;11(1):61–92.

10. Barkley RA, Murphy KR. Attention-deficit hyperactivity disorder: a clinical workbook. New York: Guilford Press; 2006.

11. Faraone S, Biederman J, Jetton JG, et al. Attention deficit disorder and conduct disorder: longitudinal evidence for a familial subtype. Psychol Med 1997;27(2): 291–300.

12. Biederman J, Newcorn J, Sprich S. Comorbidity of attention deficit hyperactivity disorder. Am J Psychiatry 1991;148(5):564–77.

13. Group MC. Moderators and mediators of treatment response for children with attention-deficit/hyperactivity disorder. Arch Gen Psychiatry 1999;56:1088–96.

14. Pliszka SR, Carlson CL, Swanson JM. ADHD with comorbid disorders: clinical assessment and management. New York: Guilford Press; 1999.

15. Pliszka S, AACAP Work Group on Quality Issues. Practice parameter for the assessment and treatment of children and adolescents with attention-deficit/ hyperactivity disorder. J Am Acad Child Adolesc Psychiatry 2007;46(7):894–921.

16. Perrin JM, Stein MT, Amler RW, et al. Clinical practice guideline: treatment of the school-aged child with attention-deficit/hyperactivity disorder. Pediatrics 2001; 108(4):1033–44.

17. Wolraich ML, Hagan JF, Allan C, et al. Clinical practice guideline for the diagnosis, evaluation, and treatment of attention-deficit/hyperactivity disorder in children and adolescents. Pediatrics 2019;144(4):e20192528.

18. Clinical practice guideline: diagnosis and evaluation of the child with attention-deficit/hyperactivity disorder. American Academy of Pediatrics. Pediatrics 2000;5:1158–70.

19. Jensen PS. A 14-month randomized clinical trial of treatment strategies for attention-deficit/hyperactivity disorder. Arch Gen Psychiatry 1999;56(12): 1073–86.

20. Blader JC, Pliszka SR, Kafantaris V, et al. Callous-unemotional traits, proactive aggression, and treatment outcomes of aggressive children with attention-deficit/hyperactivity disorder. J Am Acad Child Adolesc Psychiatry 2013;52(12): 1281–93.

21. Connor DF, Glatt SJ, Lopez ID, et al. Psychopharmacology and aggression. I: a meta-analysis of stimulant effects on overt/covert aggression–related behaviors in ADHD. J Am Acad Child Adolesc Psychiatry 2002;41(3):253–61.

22. Wolraich ML, Lambert W, Doffing MA, et al. Psychometric properties of the Vanderbilt ADHD diagnostic parent rating scale in a referred population. J Pediatr Psychol 2003;28(8):559–68.

23. Achenbach TM, Dumenci L, Rescorla LA. Ratings of relations between DSM-IV diagnostic categories and items of the CBCL/6-18, TRF, and YSR. Burlington (VT): University of Vermont; 2001. p. 1–9.

24. Chi TC, Hinshaw SP. Mother–child relationships of children with ADHD: the role of maternal depressive symptoms and depression-related distortions. J Abnorm Child Psychol 2002;30(4):387–400.

25. DuPaul GJ, Power TJ, Anastopoulos RD, et al. ADHD Rating Scale-IV: checklists, norms, and clinical interpretation. New York: Guilford Press; 1998.

26. Conners CK. Conners 3rd Edition™ manual. Toronto (Canada): Multi-Health Systems; 2008.

27. Achenbach TM, Rescorla LA. Manual for the ASEBA school-age forms & profiles. Burlington (VT): University of Vermont Research Center for Children, Youth, and Families; 2001.

28. McGoey KE, DuPaul GJ, Haley E, et al. Parent and teacher ratings of attention-deficit/hyperactivity disorder in preschool: the ADHD Rating Scale-IV Preschool Version 2007;29(4):269–76.

29. Bird HR, Yager TJ, Staghezza B, et al. Impairment in the epidemiological measurement of childhood psychopathology in the community. J Am Acad Child Adolesc Psychiatry 1990;29(5):796–803.

30. Bird HR, Shaffer D, Fisher P, et al. The Columbia Impairment Scale (CIS): pilot findings on a measure of global impairment for children and adolescents. Int J Methods Psychiatr Res 1993;3(3):167–76.

31. Bird HR, Andrews H, Schwab-Stone M, et al. Global measures of impairment for epidemiologic and clinical use with children and adolescents. Int J Methods Psychiatr Res 1996;6(4):295–307.

32. Chronis AM, Fabiano GA, Gnagy EM, et al. An evaluation of the summer treatment program for children with attention-deficit/hyperactivity disorder using a treatment withdrawal design. Behav Ther 2004;35(3):561–85.

33. Pelham WE, Burrows-MacLean L, Gnagy EM, et al. Transdermal methylphenidate, behavioral, and combined treatment for children with ADHD. Exp Clin Psychopharmacol 2005;13(2):111.

34. Hart EL, Lahey BB, Loeber R, et al. Criterion validity of informants in the diagnosis of disruptive behavior disorders in children: a preliminary study. J Consult Clin Psychol 1994;62(2):410.

35. Loeber R, Green SM, Lahey BB. Mental health professionals' perception of the utility of children, mothers, and teachers as informants on childhood psychopathology. J Clin Child Psychol 1990;19(2):136–43.

36. Brinkman WB, Epstein JN. Promoting productive interactions between parents and physicians in the treatment of children with attention-deficit/hyperactivity disorder. Expert Rev Neurother 2011;11(4):579–88.

37. Epstein JN, Langberg JM, Lichtenstein PK, et al. Use of an Internet portal to improve community-based pediatric ADHD care: a cluster randomized trial. Pediatrics 2011;128(5):e1201–8.

38. Epstein JN, Kelleher KJ, Baum R, et al. Variability in ADHD care in community-based pediatrics. Pediatrics 2014;134(6):1136–43.

39. Epstein JN, Langberg JM, Lichtenstein PK, et al. Sustained improvement in pediatricians' ADHD practice behaviors in the context of a community-based quality improvement initiative. Children's Health Care 2010;39(4):296–311.

40. Davidson KW, Cheung YK, McGinn T, et al. Expanding the role of N-of-1 trials in the precision medicine era: action priorities and practical considerations. Washington, DC: NAM Perspectives; 2018.

41. Blader JC. Nonadherence in childhood disorders: attention-deficit/hyperactivity disorder. In: Fornari VM, Dancyger I, editors. Psychiatric nonadherence: a solutions-based approach. Switzerland: Springer; 2019. p. 17–30.

42. Fornari VM, Dancyger I. Closing the gap: where do we go from here?. In: Fornari VM, Dancyger I, editors. Psychiatric nonadherence: a solutions-based approach. Switzerland: Springer; 2019. p. 213–5.

Measurement-Based Care in the Treatment of Adolescents with Substance Use Disorders

Kevin M. Simon, MD[a,b,]*, Sion Kim Harris, PhD, CPH[c,d],
Lydia A. Shrier, MD, MPH[c,d], Oscar G. Bukstein, MD, MPH[a,d]

KEYWORDS

- Adolescence • Measurement-based care • Screening tools
- Substance use disorder

KEY POINTS

- Measurement-Based Care (MBC) in adolescent substance use is one component in evidence-based care.
- Use of age-appropriate and validated measures for detecting substance use, misuse, and substance use disorders has been shown to be more effective than unvalidated tools or provider impression.
- Treatment recommendations should be tailored based on the results of the assessment and needs of the adolescent.

INTRODUCTION

Adolescence is an important developmental phase involving significant physical, cognitive, and socio-behavioral changes and vulnerabilities. Use of substances (alcohol, tobacco, cannabis, and other drugs) among adolescents ranges from experimentation, misuse (of illegal and legal substances) to substance use disorder (SUD). Adolescents are more susceptible than adults to the addictive properties of substances.[1] Although most substance use by adolescents will decrease over time, the younger an adolescent initiates substance use, the greater the risk of developing an

[a] Department of Psychiatry, Boston Children's Hospital, Harvard Medical School, 300 Longwood Avenue, Boston, MA 02115, USA; [b] Adolescent Substance Use and Addiction Program, Division of Developmental Medicine, Department of Pediatrics, Boston Children's Hospital, 300 Longwood Avenue, Boston, MA 02115, USA; [c] Center for Adolescent Behavioral Health Research, Division of Adolescent/Young Adult Medicine, Department of Medicine, Boston Children's Hospital, 300 Longwood Avenue, Boston MA 02115, USA; [d] Department of Pediatrics, Harvard Medical School, Boston, MA, USA
* Corresponding author.
E-mail address: Kevin.Simon@childrens.harvard.edu

Child Adolesc Psychiatric Clin N Am 29 (2020) 675–690
https://doi.org/10.1016/j.chc.2020.06.006
1056-4993/20/© 2020 Elsevier Inc. All rights reserved.

SUD.[2–4] Therefore, early identification of substance use and intervention for problematic use are important. To deliver the highest quality care, it is important for providers to become familiar with Measurement-Based Care (MBC) for substance use in adolescents, including administration of validated screening tools to identify level of risk associated with substance use, application of appropriate brief interventions and monitoring response to treatment.

EPIDEMIOLOGY

Alcohol continues to be the most widely used substance by adolescents. By senior year of high school, more than half (60%) of students report having ever tried alcohol in their life, 43% of whom report ever being drunk.[5] Nearly a quarter (24%) report having initiated alcohol use by eighth grade.[5]

Despite substantial prevention efforts, tobacco use (most commonly cigarette smoking) is the leading cause of preventable death in the United States. Most adults (>95%) who smoke began smoking during adolescence.[6] Fortunately, traditional cigarette smoking has decreased substantially among adolescents. In 2019, fewer than a quarter (22.3%) of high school seniors reported ever using a cigarette, down substantially from a peak of 65.4% in 1997.[5]

However, another form of tobacco use has seen a sharp rise. In 2019, an estimated 53.3% of high school students and 24.3% of middle school students reported having ever tried a tobacco product, largely due to use of electronic cigarettes (e-cigarettes).[7] Because they commonly contain nicotine derived from the tobacco plant, e-cigarettes are tobacco products.[8–10] In 2019, e-cigarettes were the most commonly used tobacco product by high school students (27.5%) and middle school students (10.5%).[7] E-cigarettes are increasingly the initial form of exposure for adolescents to nicotine, and evidence is mounting that ever using an e-cigarette predicts future cigarette smoking.[11–14]

Cannabis sativa/indica, commonly known as "marijuana," continues to be the most used illicit drug among adolescents in the United States and leading reason for their entering SUD treatment.[15] Nationally in 2019, 15.2% of 8th graders, 34% of 10th graders, and 43.7% of 12th graders had ever tried cannabis.[16] Reported adolescent marijuana vaping increased from 2018 to 2019.[17] In 2019, past 30-day prevalence of marijuana vaping was reported by 3.9% of 8th graders, 12.6% of 10th graders, and 14.0% of 12th graders.[17] There is a significant increase in the odds of using cannabis in youth who have used e-cigarettes.[12]

Use of prescription opioids began to decline in 2018 after reaching epidemic levels. The percentage of high school seniors who misused a prescription opioid in the past year declined to 3.4%.[5] Steady declines have also been observed for adolescent use of other illegal drugs, such as cocaine and methamphetamine, and of over-the-counter cough and cold medicines.[5] Using the same data set, minor decreases were seen in the use of amphetamines, LSD, and synthetic cannabinoids.

A brief summary of 2019 past 30-day substance use, by substance and grade level, among adolescents in the United States is shown in **Table 1**.[16]

SUBSTANCE USE DISORDERS

The *Diagnostic and Statistical Manual of Mental Disorders, Fifth Edition* (DSM-5) distinguishes 10 categories of substances that can become SUDs, including alcohol, stimulants (amphetamines, cocaine, and other stimulants), caffeine (intoxication and withdrawal), cannabis (with withdrawal syndrome), phencyclidine and other hallucinogens, inhalants (no withdrawal syndrome), tobacco, opioids, sedative/hypnotics/

Table 1
Past (30-day) prevalence of substance use among adolescents in the United States, 2019

Substance	Grade Level		
	8th %	10th %	12th %
Alcohol (any)	7.9	18.4	29.3
Alcohol (been drunk)	2.6	8.8	17.5
Marijuana/Hashish	6.6	18.4	22.3
Cigarettes	2.3	3.4	5.7
Smokeless tobacco	2.5	3.2	3.5
Vaping (any)	12.2	25.0	30.9
Vaping nicotine	9.6	19.9	25.5
Vaping JUUL	8.5	18.5	20.8
Vaping marijuana	3.9	12.6	14.0
Inhalants	2.1	1.1	0.9
Hallucinogens	0.6	1.3	1.8
Ecstasy (MDMA)	0.5	0.7	0.7
Cocaine	0.3	0.6	1.0
Heroin	0.1	0.2	0.3
Narcotics other than heroin	NR	NR	1.0
Amphetamines	2.2	2.4	2.0
Methamphetamine	0.1	0.3	0.3
Tranquilizers	1.2	1.3	1.3
Any prescription drug	NR	NR	3.6

Abbreviations: MDMA, methylenedioxymethamphetamine; NR, not reported.
Data from National Institute on Drug Abuse. Monitoring the future. Available at: https://www.drugabuse.gov/related-topics/trends-statistics/monitoring-future. Accessed March 15, 2020.

anxiolytics, and other substances.[18] Compared with adults, adolescents are much less likely to receive treatment for SUD, and when they do enter treatment, retention is poorer.[19,20]

RISK FACTORS

Individual, social, and familial risk factors increase likelihood of an adolescent developing substance use, misuse or SUD.[21] Teens who initiate substance use before age 14 years are at greatest risk for SUD.[1,21] Having friends who use substances is an important determinant of adolescent substance use.[22,23] Vulnerability for developing substance-related problems is especially heightened among individuals who have a family history of SUD.[24]

PSYCHIATRIC COMORBIDITY

Comorbidity is defined as having 2 or more diagnosable mental health disorders. Evidence suggests 37% to 80% of adolescents with SUD have experienced at least 1 other mental health disorder.[25,26] Co-occurring psychopathology, including depression, anxiety, and attention-deficit/hyperactivity disorder have been shown to significantly increase risk of adolescent substance use.[21,27,28] Approximately 33% of adolescents with SUD have experienced a major depressive episode.[29] There is an association between anxiety, alcohol use, and cannabis use.[30–34] Increased rates of substance use are also found in youth at risk for psychosis.[35–37]

CONFIDENTIALITY

Confidentiality plays a vital role in health care provision to adolescents. Adolescents who are aware of confidentiality and receive physician confidentiality assurances (an explanation of the legal and ethical protections and limitations of confidentiality) are more willing to seek health care services and communicate with their provider.[38–40] State laws govern minor patients' rights to confidentiality of information shared with health care providers about substance use, but states vary as to whether a minor can confidentially receive drug treatment services.[41] Providers should explain the full confidentiality policy regarding disclosure of sensitive issues directly to the adolescent at the very beginning of the assessment and each visit. It can be helpful to explain the confidentiality policy to both the adolescent and guardian simultaneously. Adolescents who are acutely at risk may need their confidentiality broken for safety.

MEASUREMENT-BASED CARE

MBC is use of patient-reported and/or other informant rating scales with evidence-based clinical practice guidelines to provide objective assessment of patient progress over time to guide a more precise care plan.[42–44] In adolescent substance use, there is also use of drug testing under certain clinical circumstances, such as being in a formal substance use treatment program.[45] We discuss MBC in terms of screening for adolescent substance use, comprehensive assessment, and monitoring treatment.

SCREENING, BRIEF INTERVENTION, AND REFERRAL TO TREATMENT

Screening, brief intervention, and referral to treatment (SBIRT) is a comprehensive and integrated approach to the delivery of early intervention and treatment services through universal screening for persons with SUDs and those at risk.[46]

SCREENING

Screening is the first step in evaluating adolescents and can involve MBC. Many adolescents who could benefit from substance treatment engagement are being missed.[19] Although several brief validated screening tools are available, providers report low rates of use of these tools, relying instead on informal nonvalidated questions and clinical impression.[47,48] Oft-cited barriers to screening for adolescence substance use are lack of time, insufficient training, and lack of familiarity with standardized tools. In addition, adolescents may not perceive need for substance use treatment. In a national survey, 94.9% of adolescents with SUD did not feel that they required treatment,[7] translating to 18.9 million adolescents lacking necessary substance use treatment.[5] However, teens do prefer being engaged and screened by their providers.[49,50] Adolescent self-report of substance use, within the context of a confidential assessment, is valid and compares favorably to bioassay results.[51–54] The American Academy of Pediatrics (AAP) and American Academy of Child and Adolescent Psychiatry recommend annual screening of adolescents for substance use.[55,56] Laboratory testing, most commonly urine drug testing or screening can be used to complement self-report when evaluating adolescent substance use; however, it is not generally supported as a stand-alone screening or assessment procedure for substance use.[45,57]

SCREENING TOOLS

The ideal screening tool is brief, easy to use, sensitive, and specific to substance use and related problems, and can guide subsequent assessment and intervention when appropriate. Brief screeners designed specifically for adolescents backed by empirical evidence include CRAFFT (both screening and brief assessment with Car, Relax, Alone, Friends/Family, Forget, Trouble items); National Institute of Alcohol Abuse and Alcoholism (NIAAA) 2-question alcohol screen; Screening to Brief Intervention (S2BI); and BSTAD (Brief Screening for Tobacco, Alcohol and Drugs) (**Table 2**).

CAR, RELAX, ALONE, FRIENDS/FAMILY, FORGET, TROUBLE

The CRAFFT has become one of the most widely used tools for detecting problematic substance use among adolescents and has substantial empirical support.[63–66] It has been validated in several countries and languages.[63,67–69] CRAFFT is an acronym created from the first letters of 6 key problems with substance use: C = ridden in a CAR driven by someone [including self] intoxicated, R = use alcohol/drugs to RELAX, A = use alcohol/drugs while ALONE, F = FORGET things you did while intoxicated, F = FAMILY or friends tell you to reduce drinking/drug use, T = gotten into TROUBLE while using alcohol/drugs (**Figs. 1** and **2**). To administer the CRAFFT, the provider begins by asking 3 questions to screen for the number of days of use during the past 12 months of (1) alcohol, (2) marijuana, and (3) any other illegal or prescription medication for the purpose of getting high. If the patient answers 0 days of use during the past 12 months for all 3 questions, the provider follows up with the "CAR" question only and provides appropriate affirmation or encouragement for continued abstinence. If the patient reports any days of use for any of the first 3 questions, then the remaining 5 (RAFFT) questions are also asked. All "yes" responses on the 6 CRAFFT items are then summed for a total score. Most CRAFFT validation studies have found a score of 2 or more to be the optimal cut point for identifying adolescents aged 18 years or younger with high risk for an alcohol or drug use disorder.[65,70,71] The CRAFFT can function as a self-report questionnaire or an interview to be administered by a provider, for more information about the manual and all versions available visit www.crafft.org.[64]

NATIONAL INSTITUTE OF ALCOHOL ABUSE AND ALCOHOLISM

The NIAAA 2-question screen has different versions based on target age group (elementary, middle, and high school age), and is designed to identify adolescent level of risk for alcohol-related problems. The past-year frequency item (number of days of drinking) was selected over the past-30-day number of drinks per day and number of days of heavy episodic drinking (5 drinks on an occasion) owing to better performance in predicting any past-year alcohol use disorder or symptoms in a large, nationally representative sample of adolescents aged 12 to 18.[60] However, optimal cut points for number of drinking days were found to vary by age and gender, resulting in different thresholds for moderate and high risk across age-gender groups.[59] The friends' use item serves both to facilitate opening a discussion about alcohol with younger adolescents as well as to identify youth at risk for any drinking and risky drinking, because peer drinking is a strong predictor of adolescent drinking behavior.[72]

Table 2
Brief description of selected adolescence substance use screening tools

Tool	Questions	Description	Cutoff	Psychometrics	Cost
CRAFFT 2.1	4–9	Asks past-12-mo number of days of use of alcohol, marijuana, and other drugs, and asks about problems associated with use	≥2 yes responses on 6 CRAFFT items	Sensitivity: 0.91 Specificity: 0.93	Free
NIAAA	2	Alcohol only: Screens for friends' use and for days of personal use in past 12 mo in children and adolescents (9–18 y old)	Age 15 or younger: 1+ days in past 12 mo Age 16–17: 6+ days in past 12 mo Age 18+: 12+ days in past 12 mo	Sensitivity: 0.89 Middle School Sensitivity: 0.88 High School Specificity: 0.91 Middle School Specificity: 0.81 High School	Free
S2BI	3–7	Asks frequency of use in past year of tobacco, alcohol, marijuana, and other drugs	Monthly single past year frequency question from the S2BI was sensitive and specific for discriminating among 4 categories of substance use experience (no past-year use, use without an SUD, mild or moderate SUD, and severe SUD) for each substance	Sensitivity: 1.00 Specificity: 0.94	Free
BSTAD	6–36	Asks past-12-mo days of tobacco, alcohol, marijuana or other substance use by person and their friends	Tobacco ≥6d Alcohol ≥2d Marijuana ≥2	Sensitivity: 0.95 Specificity: 0.97 Sensitivity: 0.96 Specificity: 0.85 Sensitivity: 0.80 Specificity: 0.93	Free

Abbreviations: BSTAD, Brief Screening for Alcohol, Tobacco, and other Drugs; CRAFFT, Car, Relax, Alone, Friends/Family, Forget, Trouble; NIAAA, National Institute of Alcohol Abuse and Alcoholism; S2BI, Screening to Brief Intervention.
Data from Refs.[58–62]

Please answer all questions **honestly**; your answers will be kept **confidential**.

During the PAST 12 MONTHS, on how many days did you:

1. Drink more than a few sips of beer, wine, or any drink containing **alcohol**? Put "0" if none.

   # of days

2. Use any **marijuana** (cannabis, weed, oil, wax, or hash by smoking, vaping, dabbing, or in edibles) or "**synthetic marijuana**" (like "K2," "Spice")? Put "0" if none.

   # of days

3. Use **anything else to get high** (like other illegal drugs, prescription or over-the-counter medications, and things that you sniff, huff, vape, or inject)? Put "0" if none.

   # of days

READ THESE INSTRUCTIONS BEFORE CONTINUING:
- **If you put "0" in ALL of the boxes above, ANSWER QUESTION 4, THEN STOP.**
- **If you put "1" or higher in ANY of the boxes above, ANSWER QUESTIONS 4-9.**

	No	Yes
4. Have you ever ridden in a **CAR** driven by someone (including yourself) who was "high" or had been using alcohol or drugs?	☐	☐
5. Do you ever use alcohol or drugs to **RELAX**, feel better about yourself, or fit in?	☐	☐
6. Do you ever use alcohol or drugs while you are by yourself, or **ALONE**?	☐	☐
7. Do you ever **FORGET** things you did while using alcohol or drugs?	☐	☐
8. Do your **FAMILY** or **FRIENDS** ever tell you that you should cut down on your drinking or drug use?	☐	☐
9. Have you ever gotten into **TROUBLE** while you were using alcohol or drugs?	☐	☐

Fig. 1. The CRAFFT Questionnaire (version 2.1) for the patient to complete. (© John R. Knight, MD, Boston Children's Hospital, 2020. Reproduced with permission from the Center for Adolescent Substance Use and Addiction Research (CeASAR), Boston Children's Hospital.)

SCREENING TO BRIEF INTERVENTION

The S2BI instrument has demonstrated high sensitivity and specificity for identifying substance use and SUD.[61,73] The single screening assessment of "past-year use" is

Begin: *"I'm going to ask you a few questions that I ask all my patients. Please be honest. I will keep your answers confidential."*

Part A
During the PAST 12 MONTHS, on how many days did you:

1. Drink more than a few sips of beer, wine, or any drink containing **alcohol**? Say "0" if none.

   # of days

2. Use any **marijuana** (cannabis, weed, oil, wax, or hash by smoking, vaping, dabbing, or in edibles) or "**synthetic marijuana**" (like "K2," "Spice")? Say "0" if none.

   # of days

3. Use **anything else to get high** (like other illegal drugs, prescription or over-the-counter medications, and things that you sniff, huff, vape, or inject)? Say "0" if none.

   # of days

Did the patient answer "0" for all questions in Part A?

Yes ☐   No ☐

↓   ↓

Ask CAR question only, then stop   **Ask all six CRAFFT* questions below**

Part B

		No	Yes
C	Have you ever ridden in a **CAR** driven by someone (including yourself) who was "high" or had been using alcohol or drugs?	☐	☐
R	Do you ever use alcohol or drugs to **RELAX**, feel better about yourself, or fit in?	☐	☐
A	Do you ever use alcohol or drugs while you are by yourself, or **ALONE**?	☐	☐
F	Do you ever **FORGET** things you did while using alcohol or drugs?	☐	☐
F	Do your **FAMILY** or **FRIENDS** ever tell you that you should cut down on your drinking or drug use?	☐	☐
T	Have you ever gotten into **TROUBLE** while you were using alcohol or drugs?	☐	☐

*Two or more YES answers suggest a serious problem and need for further assessment. See back for further instructions ⟶

Fig. 2. The CRAFFT Interview (version 2.1) for the clinician to orally administer. (© John R. Knight, MD, Boston Children's Hospital, 2020. Reproduced with permission from the Center for Adolescent Substance Use and Addiction Research (CeASAR), Boston Children's Hospital.)

quick and allows providers to administer the screen in a variety of settings. The instrument begins by asking about frequency of use of tobacco, alcohol, and/or marijuana in the past year (never, once or twice, monthly, weekly or more). If the patient endorses past-year use of any of the 3 substances, then follow-up questions are posed about use of prescription drugs, illegal drugs, inhalants, and herbs or synthetic drugs. Adolescents who report using "once or twice" in the past year are very unlikely to have an SUD. Adolescents who endorse "monthly" use are more likely to meet criteria for a mild or moderate SUD, and those who report "weekly or more" use are more likely to have a severe SUD.[74]

BRIEF SCREENER FOR TOBACCO, ALCOHOL, AND OTHER DRUGS

The BSTAD is an electronic validated high-sensitivity and high-specificity instrument for identifying substance use and SUD.[62] It is based on the NIAAA 2-question Youth Alcohol Screening Tool and expanded to include tobacco and drug use among pediatric patients. BSTAD asks a single frequency question for past year use of each of the 3 substances most commonly used by adolescents: tobacco, alcohol, and marijuana.[75] Patients who report using any of these 3 substances are then asked questions about additional substance use. The measure triages adolescents (ages 12–17) into 3 levels of risk for SUD based on their report of past year use: no reported use, lower risk, and higher risk. Consistent with the NIAAA instrument, if respondent is aged 12 to 14, "friends" questions are asked first; if aged 15 to 17 (or 14 years old in high school), "personal-use" questions are asked first.[59,62] Each risk level maps onto suggested clinical actions, summarized on the results screen.

BRIEF INTERVENTION

Brief interventions focus on encouraging healthy choices so risk behaviors are prevented, reduced, or stopped. Brief interventions may include education, counseling, or referral for intensive treatment.[76] Among adolescents presenting to an emergency department for a substance use–related problem, brief intervention has been shown to reduce subsequent alcohol use, cannabis use, and to be cost-effective compared with brief education.[77–79]

REFERRAL TO TREATMENT

The provider must be familiar with available substance use treatment services in their community. Family support and juvenile legal system mandates can play a central role in getting adolescents to enter, stay in, and complete treatment, all of which could be critical to likelihood of recovery. Substance use treatment should be tailored to the unique needs of the adolescent.

COMPREHENSIVE ASSESSMENT

A comprehensive substance use assessment is a thorough process that evaluates the onset of substance use, the quantity and frequency of use, factors contributing to and maintaining substance use, and medical and psychosocial consequences of use. The assessment process is used to identify those individuals who meet DSM-5 criteria for an SUD diagnosis. Results of a comprehensive assessment will identify which adolescents require treatment, level of care (eg, outpatient, intensive outpatient, residential) and modality of treatment, and strengths of the adolescent that may be helpful during treatment.

PROGRESS MONITORING

Monitoring clinical status of patients with SUD on a regular basis during treatment has been recommended by the Institute of Medicine since 2006.[80] Progress monitoring has been shown to improve outcomes in mental health treatment and various monitoring approaches have been successfully used as part of SUD treatment in adult populations.[81–83] There has been no randomized controlled trial comparing monitoring instruments among adolescents. See **Table 3** for description of monitoring tools.

Toxicology

Clinicians often use urine drug screens (UDS) both at assessment and during treatment. Although there are 10 substances that can lead to an SUD, many laboratories only screen urine for the "NIDA 5" (after the National Institute on Drug Abuse), cannabis, cocaine, opioids, amphetamines, and PCP; as such, several substances, notably methylenedioxymethamphetamine (MDMA), oxycodone, hydrocodone, buprenorphine, and clonazepam, are not included in many drug screen panels and must be ordered separately.[57,90] Qualitative drug screen panels indicate use by detecting a minimum concentration of a substance's metabolite in urine and thus can be used for determining abstinence, except for cannabis as cannabinoids store in adipose tissue and variably release, resulting in varying concentrations in urine. Parents/guardians should be notified that although home drug testing kits are widely available, the AAP does not endorse home drug testing without professional guidance.[57] When an adolescent is engaged in substance use treatment, clinical drug testing is routinely performed.[45] At the beginning of treatment, the provider explains the process and expectations of obtaining and testing samples. Generally, the adolescent should provide a signed consent for release of information to the parent, in this case, the results of the UDS. Contingencies for both positive UDS and negative UDS results should be discussed at the onset of treatment. The samples are collected

Table 3
Brief description of selected progress monitoring tools

Tool	Questions	Time to Complete/ Interpret (min)	Description
TLFB	Varies	15–30/5	TLFB can be administered by a provider, self-administered, or administered by computer. Involves asking patients to retrospectively estimate their substance use over the past 7 d up to 2 y prior.
Teen Addiction Severity Index (T-ASI)	157	20–45/10	Semi-structured interview that yields 70 ratings in 7 domains: substance use, school status, employment/support, family relations, social relationships, legal status, and psychiatric status.
CASI	Varies	45–90/15	Comprehensive, semi-structured, clinical assessment and outcomes interview. Composed of 10 independent modules. Modules include health, family, stressful life events, legal status, sexual behavior, mental health functioning, peer relationships, education, and use of free time. Each module assesses whether the adolescent acknowledges the presence of problems and obtains his or her rating of discomfort.

Abbreviations: CASI, Comprehensive Addiction Severity Index; TLFB, Timeline Follow back; T-ASI, Teen Addiction Severity Index.
For more information about measures, see Refs.[84–89]

randomly with the adolescent always being prepared to provide a sample. Refusal to provide a sample is considered a positive result. The provider directly views provision of the sample or takes other steps to thwart attempts to use adulterated or false samples. Drug testing can augment effectiveness of motivational interviewing, cognitive-based treatment, and contingency management approaches.[91]

SUMMARY

MBC for adolescent substance use can be viewed as an evidence-based practice that implements systematic, confidential screening for adolescents using a validated tool and additional questions, if needed, followed by an appropriate intervention, as well as drug testing. MBC for adolescence substance use is an important part of adolescent primary and specialty care. Practical, effective brief interventions can be conducted in the clinic and emergency room setting. Identifying local treatment resources can aid in referring high-risk adolescents to appropriate care.

DISCLOSURE

K.M. Simon's preparation of this article was supported in part by the National Institute on Drug Abuse and American Academy of Child and Adolescent Psychiatry Resident Training Award in Substance Use Disorders. O.G. Bukstein receives royalties from Wolters-Kluwer, Guilford Press, and Routledge Press. The other authors have no financial relationships to disclose.

REFERENCES

1. Jordan CJ, Andersen SL. Sensitive periods of substance abuse: early risk for the transition to dependence. Dev Cogn Neurosci 2017;25:29–44.

2. Chambers RA, Taylor JR, Potenza MN. Developmental neurocircuitry of motivation in adolescence: a critical period of addiction vulnerability. Am J Psychiatry 2003;160(6):1041–52.

3. Hingson RW, Heeren T, Winter MR. Age at drinking onset and alcohol dependence: age at onset, duration, and severity. Arch Pediatr Adolesc Med 2006; 160(7):739–46.

4. Casey BJ, Jones RM. Neurobiology of the adolescent brain and behavior: implications for substance use disorders. J Am Acad Child Adolesc Psychiatry 2010; 49(12):1189–201 [quiz: 1285].

5. Miech RA, Johnston LD, O'Malley PM, et al. Monitoring the Future national survey results on drug use, 1975 -2018: Volume I, Secondary school students. Ann Arbor: Institute for Social Research, The University of Michigan; 2019 Available at: http://monitoringthefuture.org/pubs.html#monographs. Accessed July 14, 2020.

6. Russell C, McKeganey N, Dickson T, et al. Changing patterns of first e-cigarette flavor used and current flavors used by 20,836 adult frequent e-cigarette users in the USA. Harm Reduct J 2018;15(1). https://doi.org/10.1186/s12954-018-0238-6.

7. Wang TW, Gentzke AS, Creamer MR, et al. Tobacco product use and associated factors among middle and high school students — United States, 2019. MMWR Surveill Summ 2019;68(12):1–22.

8. Jenssen BP, Walley SC, Groner JA, et al. E-cigarettes and similar devices. Pediatrics 2019;143(2). https://doi.org/10.1542/peds.2018-3652.

9. Brown CJ, Cheng JM. Electronic cigarettes: product characterization and design considerations. Tob Control 2014;23(SUPPL. 2). https://doi.org/10.1136/tobaccocontrol-2013-051476.

10. Walley SC, Wilson KM, Winickoff JP, et al. A public health crisis: electronic cigarettes, vape, and JUUL. Pediatrics 2019;143(6). https://doi.org/10.1542/peds.2018-2741.

11. Westling E, Rusby JC, Crowley R, et al. Electronic cigarette use by youth: prevalence, correlates, and use trajectories from middle to high school. J Adolesc Health 2017;60(6):660–6.

12. Chadi N, Schroeder R, Jensen JW, et al. Association between electronic cigarette use and marijuana use among adolescents and young adults: a systematic review and meta-analysis. JAMA Pediatr 2019;173(10). https://doi.org/10.1001/jamapediatrics.2019.2574.

13. Stanton CA, Bansal-Travers M, Johnson AL, et al. Longitudinal e-Cigarette and cigarette use among US Youth in the PATH Study (2013-2015). J Natl Cancer Inst 2019;111(10):1088–96.

14. Bold KW, Kong G, Camenga DR, et al. Trajectories of E-cigarette and conventional cigarette use among youth. Pediatrics 2018;141(1). https://doi.org/10.1542/peds.2017-1832.

15. Johnson JK. Elucidating the impact of adolescent marijuana use. J Adolesc Health 2018;63(2):129–30.

16. National Institute on Drug Abuse. Monitoring the future. Available at: https://www.drugabuse.gov/related-topics/trends-statistics/monitoring-future. Accessed March 15, 2020.

17. Miech RA, Patrick ME, O'Malley PM, et al. Trends in reported marijuana vaping among US adolescents, 2017-2019. JAMA 2020;323(5):475–6.

18. American Psychiatric Association. DSM-5 diagnostic classification. In: Diagnostic and statistical manual of mental disorders: diagnostic and statistical manual of mental disorders. 5th edition. Arlington (VA): American Psychiatric Association; 2013. https://doi.org/10.1176/appi.books.9780890425596.x00diagnosticclassification.

19. Hadland SE, Bagley SM, Rodean J, et al. Receipt of timely addiction treatment and association of early medication treatment with retention in care among youths with opioid use disorder. JAMA Pediatr 2018;172(11):1029–37.

20. Cummings JR, Wen H, Druss BG. Racial/ethnic differences in treatment for substance use disorders among U.S. adolescents. J Am Acad Child Adolesc Psychiatry 2011;50(12):1265–74.

21. Gray KM, Squeglia LM. Research Review: what have we learned about adolescent substance use? J Child Psychol Psychiatry 2018;59(6):618–27.

22. Ramirez R, Hinman A, Sterling S, et al. Peer influences on adolescent alcohol and other drug use outcomes. J Nurs Scholarsh 2012;44(1):36–44.

23. Kosterman R, Hawkins JD, Guo J, et al. The dynamics of alcohol and marijuana initiation: patterns and predictors of first use in adolescence. Am J Public Health 2000;90(3):360–6.

24. Acheson A, Vincent AS, Cohoon AJ, et al. Defining the phenotype of young adults with family histories of alcohol and other substance use disorders: studies from the family health patterns project HHS Public Access. Addict Behav 2018;77:247–54.

25. Conway KP, Swendsen J, Husky MM, et al. Association of lifetime mental disorders and subsequent alcohol and illicit drug use: results from the national comorbidity survey-adolescent supplement. J Am Acad Child Adolesc Psychiatry 2016;55(4):280–8.

26. Heradstveit O, Skogen JC, Hetland J, et al. Psychiatric diagnoses differ considerably in their associations with alcohol/drug-related problems among adolescents. A Norwegian population-based survey linked with national patient registry data. Front Psychol 2019;10. https://doi.org/10.3389/fpsyg.2019.01003.

27. Yule AM, Wilens TE. Substance use disorders in adolescents with psychiatric comorbidity: when to screen and how to treat: consider pharmacotherapy, psychotherapy when treating substance use disorders. Curr Psychiatr 2015;14(4). 36–39, 47–51.

28. Borus J, Parhami I, Levy S. Screening, brief intervention, and referral to treatment. Child Adolesc Psychiatr Clin N Am 2016;25(4):579–601.

29. Substance Abuse and Mental Health Services Administration. Results from the 2018 National survey on drug use and health: detailed tables. Rockville (MD): Center for Behavioral Health Statistics and Quality, Substance Abuse and Mental Health Services Administration; 2019. Available at: https://www.samhsa.gov/data/. Accessed December 28, 2019.

30. Ohannessian CM. Anxiety and substance use during adolescence. Subst Abus 2014;35(4):418–25.

31. Smith JP, Book SW. Comorbidity of generalized anxiety disorder and alcohol use disorders among individuals seeking outpatient substance abuse treatment. Addict Behav 2010;35(1):42–5.

32. Duperrouzel J, Hawes SW, Lopez-Quintero C, et al. The association between adolescent cannabis use and anxiety: a parallel process analysis. Addict Behav 2018;78:107–13.

33. Duffy A, Horrocks J, Milin R, et al. Adolescent substance use disorder during the early stages of bipolar disorder: a prospective high-risk study. J Affect Disord 2012;142(1-3):57–64.

34. Rusby JC, Westling E, Crowley R, et al. Associations between marijuana use and anxious mood lability during adolescence. Addict Behav 2019. https://doi.org/10.1016/j.addbeh.2018.12.029.

35. Bechtold J, Simpson T, White HR, et al. Chronic adolescent marijuana use as a risk factor for physical and mental health problems in young adult men. Psychol Addict Behav 2015;29(3):552–63.

36. Chadwick B, Miller ML, Hurd YL. Cannabis use during adolescent development: susceptibility to psychiatric illness. Front Psychiatry 2013;4. https://doi.org/10.3389/fpsyt.2013.00129.

37. Ropper AH, Marder SR, Cannon TD. Schizophrenia. N Engl J Med 2019;18:1753–61.

38. Weddle M, Kokotailo PK. Confidentiality and consent in adolescent substance abuse: an update. Virtual Mentor 2005;7(3):239–43.

39. Croft B, Parish SL. Care integration in the patient protection and affordable care act: implications for behavioral health. Adm Policy Ment Health 2013;40(4):258–63.

40. Ford CA, Millstein SG, Halpern-Felsher BL, et al. Influence of physician confidentiality assurances on adolescents' willingness to disclose information and seek future health care. A randomized controlled trial. JAMA 1997;278(12):1029–34. Available at: http://www.ncbi.nlm.nih.gov/pubmed/9307357. Accessed January 5, 2020.

41. State minor consent laws: a summary, third edition. Available at: https://www.cahl.org/state-minor-consent-laws-a-summary-third-edition/. Accessed January 21, 2020.

42. Trivedi MH, John Rush A, Wisniewski SR, et al. Evaluation of outcomes with citalopram for depression using measurement-based care in STAR*D: implications for clinical practice STAR*D study team. Vol. 163. 2006. Available at: http://ajp.psychiatryonline.org. Accessed December 29, 2019.
43. Fortney JC, Unützer J, Wrenn G, et al. A tipping point for measurement-based care. Psychiatr Serv 2017;68:179–88.
44. Marsden J, Tai B, Ali R, et al. Measurement-based care using DSM-5 for opioid use disorder: can we make opioid medication treatment more effective? Addiction 2018. https://doi.org/10.1111/add.14546.
45. Hadland SE, Levy S. Objective testing: urine and other drug tests. Child Adolesc Psychiatr Clin N Am 2016;25(3):549–65.
46. About SBIRT | SAMHSA - Substance Abuse and Mental Health Services Administration. Available at: https://www.samhsa.gov/sbirt/about. Accessed January 15, 2020.
47. Levy S, Ziemnik RE, Harris SK, et al. Screening adolescents for alcohol use: tracking practice trends of Massachusetts pediatricians. J Addict Med 2017; 11(6):427–34.
48. Agley J, Carlson JM, McNelis AM, et al. 'Asking' but not 'screening': assessing physicians' and nurses' substance-related clinical behaviors. Subst Use Misuse 2018;53(11):1834–9.
49. Knight JR, Harris SK, Sherritt L, et al. Adolescents' preference for substance abuse screening in primary care practice. Subst Abus 2007;28(4):107–17.
50. Jasik CB, Berna M, Martin M, et al. Teen preferences for clinic-based behavior screens: who, where, when, and how? J Adolesc Health 2016;59(6):722–4.
51. Knight JR, Goodman E, Pulerwitz T, et al. Reliability of the Problem Oriented Screening Instrument for Teenagers (POSIT) in an adolescent medicine clinic population (Abstract). J Adolesc Health 1996;29:125–30. Available at: http://www.ncbi.nlm.nih.gov/entrez/query.fcgi?cmd=Retrieve&db=PubMed&dopt=Citation&list_uids=11472871. Accessed January 15, 2020.
52. Levy S, Sherritt L, Harris SK, et al. Test-retest reliability of adolescents' self-report of substance use. Alcohol Clin Exp Res 2004;28(8):1236–41.
53. Walton MA, Bohnert K, Resko S, et al. Computer and therapist based brief interventions among cannabis-using adolescents presenting to primary care: one year outcomes. Drug Alcohol Depend 2013;132(3):646–53.
54. Boykan R, Messina CR, Chateau G, et al. Self-reported use of tobacco, E-cigarettes, and marijuana versus urinary biomarkers. Pediatrics 2019;143(5). https://doi.org/10.1542/peds.2018-3531.
55. Levy SJL, Williams JF. Substance use screening, brief intervention, and referral to treatment. Pediatrics 2016;138(1). https://doi.org/10.1542/peds.2016-1211.
56. Bukstein OG, Bernet W, Arnold V, et al. Practice parameter for the assessment and treatment of children and adolescents with substance use disorders. J Am Acad Child Adolesc Psychiatry 2005;44(6):609–21.
57. Levy S, Siqueira LM, Ammerman SD, et al. Testing for drugs of abuse in children and adolescents. Pediatrics 2014;133(6). https://doi.org/10.1542/peds.2014-0865.
58. Mitchell SG, Kelly SM, Gryczynski J, et al. The CRAFFT cut-points and DSM-5 criteria for alcohol and other drugs: a reevaluation and reexamination. Subst Abus 2014;35(4):376–80.
59. Patton R, Deluca P, Kaner E, et al. Alcohol screening and brief intervention for adolescents: the how, what and where of reducing alcohol consumption and related harm among young people, Alcohol and Alcoholism 2014;49(2):207–12.

60. Spirito A, Bromberg JR, Casper TC, et al. Reliability and validity of a two-question Alcohol screen in the pediatric emergency department. Pediatrics 2016;138(6). https://doi.org/10.1542/peds.2016-0691.
61. Levy S, Weiss R, Sherritt L, et al. An electronic screen for triaging adolescent substance use by risk levels. JAMA Pediatr 2014;168(9):822–8.
62. Kelly SM, Gryczynski J, Mitchell SG, et al. Validity of brief screening instrument for adolescent tobacco, alcohol, and drug use. Pediatrics 2014;133(5):819–26.
63. Harris SK, Knight JR, Van Hook S, et al. Adolescent substance use screening in primary care: validity of computer self-Administered versus clinician-Administered screening. Subst Abus 2016;37(1):197–203.
64. D'Amico EJ, Parast L, Meredith LS, et al. Screening in primary care: what is the best way to identify at-risk youth for substance use? Pediatrics 2016;138(6). https://doi.org/10.1542/peds.2016-1717.
65. Shenoi RP, Linakis JG, Bromberg JR, et al. Predictive validity of the CRAFFT for substance use disorder. Pediatrics 2019;144(2). https://doi.org/10.1542/peds.2018-3415.
66. Knight JR, Csemy L, Sherritt L, et al. Screening and brief advice to reduce adolescents' risk of riding with substance-using drivers. J Stud Alcohol Drugs 2018;79(4):611–6.
67. Wartberg L, Kriston L, Diestelkamp S, et al. Psychometric properties of the German version of the CRAFFT. Addict Behav 2016;59:42–7.
68. Skogen JC, Bøe T, Knudsen AK, et al. Psychometric properties and concurrent validity of the CRAFFT among Norwegian adolescents. Ung@hordaland, a population-based study. Addict Behav 2013;38(10):2500–5.
69. Kandemir H, Aydemir Ö, Ekinci S, et al. Validity and reliability of the Turkish version of CRAFFT substance abuse screening test among adolescents. Neuropsychiatr Dis Treat 2015;11:1505–9.
70. Pilowsky DJ, Wu LT. Screening instruments for substance use and brief interventions targeting adolescents in primary care: a literature review. Addict Behav 2013;38(5):2146–53.
71. Knight JR, Sherritt L, Harris SK, et al. Validity of brief alcohol screening tests among adolescents: a comparison of the AUDIT, POSIT, CAGE, and CRAFFT. Alcohol Clin Exp Res 2003;27(1):67–73.
72. Patrick ME, Terry-McElrath YM. High-intensity drinking by underage young adults in the United States. Addiction 2017;112(1):82–93.
73. Teens screening tool. Available at: https://www.drugabuse.gov/ast/s2bi/#/. Accessed January 15, 2020.
74. Subramaniam GA, Volkov ND. Substance misuse among adolescents: to screen or not to screen? JAMA Pediatr 2014;168(9):798–9.
75. Teens screening tool. Available at: https://www.drugabuse.gov/ast/bstad/#/. Accessed January 15, 2020.
76. D'Amico EJ, Parast L, Shadel WG, et al. Brief motivational interviewing intervention to reduce alcohol and marijuana use for at-risk adolescents in primary care. J Consult Clin Psychol 2018;86(9):775–86.
77. Tait RJ, Hulse GK, Robertson SI. Effectiveness of a brief-intervention and continuity of care in enhancing attendance for treatment by adolescent substance users. Drug Alcohol Depend 2004;74(3):289–96.
78. Bernstein E, Edwards E, Dorfman D, et al. Screening and brief intervention to reduce marijuana use among youth and young adults in a pediatric emergency department. Acad Emerg Med 2009;16:1174–85.

79. Neighbors CJ, Barnett NP, Rohsenow DJ, et al. Cost-effectiveness of a motivational intervention for alcohol-involved youth in a hospital emergency department. J Stud Alcohol Drugs 2010;71(3):384–94.

80. Institute of Medicine (US) Committee on Crossing the Quality Chasm: Adaptation to Mental Health and Addictive Disorders. Improving the Quality of Health Care for Mental and Substance-Use Conditions: Quality Chasm Series. Washington, DC: National Academies Press (US); 2006. Available from: https://www.ncbi.nlm.nih.gov/books/NBK19830/ doi: 10.17226/11470. Accessed July 14, 2020.

81. Knaup C, Koesters M, Schoefer D, et al. Effect of feedback of treatment outcome in specialist mental healthcare: meta-analysis. Br J Psychiatry 2009;195(1):15–22.

82. Poston JM, Hanson WE. Meta-analysis of psychological assessment as a therapeutic intervention. Psychol Assess 2010;22(2):203–12.

83. Goodman JD, McKay JR, DePhilippis D. Progress monitoring in mental health and addiction treatment: a means of improving care. Prof Psychol Res Pract 2013;44(4):231–46.

84. Robinson SM, Sobell LC, Sobell MB, et al. Reliability of the Timeline Followback for cocaine, cannabis, and cigarette use. Psychol Addict Behav 2014;28(1):154–62.

85. Dennis ML, Funk R, Godley SH, et al. Cross-validation of the alcohol and cannabis use measures in the Global Appraisal of Individual Needs (GAIN) and Timeline Followback (TLFB; Form 90) among adolescents in substance abuse treatment. Addiction 2004;99(SUPPL. 2):120–8.

86. Cacciola JS, Alterman AI, DePhilippis D, et al. Development and initial evaluation of the brief addiction monitor (BAM). J Subst Abuse Treat 2013;44(3):256–63.

87. Denis CM, Cacciola JS, Alterman AI. Addiction severity index (ASI) summary scores: comparison of the recent status scores of the ASI-6 and the composite scores of the ASI-5. J Subst Abuse Treat 2013;45(5):444–50.

88. Stucky BD, Edelen MO, Ramchand R. A psychometric assessment of the GAIN Individual Severity Scale (GAIN-GISS) and Short Screeners (GAIN-SS) among adolescents in outpatient treatment programs. J Subst Abuse Treat 2014;46(2):165–73.

89. Meyers K, Thomas McLellan A, Jaeger JL, et al. The development of the comprehensive addiction severity index for adolescents (CASI-A). An interview for assessing multiple problems of adolescents. J Subst Abuse Treat 1995;12(3):181–93.

90. Jaffee WB, Trucco E, Teter C, et al. Focus on alcohol & drug abuse: ensuring validity in urine drug testing. Psychiatr Serv 2008;59(2):140–2.

91. Schuler MS, Griffin BA, Ramchand R, et al. Effectiveness of treatment for adolescent substance use: is biological drug testing sufficient? J Stud Alcohol Drugs 2014;75(2):358–70.

Measurement-Based Care in the Pediatric Primary Care Setting

Barry Sarvet, MD

KEYWORDS

- Integrated care • Consultation-liaison psychiatry • Quality improvement
- General pediatrics

KEY POINTS

- Measurement-based care (MBC) practices offer the potential to improve the quality of mental health care in the pediatric primary care setting.
- The incorporation of clinical measures into the process of mental health care within a primary care practice facilitates the use of clinical algorithms, improves the accuracy of clinical assessment, and supports collaboration across a multidisciplinary team.
- MBC generates data, allowing primary care practices to address population health goals and to consequently improve performance within value-based contracting.
- Clinical measures should be used to complement, not substitute for, conventional clinical assessment techniques.

INTRODUCTION

Clinical programs supporting mental health delivery in the pediatric primary care practice have been spreading rapidly throughout the health care system over the past 15 years.[1,2] This work has been focused on improving access to care for children with psychiatric disorders amid increasing awareness of the profound suffering, disability, and economic impact of these conditions in society. These models generally provide clinical resources designed to enable pediatric primary care providers (PPCPs) and their teammates to assume responsibility for recognition, initial assessment, and management of relatively uncomplicated and common psychiatric conditions. It is important to recognize, however, that PPCPs often receive minimal training in children's mental health care during their residency[3] and that pediatric practice settings are not necessarily designed for mental health practice. Although all of the models involve specialized children's mental health professionals collaborating in some way with the primary care team, the mental health care provided in the primary

Department of Psychiatry, University of Massachusetts Medical School-Baystate, Baystate Medical Center, WG703, 759 Chestnut Street, Springfield, MA 01199, USA
E-mail address: Barry.Sarvet@baystatehealth.org

Child Adolesc Psychiatric Clin N Am 29 (2020) 691–702
https://doi.org/10.1016/j.chc.2020.06.009
1056-4993/20/© 2020 Elsevier Inc. All rights reserved.
childpsych.theclinics.com

care setting is not generally informed by the same level of knowledge and specialized experience as that provided directly by a specialist. For these reasons, it is necessary to employ strategies to ensure that mental health practices in the pediatric primary care setting are of high quality.

The term measurement-based care (MBC) refers to the practice of incorporating the collection and review of structured data describing the clinical status of patients in relation to their treatment goals.[4] There is a growing body of evidence demonstrating that MBC can significantly improve the overall quality and effectiveness of mental health care.[5] This article will consider the utilization of MBC in collaborative and integrated models of care, beginning with a brief case vignette. After this, a review of some of the general advantages of MBC will be provided, and their specific relevance in the primary care setting will be discussed. Following this, 3 broad categories of collaborative and integrated practice models will be described, and for each one, methodological aspects of applying MBC practices will be explored. Finally, the article will address unique challenges including consideration of unintended consequences or pitfalls associated with implementation of MBC in the primary care setting, barriers to adoption, and how these challenges may be addressed.

CASE

Rachel is a 13-year-old girl with major depressive disorder, which was identified upon screening at her annual checkup with her pediatrician. Her PHQ-A (Patient Health Questionnaire-9, modified for adolescents) screen showed a score of 21, with prominent symptoms of depressed mood, loss of interest, low energy, difficulty sleeping, and thoughts of self-harm. After discussion of these symptoms with her pediatrician, she was internally referred on the same day to a mental health clinician working within the pediatric practice for further evaluation. This evaluation identified several stressors including recent bullying by peers, loss of her grandmother, and being cut from the track team. The clinician confirmed the diagnosis of major depressive disorder of moderate severity and discussed her findings with a child and adolescent psychiatrist with whom she reviews her caseload on a weekly basis. On the basis of this discussion, it was decided that the patient should be offered the option of psychotherapy with or without antidepressant medication. They chose psychotherapy without medication. The clinician began weekly cognitive behavioral psychotherapy and administered the PHQ-A every 2 weeks to track progress. Although the patient reported feeling better, her scores on measures (**Fig. 1**) indicated that after an initial reduction in her PHQ-A score, she continued to experience persistent depressive symptoms that were not improving by 8 weeks after the initiation of therapy. In their weekly review, the clinician and her consulting CAP noticed that Rachel was among several patients out of a

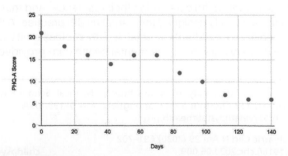

Fig. 1. Case example: Rachel.

caseload of 50 patients who appeared to be stuck in partial remission of depressive symptoms. They noted that the patient was well-engaged in therapy, addressing pertinent stressors, and complying with behavioral activation recommendations. However, she had some persistent neurovegetative symptoms including decreased energy, fatigue, and increased need for sleep along with her persistent depressed mood and anhedonia. They decided that it would be appropriate for the patient's treatment plan to be modified with a recommendation for adding a selective serotonin reuptake inhibitor (SSRI). The CAP contacted the pediatrician to convey this recommendation and to discuss the selection and dosing of the medication. The pediatrician proceeded to schedule an appointment and with the agreement of Grace and her mother, fluoxetine (10 mg/d) was begun. She continued with her psychotherapy, tolerated the medication well, and experience remission of her depression after 6 weeks.

ADVANTAGES OF MEASUREMENT-BASED CARE IN THE PEDIATRIC PRIMARY CARE SETTING
Improving Efficiency and Accuracy in Assessing Clinical Progress

Clinical measurement tools, used in conjunction with a clinical interview, offer the potential advantage of providing a more accurate and quantitative assessment of clinical change compared with an informal clinical impression on the basis of an unstructured clinical interview (**Box 1**).[6] In order to fulfill this potential, selected measures should have proven validity, reliability, and sensitivity to change for the specific age, language, and ethnicity of the patient. The selected measurement tools should be relevant to the primary goals of the patient's treatment plan. For children with a single diagnosis, the most relevant goal may simply be for the patient to achieve remission from the core symptoms of this diagnosis. In this instance, the most relevant measure is often a diagnosis-specific rating scale measuring symptoms related to the criteria for the diagnosis, such as the PHQ-A in the case example listed previously. For children who have multiple comorbid diagnoses or clinical symptoms cutting across multiple domains, the clinician must identify the goals that are most important to the child and family and develop a treatment plan based on these goals. In these situations, the most relevant measure could be focused on a particular functional impairment or a specific cluster of symptoms or behaviors related to a primary goal of the treatment plan. It is important for clinicians to be parsimonious in selecting measures. Measures do not need to be comprehensive, nor do they need to precisely match the complexity

Box 1	
Advantages of measurement-based care in the primary care setting	
Efficiency	Allows provider to focus attention in clinical interview on most pertinent issues
Accuracy of assessment	Validated measures complement impressions from clinical examination
Supports use of clinical algorithms	Quantitative data from clinical measures facilitate use of algorithms for decision support
Supports collaboration/ communication	Measure results easily shared and provides a common frame of reference for coordination of care with collaborating providers
Supports population health management	Measures can be compiled into patient registries for detecting individual needs of patients within caseloads, and for managing quality of care for groups of patients within a population

of the clinical presentation in order to be useful as an adjunct to the clinical examination.

Although the previously mentioned considerations are relevant to all clinicians regardless of their level of specialized training and degree of clinical experience, the benefit of having quantitative data to help inform treatment planning is especially relevant in the primary care setting. Primary care clinicians often lack confidence in their ability to manage mental health conditions on the basis of their limited educational preparation, especially in the context of the high-volume clinical workflow of a typical primary care setting.[7] Accordingly, when used in conjunction with a clinical interview, the use of measures may improve their confidence. Also, the review of clinical measures on a regular basis can help them to improve their clinical assessment skills by reminding them of the spectrum of symptoms about which they may not routinely inquire.

The advent of evidence-based medicine and increasing focus on quality improvement in health care delivery have led to the increasing emphasis on clinical algorithms for decision support in the management of specific medical conditions.[8] Clinical algorithms, synthesizing extensive bodies of scientific literature for practical clinical application in a user-friendly graphical format, are especially important for primary care providers, because they treat such a wide scope of health conditions. Most clinical algorithms require some quantitative measure of clinical progress in order to navigate through their branch points. By generating such quantitative data in the process of care, MBC naturally lends itself to the use of clinical algorithms, ultimately promoting the adoption of best practices in the treatment of pediatric mental health conditions.

By generating quantitative information regarding clinical progress, the use of MBC has the potential to make mental health treatment in the primary care setting more rigorous. The term clinical inertia has been used in reference to a premature shift from active to maintenance treatment, especially when patients are in partial remission from their primary condition.[9] For example, a patient with early improvement in symptoms after starting an antidepressant medication, possibly representing a placebo response, might informally report feeling much better, leading the clinician to prematurely begin tapering frequency of follow-up sessions. Such a patient, at substantial risk of relapse, could be lost to follow-up. The utilization of clinical measures, especially in conjunction with clinical algorithms, can help clinicians avoid this tendency and encourage patients and their clinicians to aim for full remission of symptomatology.

An additional important advantage to the use of clinical measures in the process of mental health treatment in the pediatric primary care setting is that they help the clinician to focus attention in the clinical interview on issues that are most pertinent to the patient's treatment. In the author's experience of providing mental health training for primary care providers, they often express feeling "at sea" when conducting clinical interviews. Within standard applications of MBC, the selected clinical measure is completed in the waiting room prior to the visit, allowing the provider to utilize the responses on the measure as an initial guide to the history of present illness. The face-to-face encounter time for primary care physicians is often much shorter than that for a mental health provider, and having a preliminary overview of the most prominent symptoms the patient is experiencing can allow the clinician to make the best use of the limited time and focus questions on the most clinically relevant symptoms. The alternative may otherwise be an inefficient fishing expedition in which the clinician, after an initial opening question about overall progress, proceeds to randomly select questions about symptoms which may or not be relevant to the patient. Limited time may be wasted, and pertinent areas of symptomatology may be missed.

Contrary to the expectation of specialists, when appropriately implemented, MBC has been demonstrated to improve rapport and engagement of patients in their treatment.[10] Improved engagement has been associated with superior outcomes, presumably by improving compliance and motivation for self-management.[11] In order to realize this benefit, the results of measures should be reviewed jointly with patients and parents, ideally with graphical display of trends, and this information should be used to inform discussion of ongoing treatment planning. This is an integral aspect of MBC that requires a suitable information technology platform with functionality for automated processing of clinical measure data in order to be practicable within a busy primary care practice setting. Fortunately, electronic medical record platforms for primary care practices are increasingly incorporating patient portal technology that include support for the administration of patient-reported outcome measures and incorporation of their results into the medical record.

Supporting Communication Between Collaborating Providers

Children's mental health treatment always requires some degree of teamwork or collaboration beyond the provider-patient relationship. Team members may include caregivers, teachers, various clinicians, allied mental health professionals, and other health care providers, many of whom are not present in the same physical location and need to communicate remotely. MBC can enable efficient communication within a team, providing a common language for reporting clinical progress. As exemplified in the previously mentioned case example, clinical measures can serve to flag patients within a shared caseload for more in-depth discussion. The specific data generated by clinical measures can help to focus treatment planning discussions between members of a clinical team in the same way that these data help a primary care provider navigate a clinical interview, making collateral discussions and consultation more streamlined and efficient.

Aggregating Measurement-Based Care Data for Population Health Management and Quality Improvement

Networks of primary care practices across the United States are increasingly engaging in value-based contracting, which has contributed to a shift in attention from exclusively focusing on individual patients to addressing the health needs of populations.[12] Accordingly, practices are striving to understand how health needs are distributed within their panels of patients and are implementing strategies to improving health outcomes for their entire panels within a fixed budget. There has been a particular interest in applying this approach to pediatric mental health needs of patients, because:

- Pediatric mental health conditions frequently go unrecognized and untreated[13]
- Untreated childhood mental health conditions have been associated with poor health outcomes[14]
- Untreated pediatric mental health conditions have been shown to result in significant increases in the utilization and cost of health care services[15]

Consequently, practices have implemented methods for detecting mental health conditions by developing systematic screening to identify patients at elevated risk for psychiatric disorders (an example is Adverse Childhood Experience [ACE] screening) and to enable early detection of psychiatric disorders (examples are screening for autism spectrum disorders in young children or depression in adolescents). Practices are also adopting clinical practice guidelines and using tools to ensure that patients with an identified health condition are receiving care in concordance with these guidelines and to monitor the clinical progress of these patients.

Patient registries are among the most important tools used by primary care practices and networks for tracking groups of patients with a common health condition. A registry is simply a list of patients defined by some criteria (eg, a list of patients between the ages of 12 and 18 who have been identified to have depression). Such a list might compile information summarizing various aspects of the treatment, including referrals made, follow-up appointments completed, utilization of other health care services, medications prescribed, and assessments of clinical progress. Naturally, MBC generates discrete, quantitative data that can be easily incorporated into such registries for tracking clinical progress. The inclusion of these clinical assessment data makes the registries much more useful than they would otherwise be if the registries were limited to data describing services. For practical reasons, the data for registries are usually consumed from existing clinical and administrative databases including registration systems, care management platforms, and discrete fields of the electronic medical record. Quantitative data from clinical measures used in MBC applications are perfectly suited for inclusion in a patient registry.

The review of a patient registry, as noted previously, can be invaluable in helping collaborating providers flag a patient who is not progressing optimally in treatment for in-depth review. But from the perspective of population health, patient registries can enable a programmatic approach within a practice for improving the quality of care for classes of patients within a primary care panel with defined mental health conditions. How many patients in a practice have been lost to follow-up after being diagnosed with major depression? How many patients being prescribed attention deficit hyperactivity disorder (ADHD) medications have had their treatment optimized with appropriate dose titration based on teacher reports of symptoms on an ADHD rating scale? Without a method of tracking, there is no ready answer. A traditional psychiatric practice with a small number of patients may be able to maintain awareness of these issues without a systematic tracking methodology; however it would be near to impossible in a high-volume primary care practice with thousands of patients.

MEASUREMENT-BASED CARE IMPLEMENTATION IN 3 MENTAL HEALTH INTEGRATION MODELS

Broadly considered, there are 3 dominant strategies or models for the delivery of mental health services in the pediatric primary care setting (**Table 1**).

Integrated Behavioral Health Clinician

In this model, a clinical social worker or psychologist is embedded in the primary care practice and functions as a member of the primary care team.[16] When a mental health concern is identified, the behavioral health clinician (BHC) is called in to conduct a brief clinical evaluation and to develop and implement a treatment plan. The primary role of the BHC is assessment and care management. Brief treatment in the form of individual, family, and/or group therapy may be provided by the BHC in the primary care setting; however, more frequently the BHC makes targeted referrals to other mental health providers for psychotherapy or other community-based services, and supports the patient and family through the referral process. This latter function is referred to as a warm hand-off. The PPCP may prescribe psychiatric medication within the scope of his or her expertise, usually limited to monotherapy for patients with uncomplicated depression, anxiety, or ADHD. The BHC may also be involved in systematic mental health screening in the practice by helping the primary care provider to administer

	Integrated Behavioral Health Clinician	Child Psychiatry Access Program	Collaborative Care Model
Table 1			
Measurement-based care in 3 models of mental health integration			
Distribution	Individual practices	Regional catchment areas	Individual practices
Mental Health Treatment	Mostly outside of practice, warm hand-offs	Psychosocial treatment usually referred out, basic psychopharmacology provided by PPCP	Both psychosocial and psychopharmacology treatment usually provided within practice
Resources to Primary Care Practice	Embedded clinician	Telephone consultation, outpatient evaluation, resource navigation	Embedded clinician plus consulting child and adolescent psychiatrist
MBC opportunity	Possible	Teach and encourage through consultation	Integral to model

and interpret screening instruments for common mental health concerns. The role of the BHC is relatively loosely defined and may vary depending on richness of staffing and priorities of the practice.

With an optimally trained BHC and adequate staffing, MBC may be implemented within this model. The BHC may be instrumental in helping to organize the administration, interpretation, and tracking of the measures, and utilizing the measures to guide ongoing care planning. The use of measures to support communication with mental health providers external to the practice is especially relevant in this model, as many of the patients are receiving their mental health care from community providers. The BHC may also assist PPCPs in compiling and reviewing patient registries for the purpose of population health management.

Child Psychiatry Access Programs

These are regional systems for helping PPCPs manage mental health needs for patients in the primary care setting by providing hotline access to telephone consultation, expedited outpatient consultations, help with resource navigation, and continuing education.[17,18] They are usually organized in a hub and spoke configuration with the specialist team working from a central location to provide these services for PPCPs within a surrounding catchment area.

Although the primary function of a child psychiatry access program (CPAP) is to educate PPCPs through patient-level consultation, another function is to provide practice-level consultation, helping affiliated practices to improve processes of mental health care. Examples of this include assisting practices in implementing mental health screening, teaching care coordinators how to navigate the system of mental health services in the community surrounding the practice, and helping the practice to adopt MBC practices including systematic use of patient-reported outcome measures and tracking of patients in a registry.[19] Use of clinical measures may be discussed and reinforced in the context of patient-level consultation (eg, when a PPCP calls a CPAP hotline with a question about the care of an adolescent patient with depression, the child psychiatry consultant may routinely ask the provider to provide information about a depression symptom severity measure such as the PHQ-A). This has the potential of reinforcing behavior change toward adoption of MBC.

Collaborative Care Model

An evidenced based model for mental health integration, the collaborative care model (CoCM) utilizes an embedded BHC/care manager (CM) to provide measurement-based mental health treatment within the practice.[20] MBC is a central pillar of the CoCM. In this model, the BHC/CM keeps track of patient progress with a patient registry, and meets with a consulting psychiatrist on a weekly basis to review the patients in treatment. The BHC/CM, psychiatrist, and the PPCP work as a team in providing patient-centered care within the practice. As described in the case example, the BHC/CM and consulting CAP review patient registries on a weekly basis. The registries are used to flag patients who are not progressing optimally in treatment for discussion and consideration for changes in the treatment plan including medication recommendations, additional diagnostic procedures including outpatient psychiatric consultation, or changes in the psychotherapy plan. The child and adolescent psychiatrist also consults directly with the PPCP regarding medication recommendations and is available to help the PPCP with additional consultation as needed throughout the course of treatment.

UNINTENDED CONSEQUENCES OF MEASUREMENT-BASED CARE

Despite its various benefits, the adoption of MBC is not without risk, especially if it is not implemented correctly. Many of these risks can be mitigated with careful planning and establishing appropriate expectations.

Administrative Burden

Primary care practices are usually busy operations, with high volumes of patient services being delivered by teams of health care professionals and support staff. Documentation of care has become more complex and time consuming with electronic health records (EHRs), and providers are held responsible for more and more functions including screening for numerous health conditions, keeping track of quality measures, and prior authorizations. Provider burnout is especially prevalent in primary care, and it is often attributed to increasing administrative burden associated with these functions.[21] The introduction of MBC into a primary care practice has the potential to increase the administrative workload of the providers, worsening the stress of their practice and reducing the finite time and energy given directly to patients. In order to avert this potential consequence, it is necessary for primary care teams to make careful plans to ensure that the function is well integrated into the workflow of the practice (**Box 2**). For example, if providers are expected to sift through file cabinets to find forms, wait for patients and parents to fill them out, manually score them, and hunt through scanned document lists to evaluate trends, the MBC practice will inevitably be unsustainable.

When there is a system in place for automated administration, scoring, and documentation of measures, it is tempting for the clinician to measure everything she or he would want to know about the patient's symptoms and functioning. This can result in a large set of measures being administered to each patient, or the use of overly comprehensive or broad band measures. This is a standard practice when conducting clinical research; however, in a clinical primary care setting, such an approach to assessment is not only burdensome to patients but becomes overwhelming and time-consuming for the provider to interpret. It can also result in providers losing sight

---

Box 2
Strategies for minimizing administrative burden of measurement-based care for pediatric primary care providers

Automated administration and scoring of clinical measures and incorporation into EHR via patient portal

Minimal provider input for launching patient-level measurement plan: selection of 1 best measure most relevant to the treatment plan, appropriate frequency of administration

Practice establishes consensus on limited set of measures for most common clinical domains

Select measures that are brief, focused, and easily interpreted

Optimal utilization of practice support staff for troubleshooting process of measure administration and ensuring that providers have results and trend lines before entering an examination room

---

of high-level clinical priorities. As noted in **Box 2**, PPCPs are encouraged to select 1 clinical measure for a given patient that best reflects the most important priority of treatment. The measure should be relevant to the patient, easy to interpret, but not necessarily comprehensive or perfectly tailored.

Over-Reliance on Measures

MBC is meant to complement and enhance a clinical interview and is a poor substitute for clinical judgment and human interaction. This is a particular risk in the primary care setting because of the limitation of time and the limited training of PPCPs in mental health assessment. Physicians are indoctrinated early in training to treat the patient, not the laboratory result. Similarly, the results of clinical self-report measures are meant to enhance or complement the clinical examination. The brief self-report measurement tools used in MBC usually measure only 1 dimension of the patient's mental health status, and the sensitivity and specificity of the best tools are well below 100%. Over-reliance on MBC in this way not only presents risk of invalid clinical assessment and poor treatment decisions, but also deprives patients of healing aspects of human connection within the provider-patient relationship.

BARRIERS TO ADOPTION

Despite a preponderance of evidence of the benefits of MBC, the practice is not yet widely disseminated.

Interfering Beliefs

Despite evidence to the contrary,[22] many psychiatrists believe that the information generated from patient-reported outcome measures does not substantially enhance the accuracy of their clinical assessment. This may be less so for primary care providers; however, lack of interest among consulting and embedded mental health specialists to whom PPCPs turn for advice may either influence their attitudes directly or represent a missed opportunity for educating them about their value.

Logistical Challenges

The potential administrative burdens discussed previously as unintended consequences also function as barriers to MBC adoption. PPCPs often feel inundated with forms and information, and worry that their patients will be annoyed with repeatedly completing clinical measures. This is a realistic concern for busy primary care offices; therefore it is essential to consider this at the outset of planning. One way of mitigating this barrier is to start small, beginning with 1 measure for 1 disorder, and testing it with 1 provider and a small number of patients. This approach, described more fully as the PDSA model of rapid cycle process improvement,[22] allows practices to introduce a new function on a small scale, with minimal initial investment of resources and limited risk of adverse consequences. After reviewing the experience of providers, patients, and office staff, adjustments can be made easily to optimize the new process, and then the process can be gradually scaled to include more patients, more providers, and additional measures for other diagnostic groups.

Resource Limitations and Cost

Dedicating time for planning, adding tasks to staff and providers, and developing the necessary information technology resources costs money that is not readily available to practices. This may be less of a barrier for large primary care networks that may already have robust information technology platforms with patient portals, but it is a valid concern for all practices grappling with substantial financial risk and limited staffing and technology resources. There are current procedural terminology (CPT) codes for the administration, scoring, and review of clinical measures that can help support the costs associated with MBC, however this type of reimbursement does not benefit practices that have shifted to capitated contracting and value-based reimbursement. For these practices, the return on investment may be derived from payments associated with improved performance on behavioral health quality measures. Beyond the initial investment associated with the adoption and optimization of MBC processes, MBC has the potential of creating efficiencies; however, the start-up cost represents an especially challenging barrier and may need to be addressed directly through dedicated financing programs by governmental and commercial payers.

SUMMARY

Challenges associated with the integration of pediatric mental health care in the primary care setting include limitations of training and time, high volume of patients, need for coordination with external specialists, limited infrastructure, and limited funding. All of these issues can negatively influence the quality of mental health service delivery. When correctly implemented, MBC processes have the potential to mitigate many of these challenges, and perhaps more importantly, generate data allowing practices to evaluate and improve the performance of integrated mental health processes. Implementing MBC requires initial investment of staff resources for planning, training, and information technology resources, which will need to be supported by practice organizations, payers, and/or state and federal government. CAPs and other children's mental health professionals involved in collaborative and/or integrated mental health service delivery may be instrumental in promoting and supporting the adoption of MBC in the primary care setting.

DISCLOSURE

The author has nothing to disclose.

REFERENCES

1. The National Network of Child Psychiatry Access Programs. Available at: https://nncpap.org/thenetwork.html. Accessed February 21, 2020.

2. American Academy of Child and Adolescent Psychiatry. Pediatric Integrated Care Resources Center. Available at: http://www.integratedcareforkids.org. Accessed February 21, 2020.

3. McMillan J, Land M, Leslie L. Pediatric residency education and the behavioral and mental health crisis: a call to action. Pediatrics 2017;139(1). https://doi.org/10.1542/peds.2016-2141.

4. Harding K, Rush A, Arbuckle M, et al. Measurement-based care in psychiatric practice: a policy framework for implementation. J Clin Psychiatry 2011;72(8):1136–43.

5. de Jong R, Snoek H, Staal W, et al. The effect of patients' feedback on treatment outcome in a child and adolescent psychiatric sample: a randomized controlled trial. Eur Child Adolesc Psychiatry 2019;28(6):819–34.

6. Hatfield D, McCullough L, Frantz SH, et al. Do we know when our clients get worse? An investigation of therapists' ability to detect negative client change. Clin Psychol Psychother 2010;17(1):25–32.

7. Horwitz S, Storfer-Isser A, Kerker B, et al. Barriers to the identification and management of psychosocial problems: changes from 2004 to 2013. Acad Pediatr 2015;15(6):613–20.

8. Djulbegovic B, Guyatt G. Progress in evidence-based medicine: a quarter century on. Lancet 2017;390(10092):415–23.

9. Henke RM, Zaslavsky AM, McGuire TG, et al. Clinical inertia in depression treatment. Med Care 2009;47(9):959.

10. Dowrick C, Leydon G, McBride A, et al. Patients' and doctors' views on depression severity questionnaires incentivised in UK quality and outcomes framework: qualitative study. BMJ 2009;338:b663.

11. Krupnick J, Sotsky S, Simmens S, et al. The role of the therapeutic alliance in psychotherapy and pharmacotherapy outcome: findings in the National Institute of Mental Health Treatment of Depression Collaborative Research Program. J Consult Clin Psychol 1996;64(3):532–9.

12. Cattel D, Eijkenaar F. Value-based provider payment initiatives combining global payments with explicit quality incentives: a systematic review. Med Care Res Rev 2019. https://doi.org/10.1177/1077558719856775. 1077558719856775.

13. Whitney DG. Peterson MD US National and State-Level Prevalence of Mental Health Disordes and Disparities of Mental Health Care Use in Children. JAMA Pediatr 2019;173(4):389–91.

14. Goodman A, Joyce R, Smith JP. The long shadow cast by childhood physical and mental problems on adult life. Proc Natl Acad Sci U S A 2011;108(15):6032–7.

15. Soni A. Top five most costly conditions among children, ages 0-17, 2012: estimates for the U.S. civilian noninstitutionalized population. Rockville (MD): Agency for Healthcare Research and Quality, Medical Expenditure Panel Survey; 2015. Statistical Brief #472.

16. Gunn W, Blount A. Primary care mental health: a new frontier for psychology. J Clin Psychol 2009;65(3):235–52.

17. Sarvet B, Gold J, Bostic JQ, et al. Improving access to mental health care for children: the Massachusetts Child Psychiatry Access Project. Pediatrics 2010;126(6):1191–200.

18. Hilt RJ, Romaire MA, McDonell MG, et al. The partnership access line: evaluating a child psychiatry consult program in Washington State. JAMA Pediatr 2013;167(2):162–8.

19. Sarvet B, Ravech M, Straus J. Massachusetts child psychiatry access project 2.0: a case study in child psychiatry access program redesign. Child Adolesc Psychiatr Clin N Am 2017;26(4):647–63.
20. Raney L. Integrating primary care and behavioral health: the role of the psychiatrist in the collaborative care model. Focus (Am Psychiatr Publ) 2017;15(3): 354–60.
21. Rao S, Kimball A, Lehrhoff S, et al. The impact of administrative burden on academic physicians: results of a hospital-wide physician survey. Acad Med 2017; 92(2):237–43.
22. Hannan C, Lambert M, Harmon C, et al. A lab test and algorithms for identifying clients at risk for treatment failure. J Clin Psychol 2005;61(2):155–63.

Section III: Special Considerations

Measurement-based Data to Monitor Quality: Why Specification at the Population Level Matter?

Bonnie T. Zima, MD, MPH

KEYWORDS

- Routine outcome monitoring • Performance measurement • Quality measures
- Child mental health

KEY POINTS

- Specification of the population level has implications for the purpose, proposed target mechanisms that drive quality improvement, methodologic challenges, and implications for program evaluation and data interpretation.
- Populations levels for measurement-based care can be conceptualized at the individual (tier 1), clinical aggregate (tier 2), and national level (tier 3).
- Methodologic challenges and their implications underscore the complexity of developing a data infrastructure to measure the delivery of recommended care and its association to clinical outcomes.
- Findings support the Institute of Medicine's national call for federally funded research almost 3 decades ago.

Measuring the quality of care is envisioned as a key driver to transforming the US health care system.[1] The landmark Institute of Medicine's 2001 report, Crossing the Quality the Chasm: A New Health System for the 21st Century, conceptualizes quality improvement to be guided by 6 aims, namely that care be safe, effective, timely, efficient, equitable, and patient-centered.[2] Adaptation of this national framework for mental health care further underscored the public health significance to improve the quality of care for behavioral health disorders, as evidenced by high prevalence, direct and societal costs, and substantial gaps in recommended and actual care.[3] A national call for transformation of the US healthcare system in 2008 proposed the simultaneous pursuit of 3 aims: improving the experience of care, improving population health, and reducing health care per capita costs.[4] This triple aim became the foundation for the

UCLA-Semel Institute for Neurosciences and Human Behavior, University of California at Los Angeles, UCLA Center for Health Services & Society, 10920 Wilshire Boulevard #300, Los Angeles, CA 90024, USA
E-mail address: bzima@mednet.ucla.edu

Child Adolesc Psychiatric Clin N Am 29 (2020) 703–731
https://doi.org/10.1016/j.chc.2020.06.008
1056-4993/20/© 2020 Elsevier Inc. All rights reserved.

childpsych.theclinics.com

National Quality Strategy, an early requirement of the 2010 Affordable Care Act.[5] Within the triple aim, the population levels and corresponding units of analyses are purposively muddled to provide a health policy goal that is encompassing, transactional, and will stimulate change. However, as efforts to implement and scale up measurement-based care (MBC) are underway, the importance of specifying which population level one wishes to measure and clarification of the purpose for measuring are increasingly apparent.

To demonstrate the significance of conceptualizing MBC by population level, this article provides an overview of the different purposes, proposed mechanisms, and early lessons learned for MBC at the individual (tier 1), clinical aggregate (tier 2), and national (tier 3) levels. Within tier 2, there is fertile ground to test measurement approaches in preparation of scaling up to statewide tracking of quality indicators, and several examples are shared. For each tier, methodologic challenges and implications for program evaluation or data interpretation are presented to safeguard against premature judgements about patient treatment resistance or provider, clinic, agency, health care system, or state Medicaid agency performance. Select details are provided to demonstrate some of the nuances that may be missed if only descriptive data are presented. To begin, a brief overview of the health policy context for measuring child behavioral health quality and its unique challenges is provided.

MEASURING CHILD BEHAVIORAL HEALTH QUALITY: POLICY CONTEXT AND UNIQUE CHALLENGES

For children, provisions in the Children's Health Insurance Program Reauthorization Act (CHIPRA) of 2009 stipulated improvements to the quality of care and health outcomes for children enrolled in the Child Health Insurance Program (CHIP) and Medicaid state programs,[6] impacting more than 35 million children, comprising 50.6% of all CHIP and Medicaid beneficiaries.[7] Under the auspices of the Agency for Healthcare Research and Quality, an initial core set of 24 quality measures was submitted to the secretary of the Department of Health and Human Services (DHHS) on Jan. 1, 2010. Every year starting in 2013, the core set of measures is reviewed, and measures are considered for addition or removal.[8] In 2020, state Medicaid agencies will be asked to voluntarily report adherence rates for up to 24 quality measures, of which 4are related to child mental health. Beginning in 2024, State reporting of quality measures from the core set will be mandatory, as stipulated by the 2018 Bipartisan Budget Act.[9]

These policy levers have accelerated the urgency to establish a nationwide data infrastructure system to monitor and track improvement in quality of care.[2] This timeline also underscores the need to earmark federal funding for research to develop, further refine, and create innovative solutions to measure the quality of behavioral health care.[10–13] With the expansion of electronic health care record (EHR) systems and advances in EHR data science (eg, EHR phenotyping, natural language processing, and predictive modeling), identification of more granular predictors of improved care is promising.[14]

Nevertheless, the task of improving existing data infrastructure to assess the quality of child behavioral health care poses additional challenges. One of the foundations for a quality measure is rigorous scientific evidence to support the relationship between recommended care and improved clinical outcomes that are meaningful. However, the scientific evidence underlying recommended care for child psychiatric disorders, especially long term and among more diverse populations, is sparse.[15,16] There are also limitations of administrative data that impede assessment of whether recommended care was provided (eg, lack of procedure codes for evidence-based psychotherapies)[13,17] and reliance on adjudicated pharmacy claims data as a proxy for medication adherence.[18,19]

For children, the priority is placed on the prevention and early detection of mental health problems, including risk for suicide.[20–22] Thus demonstration of the value of high-quality child mental health care requires an association between receipt of recommended care processes with a continuum of corresponding outcomes. For preventive care, proximal outcomes may be improvement in child and/or family resilience or reduction in risk factors that over time are associated with the lack of progression from symptoms to psychiatric disorder to adverse adult outcomes. Further, quality measurement of child behavioral health care requires additional case mix adjustment to account for variation in development, parent- and family-level contextual factors (eg, maternal depression), and service use across multiple child-serving care sectors (eg, schools, child welfare). With these challenges in mind, examples of different uses of MBC data by 3 population levels and related caveats for program evaluation and data interpretation are described.

MEASUREMENT-BASED CARE DATA BY POPULATION LEVEL
Tier 1: Individual Level

At the individual level (tier 1), the main purpose of MBC is to inform clinical decision making (**Table 1**). MBC is conceptualized as routinely collecting patient-reported outcomes measures, with priority placed on symptom rating scales. The target mechanisms for change include improving early detection of nonresponse to treatment and patient-provider communication.[23–25] Routine outcome monitoring (ROM) may be especially effective for monitoring patients who are not clinically improving in therapy.[25,26]

Implementation of MBC at the individual level, mostly for adults, has yielded several early lessons learned. To be effective, symptom ratings scale data must be current, interpretable, and readily available during clinical encounters.[23] The data should be presented in clinically meaningful categories (eg, response, remission, nonresponse, relapse and recurrence) to align with treatment guidelines[23,27] and be actionable.[28] To detect real change in adolescent depression symptoms using the Patient Health Questionnaire-9 items (PHQ-9), a promising approach is to calculate the reliable change index, a statistical approach that accounts for the standard error of measurement.[29,30]

For tier 1 MBC, there are several methodologic challenges with implications for data interpretation at the patient and clinician levels (**Table 2**). The main outcome for individual level MBC is timeliness of change in the clinician's treatment approach, with the underlying assumptions that the clinician is given reliable and valid patient-reported data that are easily interpretable and he or she selects a treatment option for which evidence supports more benefit than risk. This is a high bar, especially for child mental health care in community-based treatment settings for which parents may be the main informants, and there is a paucity of scientific evidence for recommended care and its long-term benefit.[31,32]

For monitoring change in child clinical outcomes over time, the Achilles' heel is the reliance on parent and/or youth report of symptoms. Findings from rating scales are not a substitute for clinical judgment.[23] In busy clinic settings, fidelity of parent or youth responses to a mental health screen may vary with informant and over time. Parent ability to detect and report target symptoms may also vary with parent by

Table 1
Measurement-based care by population levels: primary goal, proposed mechanisms of action, and early lessons learned

Primary Goal	Proposed Mechanisms	Early Lessons Learned
Tier 1: individual		
Inform clinical decisions	Improved early detection of nonresponse to treatment; Improved patient-provider communication	Symptom rating scale data must be current, interpretable, and available during the clinical encounter, assessed frequently, and be actionable
Tier 2: clinical aggregate		
Monitor performance	Feedback on variation in clinical outcomes by provider, clinic, hospital, or agency level will identify target areas for quality improvement and guide resource allocation decisions	Collaborative care models, predominantly for adult major depression, that employ care managers to monitor target symptoms and communicate to the primary care provider or consulting psychiatrist are effective in improving quality of care; Measurement-based feedback systems have relatively poor and inconsistent clinician uptake; Mandating clinician completion of rating forms to track clinical outcomes is not sufficient; Poor data quality undermines capacity to identify target areas for improvement and weakens rationale for financial incentives or penalties; Public investment in the development and maintenance of data infrastructure to measure the delivery of recommended care processes and association with clinical outcomes is needed

(continued on next page)

Table 1 (*continued*)		
Primary Goal	**Proposed Mechanisms**	**Early Lessons Learned**
Tier 3: state Medicaid agency		
Monitor change in adherence rates to national quality measures	Public reporting of quality measure adherence rates drives improvement by identifying target areas for improvement that health plans can be held accountable to change	Scientific evidence supporting the clinical validity of the 4national child mental health quality measures is sparse Wide variation in state adherence rates signals the need for more standardized methods for data collection, analysis, and reporting Federal investment in research is needed to further refine child behavioral health quality measures to improve clinical validity and identify predictors of significant change in adherence rates

type of symptom (eg, internalizing vs externalizing), across parents within a family, and change over time in either direction, potentially influenced by parent-child relationships, patient education, or respondent fatigue.[33–35] For youth, there may be disagreement with parent report that requires additional time to reconcile to determine the diagnosis or judge whether there is clinical improvement.

In addition, time points for clinically monitoring symptoms vary. At the individual level, there is an inherent trade-off between personalizing treatment at the expense of diminishing capacity to compare across patients. The time points for monitoring symptoms may vary within a patient's episode of care. The advantage is that clinician feedback is in real time, allowing for tailoring of the treatment plan. However, customization reduces the capacity to compare clinical improvement across patients, even with the same provider.

The number of times standardized clinical information is obtained also differs, yielding different amounts of data for each patient. The extent of data per patient may be influenced beyond clinician-level factors, such as organization characteristics that reduce clinician burden, improve team communication (eg, the care manager monitors and reports aggregated target symptoms to the primary care provider), and support documentation (eg, integration of patient-reported ratings into the EHR). The extent of symptom monitoring may also differ by provider characteristics (eg, training or discipline) and patient clinical status (eg, severity or psychosocial complexity). Among adolescents in a large provider networks, use of the PHQ-9 was related to an increase in depression diagnoses in primary care,[36] and predictors of clinician use of depression screening included more severe initial depressive symptoms.[37] In addition, early treatment trajectory may positively or negatively influence data collection. Early positive response to treatment may reduce the likelihood of

Table 2
Measurement-based care at the individual level (tier 1): methodologic challenges and implications for data interpretation by patient and clinician levels

Methodologic Challenges	Implications for Data Interpretation
Patient-level	
Reliance on parent and/or youth report of symptoms	Parent or youth fidelity to instructed use of an outcome measure is not usually assessed, making it difficult to separate out potential reporting and measurement errors from reported clinical change or stability in target symptoms Parent ability to detect and report target symptoms may vary with parent by type of symptom (eg, internalizing vs externalizing), across parents within a family, and change over time in either direction (ie, patient education may enhance accuracy of symptom reporting, respondent fatigue may reduce accuracy) For youth, disagreement between parent and youth report of symptoms may require additional clinician time to judge whether there is clinical improvement
Variable time points	Time points for assessing clinical improvement varies within each patient's unique episode of care A trade-off is made to personalize treatment at the expense of diminishing capacity to compare across patients.
Variable number of times standardized clinical information is collected	Amount of data for each patient varies Influential factors include: Patient's clinical status • Clinical severity and psychosocial complexity • Early treatment trajectory (positive or negative) Provider differences • Training • Discipline Organizational factors • Care manager support to monitor target symptoms • Integration of patient-reported ratings into EHR
Time window and target area for improvement vary by type of intervention	The time window and type of desired outcome for an 8 to 12-wk parent training or evidence-based therapy should be tailored to the intervention The time window for assessing the efficacy of a new medication, change in medication (type, dose) will vary by type of medication with priority placed on medication safety and reduction in target symptoms

(continued on next page)

Table 2
(continued)

Methodologic Challenges	Implications for Data Interpretation
Timeliness of improvement may vary by type of clinical outcome	Acute symptom reduction may be more likely in a shorter period of time than changes in functioning (eg, improvement in academic achievement, peer relationships, family functioning). Long-term improvement in child functioning may be missed if data source is limited to claims data for acute-care episode (ie, Medicaid reimbursement for outpatient mental health care) and not individually linked to other data sources (ie, school records)
Clinician-level	
Poor clinician uptake and inconsistent use of baseline and follow-up measures	Missing data at baseline and follow-up time points make it problematic to track clinical improvement over time
Potential disparities in clinician use of a measurement feedback system by patient insurance status	Potential selection effects that may underestimate indicators of clinical improvement or clinician responsiveness to change treatment approach among publicly insured patients
Variable strength of scientific evidence for recommended care processes or treatment guidelines for child psychiatric disorders	Treatment options at clinical decision points have variable levels of scientific evidence to support appropriate care recommendations. Clinical judgment and patient preferences (parent, child, youth), which are more time- and labor intensive to measure, are likely influential factors at these decision points and are also components of acceptable care

clinician monitoring of symptoms, whereas early signs on nonresponse or lack of continued clinical improvement may stimulate more frequent symptom monitoring.

For children, first-line treatment may include a trial of an evidence-based therapy prior to psychotropic medication treatment. The time window and target area for these interventions vary. Parent training, for example, may require completion of 8 to 12 sessions with monitoring of changes in parenting skills that align with the content of teaching modules. The time window for assessing the efficacy of medication treatment differs by medication type or dose, and reduction in target symptoms is usually the clinical outcome. Timeliness of clinical improvement may also vary by type of clinical outcome. Acute symptom reduction may occur within a shorter time period compared with improved child functioning. Data collection methods may also vary, introducing differences in data quality, timing, and clinician feedback, potentially influencing patient-provider communication and clinical decision making.

At the clinician level, poor uptake of MBC and inconsistent use of baseline and follow-up measures can yield missing data that make it impossible to systematically track clinical improvement over time at the individual level. Potential explanations include clinician burden, lack of provider training and resources, clinician perception of the limitations of existing measures, lack of regular feedback on outcome data, and poor reimbursement.[38–40]

Further, an underlying assumption in MBC at the individual level is that clinical decision points include alternative evidence-based practices. Scientific evidence to support decision points, particularly for psychotropic medication treatment for children, may be less robust or equivocal.[31,32] The need for additional research to inform treatment guidelines leaves greater room for clinical judgment, parent and youth preferences, accommodating to logistical issues to support continuity of care (ie, drug formulary), and other unmeasurable factors that influence clinical decision making. Clinical judgment and parent preferences, which are more time- and labor–intensive to measure, are likely influential factors at these decision points and are components of acceptable care.

Tier 2: Clinical Aggregate Level

The main purpose of MBC at the clinical aggregate level is to monitor performance with the underlying assumption that provision of recommended care will be associated with improvement in clinical outcomes that are meaningful (ie, effective and align with parent, provider, and system priorities) (see **Table 1**). The proposed mechanism of change is that feedback on variation in clinical outcomes by provider, clinic, hospital, or agency will identify target areas for quality improvement and guide resource allocation decisions.[41,42] Tier 2 is conceptualized as the clinical aggregate level to encompass common methodologic challenges in program evaluation at the patient, provider, clinician, clinic, hospital, or agency (county or state) level. Program evaluation is a broad term that spans examining the match between program structure and contract, engagement of peer coaches (eg, to support self-management, continuity of care), and patient satisfaction to decreased health care costs.[43] Within this continuum, priority is placed on methods that measure provider adherence to recommended care processes and clinical outcomes.

Data at tier 2 are also a key source of pilot data to inform the development, testing, and refinement of approaches to deliver care and measure quality of care prior to large-scale use (tier 3). In efforts to scale up MBC at the clinical aggregate level, stepped care models have proven to be effective, especially for adult major depression. To reduce clinician burden and standardize implementation of stepped care (ie, care tailored to the clinical need of the patient), rating scale data are collected by a care manager for a specific psychiatric disorder (eg, major depression), and these findings are shared with the primary care provider and consulting psychiatrist.[41] For adults receiving care in collaborative care for major depression, findings from numerous randomized clinical trials suggest that frequent and timely feedback of patient reported symptoms to the provider during medication management and psychotherapy encounters significantly improve clinical outcomes.[23,41] For adolescents, adaptation of a collaborative care model for depression, using an initial in-person engagement session and regular follow-up by master's level clinicians, was also found to significantly reduce depressive symptoms at 12 months compared with usual care using a randomized clinical trial design.[44] In addition, among a large sample of youths receiving home-based mental health care, weekly feedback to clinicians was associated with faster treatment response, and findings suggested a dose-response relationship when clinicians viewed more feedback reports.[28]

Implementation trials of measurement feedback systems in select clinics suggest clinician uptake is relatively poor, and additional support is required to achieve promising results. Among 4 community-based mental health clinics in New York, clinic uptake of a measurement feedback system, the Contextual Feedback System, was

50%. Two clinics discontinued use, and the remaining two required further refinement (eg, modify clinic work flows to integrate use, local project plans to implement) and support (eg, weekly consultation calls or coaching) to implement.[45] Nevertheless, pilot data suggest among youth who received care using more of the measurement feedback system, improvement during the treatment phase was faster.[45] In addition, among one of the few 5-year implementation trials of integrating a digital MFS into the work flow in a child psychiatry department within a pediatric tertiary care center, clinician ratings of system usability were below industry standards, and uptake by clinicians was poor but improved with daily reminders and incentives.[24] At the patient level, striking disparities were found, such that patients enrolled in Medicaid were approximately half as likely to be provided a measurement feedback account and approximately 60% less likely to complete any measures compared with their privately insured counterparts.

At the state mental health agency level, efforts for statewide implementation of MBC are highly variable. In 2013, only 29 state Medicaid behavioral health agencies provided online information related to measuring behavioral health care quality; use of quality measures varied widely by state, with few targeting care for children.[46] Findings from Minnesota's Community Measurement Program suggest that use of PHQ-9 for screening and monitoring at 6 and 12 months widely varies by medical group and clinic. For adults, use of the PHQ-9 varies from 0% to 100% by medical group and clinic; 6-month follow-up screening varies between 1.8% to 54.6% for medical groups and 1.9% to 73.4% for clinics, and 12-month screening rates vary from 0% to 48.0% for medical groups and 0% to 49.8% for clinics.[47] Among adolescents, reported use of PHQ-9 screening ranges from 0% to 100% for both medical groups and clinics.[47] In New York, the Office of Mental Health utilizes a Web-based tool to monitor psychotropic medication prescribing practices, based on Medicaid claims and encounter data. The quality indicator set for children examines trends in psychotropic polypharmacy, high-dose psychotropic prescriptions, and psychotropic medication prescriptions among children 5 years or younger.[45] Findings are used to examine clinic and prescriber performance compared with state and regional comparators, develop lists of youth with quality flags for provider review, and describe child psychotropic medication treatment patterns over time.[45]

In California, since 1991, there have been several state legislative mandates for publicly reporting the quality of mental health care and clinical outcomes,[48–51] but funds are not earmarked for the development and maintenance of the data infrastructure required to meet these policy goals. The state is left to mandate mental health county agencies to collect, submit, and report clinical outcome data, yielding at best inconsistent data and underscoring the need for a robust quality monitoring system for child mental health care.[42,52–54]

Examples of some of the methodologic challenges and implications for program evaluation of child mental health care are summarized in **Table 3**. Together with university-based researchers, clinic, agency, or health care system partners must comply with the Health Insurance Portability and Accountability Act (HIPAA), as well as their home institution's policies and procedures related to data privacy and security. As there is no boiler-plate administrative mechanism, written agreements for data access, transfer, use, analysis, linking, and reporting are often unique to the project and require consultation from compliance officers, contracts and grants office, legal counsel, and/or institutional review boards. In developing proposals to examine quality of care, existing data sources should be carefully reviewed, because most were not developed to examine quality of care and may lack procedure codes that align with evidence-based practices. Likewise, Medicaid claims data are often difficult to

Table 3
Measurement-based care at the clinical aggregated level (tier 2): examples of methodologic challenges and implications for program evaluation

Methodologic Challenges	Implications for Program Evaluation
Ethics	
Data privacy and security	Consultation with agency and university compliance officers, institutional review boards, contracts and grants office, and legal counsel is often required to develop administrative mechanisms for data access, transfer, analysis, linking, and reporting that are compliant with Health Insurance Portability and Accountability Act (HIPAA) and other agency and university policies and procedures
Data source	
Primary purpose of data source (eg, Medicaid claims) may not be able to examine quality of care	Careful review of existing data source methods and study variables is critical to understanding the capacity of the data source to address research question and identify limitations that can safeguard against overgeneralization of findings
Procedure codes in claims data may not specify evidence-based practices	Receipt of psychosocial treatment may be counted if there is billing for individual, family, or group therapy, making it impossible to identify if evidenced-base therapies were provided and their extent of fidelity
Linkage between Medicaid claims and other child-serving public agencies data at individual level	Individual linkage between claims data for outpatient child mental health care and other child-serving care sectors (eg, schools, child welfare, juvenile justice, or primary care) may not be feasible, reducing capacity to link receipt of recommended mental health prevention, early intervention, or treatment to improved child societal outcomes (eg, academic achievement or family preservation)

(continued on next page)

Table 3
(continued)

Methodologic Challenges	Implications for Program Evaluation
Study design	
Match study design and methods to research question	Various study designs and methods could be used, but the final study design and methods (eg, quantitative and/or qualitative) must have the potential to address the specific aims of the study a priori Define eligibility criteria (inclusion or exclusion) and study time period For administrative data: • Clarify whether cross-sectional study within number of years in study time period (include all eligible subjects) or longitudinal cohort study (follow select group over time). • If longitudinal cohort study, must define time window for "looking back" to define new episode of care and apply generally accepted rule from prior research (eg, 3, 6, 12 mo). • Explore if a patient had more than one episode of care during study time period, examine frequency distributions, and consider feasibility of examining frequent, repeat users of care and/or high cost subpopulations.
Sample	
Adequate representation of diverse and understudied child populations	Examine distribution of child sociodemographic characteristics in data source. Review data weighting methods if applicable. Consider options to ensure adequate sample size of sociodemographic groups (eg, oversample all girls for quality of care for ADHD) to examine disparities in care a priori.
Insurance status may not be constant	Include only continuously enrolled patients during the study year and use generally accepted rule for definition for continuous enrollment (eg, 11 mo coverage/year).

(continued on next page)

Table 3 (*continued*)	
Methodologic Challenges	**Implications for Program Evaluation**
Insurance benefits may vary	Assess potential variation insurance benefits across health plans and conduct sensitivity analysis to explore influence on findings.
Study Variables	
Patient-level Proximal Outcomes: Receipt of 1Recommended Care	
Operationally define receipt of recommended care processes	If examining adherence to recommended care processes (eg, treatment-guideline concordant care, adherence to quality measure) technical specifications for index start and end dates, numerator and denominator must be clearly described. This process should also identify limitations of existing data source(s) that have implications for data interpretation and recommendations for future research.
Episode of care varies by patient	Must identify index start and end date using operational definitions. Definition of end date may be dependent upon clinic policies regarding when to discharge patient or close case, or clinical judgment that care is no longer indicated.
Implementation of recommended care varies	Consider options to build in capacity to assess how recommended care is delivered over a continuum of steps (eg, uptake, engagement, adoption, acceptability, feasibility, penetration, sustainability). These data may identify target mechanisms to explain change or lack of change in clinical outcomes and can inform target areas for quality improvement.

(*continued on next page*)

Table 3
(continued)

Methodologic Challenges	Implications for Program Evaluation
Patient-level Distal Outcomes: Clinical Outcomes	
Sparse evidence to support the reliability and validity of clinical outcome measures for children receiving care in community-based treatment settings.	Difficult to separate out measurement error from clinical change or stability in reported symptoms.
Variation in the availability and established psychometric properties for child clinical outcome measures that are not in English.	Potential for greater measurement error for non-English speaking parents or youth and direction of potential bias is unclear. Reduce capacity to accurately assess disparities in care.
Use of combined parent and youth report for adolescents	Disagreement is common between parent and youth report of symptoms. Explore variation in main findings by combined, either, parent-only, youth-only reported symptoms.
Data may be missing at baseline and prescribed follow-up time points (eg, 3, 6, 12 mo)	Questions are raised as to whether incomplete cases should be excluded that would reduce sample size, especially if statistical approaches to address missing data problems are not feasible.
Time points for assessing clinical improvement may vary by patient	Potential influential factors include: • Mandate to collect clinical outcome measure when patient clinically deemed to complete therapy • Use clinical outcome measure collected nearest to last mental health contact (drop out or completed care?) • Poor alignment between time of follow-up and follow-up time points

(continued on next page)

Table 3
(continued)

Methodologic Challenges	Implications for Program Evaluation
There is a potential selection bias when follow-up outcome data is dependent upon contact with services.	Early termination of care with no follow-up outcome data may imply improvement with brief intervention or poor continuity of care with persistent or worsening of target symptoms. Continued care with little change in clinical outcomes may signal clinical need for on-going care of a chronic condition which could be classified as acceptable care.
Variation in data collection methods	Assess extent of missing data by data collection method. Examples include: • Entry on tablet in waiting room with integration into EHR • Patient portal use of registry • Paper survey included with other patient registration forms • By care manager or clinician during clinical encounter Explore potential variation in data quality by data collection method if a program allows for flexibility in reporting or changes in data collection approach over time within a clinic, division, hospital or agency.
Defining "avoidable" or "unnecessary" repeat ED use or inpatient psychiatric hospitalizations	Repeated or more frequent ED use for a primary mental health problem or inpatient psychiatric hospitalization may be an indicator of poor quality or improved early detection and access to more timely intensive clinical care. The challenge is how to operationally define avoidable or unnecessary ED use or inpatient psychiatric care. This task raises questions related to who is to be held accountable (ie, health plan, hospital, physician) and limitations of existing data sources to identify potential target areas for

(continued on next page)

Table 3
(continued)

Methodologic Challenges	Implications for Program Evaluation
	prevention (ie, third-payer policies that may impede timely filling of medication prescription following hospital discharge).
Patient-level Independent Variables	
Baseline clinical severity varies by patient	Baseline data should include generally accepted broad indicators of clinical severity (ie, prior inpatient psychiatric hospitalizations, prior suicide attempts, comorbid disorders (physical, mental) to build capacity for case-mix adjustment.
Baseline psychosocial complexity varies by patient	Baseline data ideally should include indicators of psychosocial complexity (eg, adverse childhood exposures, parental risk factors, social determinants of health) to build capacity to adjust for factors that may influence child clinical outcomes but are beyond the control of the provider, clinic, agency, or health plan.
Comorbidities and psychosocial complexity may vary over time	Periodic assessment of change in common comorbid conditions (eg, substance use: new onset, continued, relapse, remission) and social determinants of health (ie, removal from home, family homelessness, parental unemployment) could build capacity to assess contextual factors that may explain lack of improvement or worsening of clinical outcomes despite delivery of recommended care or more intensive treatment.
Provider-level Independent Variables	
Variation in training and disciplines	Obtain baseline information on providers that may be influential in type of care and how care is delivered: • Discipline • Years of clinical experience

(continued on next page)

Table 3
(continued)

Methodologic Challenges	Implications for Program Evaluation
Variation in provider case load	Report average provider caseload but also consider creating study variables that may stratify provider caseloads that are administratively meaningful, especially if preliminary data suggests there are relatively consistent differences by provider. Consider feasibility to adjust for patient clustering by provider in the data analysis.
Variation in extent of multi-disciplinary team integration	Extent of contact with multidisciplinary team members by vary by patient and over time by patient. Roles within the mental health team may vary by clinic care model and change over time. As mental health teams mature, task shifting may occur, such as: • Primary care provider assumes lead for psychotropic medication treatment following stabilization by referred psychiatrist. • Crisis mental health team may reduce involvement of law enforcement
Clinic-level Independent Variables	
Variation in organizational culture and climate	Organizational climate and culture may be influential in successfully delivering recommended care and is often understudied.
Variation in staff mix and turn-over	Number of persons employed by role, full-time equivalents by role, extent of match in sociodemographic characteristics with community served, and staff turn-over are examples of factors at the staffing level which may influence the quality of care delivered.

(continued on next page)

Table 3 (continued)	
Methodologic Challenges	**Implications for Program Evaluation**
System-level Independent Variables	
Variation in care models within or across clinics	How care is delivered may substantially differ by clinic or mental health programs within clinics, making it problematic to compare clinical improvement across clinics or programs. Work flow analyses are useful tools to operationalize clinic work flows to identify common and unique elements of care models. A relatively large number of comparable care models (ie, telehealth-enhanced vs usual care) with ideally similar organizational (ie, publicly-funded) and patient characteristics would be needed to test variation in quality of care by type of care model.
Variation in number of clinics within an organization	Baseline survey data from clinic administrators and providers can be used to describe the health care system to be evaluated and provide rationale for testing variation in quality by shared organizational characteristics. Statistical analysis may include adjustment for clustering at the clinic level within a closed health care system or agency.

Abbreviations: ED, emergency department.

individually link with data from other child-serving care sectors (eg, schools, child welfare, or juvenile justice), reducing the capacity to examine the association between receipt of recommended care in publicly funded outpatient mental health care and improved societal child outcomes such as reduction in rates of removal from home or school failure.[17,55,56]

Following selection of a data source(s), statistical consultation should ideally be sought out early to clarify the study design and troubleshoot costly errors that will affect data quality and interpretation. Various study designs and methods, including combining quantitative and qualitative data, could be used. However, the key is a priori matching the study design and methods to the research questions. If provided with several years of claims data, for example, is it feasible to conduct a cross-sectional study that combines data across years. Alternatively, is the research question better addressed if following a cohort of children or youth over time, retrospectively or prospectively? How will new-onset cases be defined? Likewise, the parameters for developing the final sample should be specified a priori. Are children from racial/ethnic minority groups adequately represented to test for health care disparities? Can insurance status be held constant, and if so, what are the trade-offs (eg, generalizability)?

Clinical outcomes can be conceptualized as proximal, corresponding to receipt of recommended care, and distal, corresponding to clinical outcomes, to build capacity to measure the extent recommended care is delivered prior to examining the relationship to clinical outcomes. Challenges remain on how to operationally define receipt of recommended care that aligns with treatment guidelines, and operational definitions for the data source will likely identify limitations that have implications for data interpretation. In addition, a child's episode of care should be explicitly defined, which may also identify limitations in the data source of how the index start and end date can be defined. Implementation of recommended care also varies. Change in clinical outcomes in either direction (or stability) may be influenced by how recommended care is delivered.[57]

In addition, most symptom rating scales for children were originally designed to detect need for a mental health evaluation. There is sparse evidence to support the reliability and clinical validity of mental health screening measures if used as a clinical outcome measure in community-based mental health programs, especially for children, youth, and their parents whose primary language is not English.[42] In anticipation of disagreement between informants, a sensitivity analysis that explores variation by combined, parent-only, and youth-only reported symptoms should be part of the preliminary data analyses.

Data attrition, particularly in community-based populations, is especially a problem when monitoring clinical outcomes over time. Data may be missing at baseline, and prescribed follow-up time points, time points for collecting follow-up rating scales, may not align with a child's appointment. Additionally, there is a selection bias when follow-up outcome data depend on service user data. If clinical outcome data are missing among children who drop out of care, it is impossible to tell if a brief intervention at baseline led to no further need for clinical care or poor continuity of care related to persistent or worsening of target symptoms. Continued care with little change in clinical outcomes may also signal the need for on-going care of a chronic condition that could be classified as acceptable care.[18] During data analysis, statistical consultation on approaches to address missing data problems (eg, multiple imputation or propensity score analysis) is warranted. Among programs that routinely collect rating scale data, methods may vary, and extent of missing data may differ by data collection method. Little is known how data collected by entry on a tablet, patient portal use, or paper survey as part of the patient registration process influence data quality. Thus, for program evaluations that combine clinical outcome data across multiple sources, exploratory analyses should be conducted to assess potential selection bias.

In addition, there is much interest in linking the receipt of recommended mental health care to the reduction of more costly care, such as emergency department use and inpatient psychiatric hospitalization.[58–61] The challenge, however, is defining avoidable or unnecessary use. Repeated use of these more expensive interventions may be related to poor access or quality of outpatient mental health care or an indicator that there was better detection of clinical need for more intensive treatment because of receiving continuous outpatient mental health care.

Independent variables can be conceptualized at the patient, provider, clinic, agency, and system level. Patient clinical characteristics are often used to adjust for case mix. In addition to clinical severity, data sources should be explored for indicators of psychosocial complexity (eg, poverty, foster care placement, or parental incarceration) to build capacity of how social determinants may influence quality of care.

Examples of provider-level differences that may influence care delivery include training, discipline, caseload, and extent of team integration. At the clinic level, examples are variation in organizational culture and climate and staffing.[62,63] At the system level, some examples of study variables are types of care models and number of clinics within the organization.[64] **Table 3** is not comprehensive but instead demonstrates some of the nuances in study design and methods necessary to build in capacity to interpret performance measurement data.

Tier 3: National Level

At the national level (tier 3), the main purpose is to monitor change in adherence rates to national quality measures (see **Table 1**). The core sets of quality measures are used to assess the quality of care provided by states to Medicaid and CHIP beneficiaries. State reporting on a uniform set of measures is envisioned to facilitate state and national analyses and track performance over time. The proposed mechanism of change is public reporting on quality measure adherence rates will drive quality improvement by identifying target areas that state Medicaid agencies can be held accountable to address. Incremental increases in measure adherence rates over time are interpreted as improvement in quality of care.

In the 2020 child core set, 4 quality measures are related to child mental health (**Table 4**). Two of the measures are from the initial core set and thus have additional data to track improvement over time.[8] The original 2 measures are related to follow-up care for stimulant medication treatment for children with attention deficit hyperactivity disorder (ADHD) and follow-up care after hospitalization for mental illness at 7 and 30 days. The newly added measures focus on trial of any first-line, broadly defined psychosocial care prior to prescription of an antipsychotic medication and metabolic monitoring for children and adolescents on antipsychotic medication. The data sources for these measures are predominantly administrative, and thus adherence rates indicate the extent recommended care processes are documented and/or billed. Details of the technical specifications are publicly available.[65] The core set is reviewed annually, and measures are selected to capture of wide breadth of disorders and care processes.

Yet despite national use, scientific evidence supporting the clinical validity of these measures is sparse,[14,15] consistent with adult mental health quality measures,[13,17,66] and state-reported adherence rates vary widely. Using reported adherence rates from state Medicaid agencies across 40 states,[67] the national average was 48% of children with a new stimulant medication prescription had at least 1 follow-up visit in the first 30 days. The mean percentage varied widely by states, ranging from 13.9% in Iowa to 66.7% in Wyoming, which cautiously reported challenges in tracking continuous enrollment, which is required in the measure specifications. For the C&M phase, an average of 58.6% of children nationally had at least 2 follow-up visits, ranging from an average of 34.4% in Colorado to 97.5% in Alabama. Overall, the average improvement in adherence to this measure was slightly less than 6% for both phases.

For the follow-up visit after hospitalization for mental illness measure, on average of 47.5% of children nationally had a follow-up visit within 7 days of discharge, and 66.7% had at least 1 visit within 30 days of discharge. Statewide variation was wide, ranging from 6.4% in Alaska to 88.9% in Alabama for the 7-day follow-up visit and 28.1% to 93.2% in these respective states for the 30-day follow-up visit. Since fiscal year 2012, the mean adherence rate for the 7 day follow-up decreased slightly by 2.5%, and there was little change in the difference in the 30-day follow-up visit rate (−0.2) over the past 5 years. Data on publicly reported state adherence rates for the

Table 4
National child behavioral health quality measures in 2020 Child Core Set

NQF #	Steward	Measure Description	Data Source(s)
0108	NCQA	Follow-Up Care for Children (6–12 y) Prescribed ADHD Medication Percentage of children newly prescribed attention-deficit/hyperactivity disorder (ADHD) medication who had at least three follow-up care visits within a 10-month period, one of which was within 30 d of when the first ADHD medication was dispensed. Two rates are reported. Initiation Phase: Percentage of children ages 6–12 as of the Index Prescription Start Date (IPSD) with an ambulatory prescription dispensed for ADHD medication, who had one follow-up visit with practitioner with prescribing authority during the 30-d Initiation Phase. Continuation and Maintenance (C&M) Phase: Percentage of children ages 6–12 as of the IPSD with an ambulatory prescription dispensed for ADHD medication who remained on the medication for at least 210 d and who, in addition to the visit in the Initiation Phase, had at least two follow-up visits with a practitioner within 270 d (9 mo) after the Initiation Phase ended. Numerator: Among children newly prescribed ADHD medication, those who had timely and continuous follow-up visits. Denominator: Children 6–12 y of age newly prescribed ADHD medication.	Administrative EHR
0576	NCQA	Follow-Up After Hospitalization for Mental Illness Percentage of discharges for children ages 6–17 who were hospitalized for treatment of selected mental illness or intentional self-harm diagnoses and who had a follow-up visit with a mental health practitioner. Two rates are reported: Percentage of discharges for which the child received follow-up within 30 d after discharge. Percentage of discharges for which the child received follow-up within 7 d after discharge. Numerator: An outpatient visit, intensive outpatient visit or partial hospitalization with a mental health practitioner within 30 d after discharge. Include outpatient visits, intensive outpatient visits or partial hospitalizations that occur on the date of discharge. Numerator: An outpatient visit, intensive outpatient visit or partial hospitalization with a mental health practitioner within 7 d after discharge. Include outpatient visits, intensive outpatient visits or partial hospitalizations that occur on the date of discharge. Denominator (for both time points): Patients 6 y and older as of the date of discharge who were discharged from an acute inpatient setting (including acute care psychiatric facilities) with a principal diagnosis of mental illness during the first 11 mo of the measurement year (eg, January 1 to December 1).	Administrative

(continued on next page)

Table 4 (*continued*)			
NQF #	**Steward**	**Measure Description**	**Data Source(s)**
2801	NCQA	Use of First-Line Psychosocial Care for Children and Adolescents on Antipsychotics Percentage of children and adolescents ages 1–17 who had a new prescription for an antipsychotic medication and had documentation of psychosocial care as first-line treatment. Numerator: Children and adolescents from the denominator who had psychosocial care as first-line treatment prior to (or immediately following) a new prescription of an antipsychotic. Denominator: Children and adolescents who had a new prescription of an antipsychotic medication for which they do not have a U.S Food and Drug Administration primary indication.	Administrative
2800	NCQA	Metabolic Monitoring for Children and Adolescents on Antipsychotics Percentage of children and adolescents with ongoing antipsychotic medication use who had metabolic testing during the year. Numerator: At least one test for blood glucose or HbA1c and at least one test for LDL-C or cholesterol during the measurement year. Denominator: Children and adolescents age 1–17 y who have had two or more antipsychotic medications dispensed on separate dates of service during the measurement year.	Administrative

Abbreviations: ADHD, attention deficit/hyperactivity disorder; EHR, electronic health record; NCQA, National Committee on Quality Assurance; NQF, National Quality Forum.

remaining national child behavioral health measures are limited given that they are relatively new to the 2020 child core set.

Overall, these publicly reported adherence rates by states should be interpreted cautiously, because methods for data collection and reporting varied widely by state.[66] States differed by types of public insurance (eg, Medicaid: fee for service, managed care, primary care case management, CHIP), data capture approach, operational definitions of some of the specifications, and whether they reported data from the state's external quality review organization. Nevertheless, these findings suggest that development of more standardized methods for data collection, analysis, and reporting is needed to more accurately compare quality measure adherence rates by state. Federal investment in research is needed to further refine child behavioral health quality measures to improve clinical validity and identify predictors of significant change in adherence rates.[2,3,13,15–17]

Some of the implications for data interpretation of the national quality measure adherence rates are summarized in **Table 5**. All 4 national quality measures for child mental health care were originally from the Healthcare Effectiveness Data and Information Set (HEDIS) developed by the National Committee for Quality Assurance, a national leader in health care system accreditation. Thus, the measures were developed with the intention to assess quality of care at the health plan level. Examples of the

Table 5
Measurement-based care at the State Medicaid agency level (Tier 3): methodologic challenges and implications for data interpretation by national quality measure

Methodologic Challenges	Implications for Data Interpretation
Follow-Up Care for Children (6–12 y) Prescribed ADHD Medication	
Developed for use at the health plan level.	Not easily adapted to examine quality at the provider, clinic or hospital level.
Restricted to children ages 6–12 y	Unable to comment on ADHD medication treatment for teens or adults.
Relies on prescription fill rates using adjudicated pharmacy claims data.	Medication prescription persistence does not equate to medication adherence.
The prescriber may be a psychiatrist, primary care physician, or physician assistant.	Unable to differentiate whether rates vary by provider type. In integrated care models, there may be shifting of the provider within a child's episode of care.
The C&M phase excludes a substantial proportion of children who do not meet criteria for continuous medication treatment.	The denominators change between the initiation and C&M phase. If only the rates are reported for each phase, it is difficult to assess the actual proportion of children who do not receive on-going medication treatment which is common target area for quality improvement.
A minimum of one follow-up visit and one telephone contact with a prescriber over a 9 month period is not sufficient to monitor medication safety, especially for a Schedule II drug.	Even if a child passes this measure, questions are raised regarding whether medication safety is being adequately monitored, especially for a Schedule II drug. The Department of Justice limits multiple prescriptions to the combined effect of allowing a patient to receive, over time, up to a 90-d supply of a particular schedule II controlled substance.
Treatment is limited to medication treatment.	Unable to assess whether children or parents are also receiving evidence-based therapies, such as parent training, or timing of trial of an evidence-based therapy prior to trial of stimulant medication.
Follow-Up After Hospitalization for Mental Illness	
Developed for use at the health plan level.	Applying this measure to a health care system, hospital or clinic presents an attribution problem. Even if discharge planning includes follow-up care in a community-based mental health program, the inpatient provider, team, or hospital may not have any authority or power to improve access to and timeliness of follow-up outpatient mental health care.

(continued on next page)

Table 5
(continued)

Methodologic Challenges	Implications for Data Interpretation
Primary care providers are excluded.	Contact with primary care providers for follow-up care for mental health condition is underestimated. With increases in pediatric integrated care models, rates of measure adherence may appear to decline.
Type of mental health practitioner may include a physician, psychologist, registered nurse, clinical social worker, marriage and family therapist or professional counselor.	Among children who pass this measure, it is impossible to assess type of provider. For children discharged with medication prescriptions, timely access to a psychiatrist cannot be assessed.
The follow-up visit may be for an outpatient visit, an intensive outpatient encounter or partial hospitalization, a community mental health center visit, electroconvulsive therapy, an observation visit, transitional care management service with a mental health practitioner, or telehealth visit.	Unable to assess if care provided during a follow-up visit aligned with a child's clinical needs.
Follow-up contact with outpatient mental health care does not include services delivered on the hospital discharge date.	Contact with an on-site mental health clinic on day of hospital discharge is not counted, but could be influential in the likelihood to successful receive timely outpatient mental health care.
Use of First-Line Psychosocial Care for Children and Adolescents on Antipsychotics	
Developed for use at the health plan level.	Unable to assess performance at the provider or hospital level.
Lack of procedure codes in administrative data for evidence-based therapies.	Unable to assess whether an adequate trial of an evidence-based therapy was provided prior to starting antipsychotic medication treatment. Unable to assess whether child is receiving special education services that may include evidence-based therapies.
Clinical indications for starting antipsychotic medication are not specified in administrative data and may not be consistently documented in progress notes.	Unable to assess whether concerns about safety (eg, reduction in self-injurious behaviors or aggression) were related to starting antipsychotic medication prior to trial of individual, family or group therapy. Record abstraction is time- and labor-intensive and there may be a documentation effect. Research is needed to apply advances in EHR data science to assess quality measure adherence.

(continued on next page)

Table 5 (continued)	
Methodologic Challenges	**Implications for Data Interpretation**
Metabolic Monitoring for Children and Adolescents on Antipsychotics	
Developed for use at the health plan level.	Unable to assess performance at the provider or hospital level.
Timing of either laboratory test may occur any time during the measurement year and may not align with baseline or follow-up medication visits.	Unable to assess whether metabolic screening was at baseline or follow-up to assess medication safety monitoring during antipsychotic medication treatment.

Abbreviations: ADHD, attention deficit/hyperactivity disorder; C&M, continuation and maintenance; EHR, electronic health record.

implication for data interpretation for each measure related to this restriction are provided.

In addition, for the follow-up care for ADHD measure, the age range is restricted to children ages 6 to 12, limiting the capacity to comment on quality of care for youth or adults with ADHD. Although stimulant medication prescription persistence is poor in managed care Medicaid programs,[18] this measure does not directly report the substantial proportion of children who do not receive ongoing stimulant medication treatment. Concerns about adequate medication safety monitoring have also been raised, given that a minimum of 1 follow-up visit and a telephone contact with a prescriber during a 9-month period is sufficient to pass, and this level of contact is inconsistent with federal rules for prescription of Schedule II drugs.[68,69]

For the follow-up after hospitalization for mental illness, the attribution problem is demonstrated. Even if hospital discharge planning includes a referral to outpatient mental health care, the provider, inpatient team, or hospital may not have the authority or power to improve access to or timeliness of follow-up care. As more care is provided in integrated pediatric care models, adherence rates may be increasing underestimated, because primary care providers are not included in the specifications for allowed providers. Contact with follow-up care is also broadly defined, making it impossible to assess whether care provided aligned with the child's clinical needs (eg, medication follow-up with a psychiatrist).

For the 2 measures related to antipsychotic medication, lack of procedure codes make it impossible to assess whether evidence-based therapy was provided prior to medication trial or there was an adequate trial of therapy prior to starting antipsychotic medication. Conclusions regarding appropriate use of antipsychotic medication also cannot be made. For example, starting an antipsychotic medication to reduce self-injurious behaviors or severe agitation cannot be determined from solely the adherence rate. For the metabolic monitoring measure, the timing for at least one of the laboratory tests is purposively broad to include any time during the measurement year, which does not equate to obtaining baseline and follow-up laboratory testing at prescribed time points for children on more long-term antipsychotic medication that is consistent with treatment guidelines.

SUMMARY

Although the triple aim of the National Quality Strategy purposively combines population levels, the specification of the population level to apply MBC is important. To demonstrate this, population levels are conceptualized at the individual (tier 1), clinical aggregate (tier 2), and national level (tier 3). Under this conceptual framework, the population level has implications for the purpose, proposed target mechanisms that drive quality improvement, methodologic challenges, and implications for program evaluation and data interpretation. Some of the detailed methodologic issues and their implications underscore the complexity of developing a data infrastructure that ideally includes safeguards against premature judgements of a patient's treatment resistance, or provider, clinic, hospital or agency, or state Medicaid performance. Without these safeguards in place, descriptive data on adherence rates to recommended care processes or change in clinical outcomes should be viewed as preliminary, and used to support the Institute of Medicine's national call for federally funded research almost 3 decades ago.

DISCLOSURE

The author has nothing to disclose.

REFERENCES

1. Conway PH, Clancy C. Transformation of health care at the front line. JAMA 2009; 310:763–5.
2. Institute of Medicine. Crossing the quality chasm: a new health system for the 21st century. Washington, DC: National Academies Press; 2001.
3. Institute of Medicine. Improving the quality of health care for mental and substance use conditions. Washington, DC: National Academies Press; 2006.
4. Berwick DM, Nolan TW, Whittington J. The triple aim: care, health, and cost. Health Aff 2008;27(3):759–69.
5. Patient Protection and Affordable Care Act, 42 U.S.C. § 18001 (2010). Patient Protection and Affordable Care Act, 42 U.S.C. § 18001 et seq. 2010.
6. Children's Health Insurance Program. Reauthorization Act of 2009. Available at: https://www.congress.gov/bill/111th-congress/house-bill/2. Accessed January 2, 2020.
7. Centers for Medicare and Medicaid. Keeping America Healthy: July 2018 Medicaid & CHIP enrollment data highlights. Available at: https://www.medicaid.gov/medicaid/program-information/medicaid-and-chip-enrollment-data/report-highlights/index.html. Accessed January 2, 2020.
8. Centers for Medicare & Medicaid Services. 2020 Core Set of Children's Health Care Quality Measures for Medicaid and CHIP (Child Core Set). Available at: https://www.medicaid.gov/medicaid/quality-of-care/downloads/performance-measurement/2020-child-core-set.pdf. Accessed December 10, 2019.
9. H.R. 1892 One Hundred Fifteenth Congress of the United States of America. Available at: https://www.congress.gov/115/bills/hr1892/BILLS-115hr1892enr.pdf. Accessed January 2, 2020.
10. Hermann RC, Chan JA, Zazzali JL, et al. Aligning measurement-based quality improvement with implementation of evidence-based practices. Adm Policy Ment Health 2006;33(6):636–45.
11. Ranallo PA, Kilbourne AM, Whatley AS, et al. Behavioral health information technology: from chaos to clarity. Health Aff 2016;35:1106–13.
12. Prince M, Yuen EK, Goetter EM, et al. MHealth: a mechanism to deliver more accessible, more effective mental health care. Clin Psychol Psychother 2014; 21:427–36.

13. Pincus HA, Spaeth-Rublees B, Watkins K. The case for measuring quality in mental health and substance abuse care. Health Aff 2011;30(4):730–6.
14. Edgcomb JB, Zima B. Machine learning, natural language processing, and the electronic health record: innovations in mental health services research. Psychiatr Serv 2019;70(4):346–9.
15. Zima BT, Murphy JM, Scholle SH, et al. National quality measures for child mental health care: background, progress and next steps. Pediatrics 2013;131:S38–49.
16. Zima BT, Edgcomb JB, Shugarman SA. National child mental health quality measures: adherence rates and extent of evidence for clinical validity. Curr Psychiatry Rep 2019;21(1):6.
17. Kilbourne AM, Keyser D, Pincus HA. Challenges and opportunities in measuring the quality of mental health care. Can J Psychiatry 2010;55(9):549–57.
18. Zima BT, Bussing R, Tang L, et al. Quality of care for childhood attention-deficit/hyperactivity disorder in a managed care Medicaid program. J Am Acad Child Adolesc Psychiatry 2010;49(12):1225–37.
19. Cummings JR, Ji X, Allen L, et al. Racial and ethnic differences in ADHD treatment quality among Medicaid-enrolled youth. Pediatrics 2017;139(6):e20162444.
20. American Academy of Pediatrics. Mental Health Initiatives. Available at: https://www.aap.org/en-us/advocacy-and-policy/aap-health-initiatives/Mental-Health/Pages/default.aspx. Accessed December 19, 2019.
21. American Academy of Child and Adolescent Psychiatry. Policy statement on mental health screening in primary care. Available at: https://www.aacap.org/AACAP/Policy_Statements/2019/Mental-Health-Screening-Primary-Care.aspx. Accessed December 19, 2019.
22. American Academy of Child and Adolescent Psychiatry. Policy statement on suicide prevention. Available at: https://www.aacap.org/AACAP/Policy_Statements/2019/AACAP_Policy_Statement_on_Suicide_Prevention.aspx. Accessed December 19, 2019.
23. Fortney JC, Unützer J, Wrenn G, et al. A tipping point for measurement-based care. Psychiatr Serv 2016;68(2):179–88.
24. Liu FF, Cruz RA, Rockhill CM, et al. Mind the gap: considering disparities in implementing measurement-based care. J Am Acad Child Adolesc Psychiatry 2019;58(4):459–61.
25. Carlier IV, Meuldijk D, Van Vliet IM, et al. Routine outcome monitoring and feedback on physical or mental health status: evidence and theory. J Eval Clin Pract 2012;18(1):104–10.
26. Lambert MJ, Whipple JL, Hawkins EJ, et al. Is it time for clinicians to routinely track patient outcome? A meta-analysis. Clinical Psychology: Science and Practice PR 2003;10(3):288–301.
27. Frank E, Prien RF, Jarrett RB, et al. Conceptualization and rationale for consensus definitions of terms in major depressive disorder: remission, recovery, relapse, and recurrence. Arch Gen Psychiatry 1991;48(9):851–5.
28. Bickman L, Kelley SD, Breda C, et al. Effects of routine feedback to clinicians on mental health outcomes of youths: results of a randomized trial. Psychiatr Serv 2011;62(12):1423–9.
29. Liu FF, Adrian MC. Is treatment working? Detecting real change in the treatment of child and adolescent depression. J Am Acad Child Adolesc Psychiatry 2019;58(12):1157–64.
30. Jacobson NS, Truax P. Clinical significance: a statistical approach to defining meaningful change in psychotherapy research. J Consult Clin Psychol 1991;59(1):12–9.

31. Ignaszewski MJ, Waslick B. Update on randomized placebo-controlled trials in the past decade. J Child Adolesc Psychopharmacol 2018;28(10):668–75.
32. Schweren L, Hoekstra P, Van Lieshout M, et al. Long-term effects of stimulant treatment on ADHD symptoms, social–emotional functioning, and cognition. Psychol Med 2019;49(2):217–23.
33. Wren FJ, Bridge JA, Birmaher B. Screening for childhood anxiety symptoms in primary care: integrating child and parent reports. J Am Acad Child Adolesc Psychiatry 2004;43(11):1364–71.
34. Kazdin AE. Informant Variability in the Assessment of Childhood Depression. In: Reynolds WM, Johnston HF, editors. Handbook of depression in children and adolescents. Issues in Clinical Child Psychology. Boston: Springer; 1994.
35. Lifford KJ, Harold GT, Thapar A. Parent–child relationships and ADHD symptoms: a longitudinal analysis. J Abnorm Child Psychol 2008;36(2):285–96.
36. Lewandowski RE, O'Connor B, Bertagnolli A, et al. Screening for and diagnosis of depression among adolescents in a large health maintenance organization. Psychiatr Serv 2016;67(6):636–41.
37. O'Connor BC, Lewandowski RE, Rodriguez S, et al. Usual care for adolescent depression from symptom identification through treatment initiation. JAMA Pediatr 2016;170(4):373–80.
38. Norman S, Dean S, Hansford L, et al. Clinical practitioner's attitudes towards the use of routine outcome monitoring within child and adolescent mental health services: a qualitative study of two child and adolescent mental health services. Clin Child Psychol Psychiatry 2014;19(4):576–95.
39. Batty MJ, Moldavsky M, Foroushani PS, et al. Implementing routine outcome measures in child and adolescent mental health services: from present to future practice. Child Adolesc Ment Health 2013;18(2):82–7.
40. O'Donnell AN, Williams M, Kilbourne AM. Overcoming roadblocks: current and emerging reimbursement strategies for integrated mental health services in primary care. J Gen Intern Med 2013;28(12):1667–72.
41. Unützer J, Park M. Strategies to improve the management of depression in primary care. Prim Care 2012;39(2):415–31.
42. Zima BT, Marti FA, Lee CE, et al. Selection of a child clinical outcome measure for statewide use in publicly funded outpatient mental health programs. Psychiatr Serv 2019;70(5):381–8.
43. Agency for Healthcare Research and Quality. Patient self-management support programs: an evaluation: program evaluation. Available at: https://www.ahrq.gov/research/findings/final-reports/ptmgmt/evaluation.html. Accessed January 2, 2020.
44. Richardson LP, Ludman E, McCauley E, et al. Collaborative care for adolescents with depression in primary care: a randomized clinical trial. JAMA 2014;312(8):809–16.
45. Hoagwood KE, Olin SS, Horwitz S, et al. Scaling up evidence-based practices for children and families in New York State: toward evidence-based policies on implementation for state mental health systems. J Clin Child Adolesc Psychol 2014;43(2):145–57.
46. Seibert J, Fields S, Fullerton CA, et al. Use of quality measures for Medicaid behavioral health services by state agencies: implications for health care reform. Psychiatr Serv 2015;66:585–91.
47. Minnesota Community Measurement Program. 2018 Minnesota health care quality report, detailed medical group and clinic level tables. Available at: https://

mncm.org/wp-content/uploads/2019/02/mncm-quality-report-2019-appendix-tables-depression.pdf. Accessed January 2, 2020.

48. State of California, Legislative Analyst Office. Realignment revisited: an evaluation of the 1991 experiment in state-county relations. 2001. Available at: http://www.lao.ca.gov/2001/realignment/020601_realignment.html. Accessed January 2, 2020.

49. State of California, Legislative Analyst Office. Mental health realignment, January 26, 2011. Available at: http://www.lao.ca.gov/handouts/Health/2011/Mental_Health_1_26_11.pdf. Accessed January 2, 2020.

50. Arnquist S, Harbage P. A complex case: public mental health delivery and financing in California. Oakland (CA): California HealthCare Foundation; 2013. Available at: https://www.chcf.org/publication/a-complex-case-public-mental-health-delivery-and-financing-in-california/. Accessed January 2, 2020.

51. Performance outcomes system statute: welfare and institutions code, section 14707.5. Available at: https://codes.findlaw.com/ca/welfare-and-institutions-code/wic-sect-14707-5.html./. Accessed January 2, 2020.

52. Meisel J. Mental Health Services Oversight and Accountability Commission Evaluation Master Plan. Available at: http://archive.mhsoac.ca.gov/Evaluations/docs/EvaluationMasterPlan_Final_040413.pdf. Accessed January 2, 2020.

53. Little Hoover Commission. Promises still to keep: a decade of the mental health services act. 2015. Available at: https://mentalillnesspolicy.org/wp-content/uploads/LittleHooverCommish.pdf. Accessed January 2, 2020.

54. Ashwood JS, Kataoka SH, Eberhart NK, et al. Evaluation of the Mental Health Services Act in Los Angeles County: implementation and outcomes for key programs. Santa Monica (CA): RAND Corporation; 2018. Available at: https://www.rand.org/pubs/research_reports/RR2327.html. Accessed January 2, 2020.

55. Deans KJ, Minneci PC, Nacion KM, et al. Health care quality measures for children and adolescents in foster care: feasibility testing in electronic records. BMC Pediatr 2018;18(1):79.

56. Geierstanger SP, Amaral G, Mansour M, et al. School-based health centers and academic performance: research, challenges, and recommendations. J Sch Health 2004;74(9):347–52.

57. Proctor EK, Powell BJ, McMillen JC. Implementation strategies: recommendations for specifying and reporting. Implement Sci 2013;8(1):139.

58. Plemmons G, Hall M, Doupnik S, et al. Hospitalization for suicide ideation or attempt: 2008–2015. Pediatrics 2018;141(6):e20172426.

59. Gay JC, Agrawal R, Auger KA, et al. Rates and impact of potentially preventable readmissions at children's hospitals. J Pediatr 2015;166(3):613–9.

60. Bardach NS, Coker TR, Zima BT, et al. Common and costly hospitalizations for pediatric mental health disorders. Pediatrics 2014;133(4):602–9.

61. Zima BT, Rodean J, Hall M, et al. Psychiatric disorders and trends in resource use in pediatric hospitals. Pediatrics 2016;138(5):e20160909.

62. Aarons GA, Glisson C, Green PD, et al. The organizational social context of mental health services and clinician attitudes toward evidence-based practice: a United States national study. Implement Sci 2012;7(1):56.

63. Glisson C, Dukes D, Green P. The effects of the ARC organizational intervention on caseworker turnover, climate, and culture in children's service systems. Child Abuse Negl 2006;30(8):855–80.

64. Coker TR, Porras-Javier L, Zhang L, et al. A telehealth-enhanced referral process in pediatric primary care: a cluster randomized trial. Pediatrics 2019;143(3):e20182738.

65. Centers for Medicare & Medicaid Services, Center for Medicaid and CHIP Services, core set of children's health care quality measures for Medicaid and CHIP (child core set) technical specifications and resource manual for federal fiscal year 2019 reporting. 2019. Available at: https://www.medicaid.gov/medicaid/quality-of-care/downloads/medicaid-and-chip-child-core-set-manual.pdf. Accessed January 3, 2020.
66. Kilbourne AM, Beck K, Spaeth-Rublee B, et al. Measuring and improving the quality of mental health care: a global perspective. World Psychiatry 2018; 17(1):30–8.
67. Centers for Medicare and Medicaid. 2017 annual reporting on the quality care for children in Medicaid and CHIP (FFY 2016): performance on the child core set measures for FFY 2016, 2015, 2014, 2013 (zip file). Available at: https://www.medicaid.gov/medicaid/quality-of-care/performance-measurement/child-core-set/index.html. Accessed January 3, 2020.
68. Zima BT, Norquist GS, Altchuler SI, et al. Office visits to monitor stimulant medication safety and efficacy: recommended care. J Am Acad Child Adolesc Psychiatry 2018;57(6):438–9.
69. Department of Justice, Drug Enforcement Administration, Diversion Control Division. Issuance of multiple prescriptions for Schedule II controlled Substances. Available at: https://www.deadiversion.usdoj.gov/faq/mult_rx_faq.htm. Accessed January 3, 2020.

Using Measurement-Based Care Data in Population Health Management

Cody A. Hostutler, PhD[a,b], Ujjwal Ramtekkar, MD, MPE, MBA[c,d],*

KEYWORDS

- Pediatric • Primary care • Measurement-based care • Clinical registries
- Population health

KEY POINTS

- There is no evidence supporting screening alone as an effective intervention for improving mental health outcomes.
- Clinical registries informed by principles of measurement-based care and population health have been effective at improving outcomes in adults and with some pediatric physical health conditions, but little attention has been afforded to youth pediatric mental health registries in primary care.
- Clinical registries can range from a simple password-protected Excel file to complex, dynamic clinical registries integrated into electronic health records, and, despite barriers, should be used and evaluated in pediatric mental health care within primary care.

Identifying children with developmental, behavioral, and emotional needs in childhood is an important component of comprehensive primary care service delivery. Approximately half of all lifetime mental health conditions begin by age 14,[1] and the average time between symptom onset and treatment is almost 11 years.[2] Although there is a myriad of factors contributing to this significant delay in obtaining treatment, 1 important factor is the difficulty primary care providers (PCPs) have in identifying the presence of mental health disorder during their brief encounters.[3] Sheldrick and colleagues[4] found that the sensitivity of PCPs' identification of mental health conditions is approximately 14% to 54%, and specificity ranged from 69% to100% when relying on clinical judgment alone. Although use of screening tools can improve early identification,[5] there is limited evidence that screening alone leads to improved outcomes.[6,7] Even when enhancing screening procedures to include alerting PCPs to

[a] Department of Pediatric Psychology and Neuropsychology, Nationwide Children's Hospital; [b] Department of Pediatrics, The Ohio State University; [c] Department of Child and Adolescent Psychiatry, Nationwide Children's Hospital; [d] Department of Psychiatry, The Ohio State University
* Corresponding author. 700 Children's Drive, Columbus, OH 43205.
E-mail address: Ujjwal.ramtekkar@nationwidechildrens.org

Child Adolesc Psychiatric Clin N Am 29 (2020) 733–741
https://doi.org/10.1016/j.chc.2020.06.010
1056-4993/20/© 2020 Elsevier Inc. All rights reserved.

childpsych.theclinics.com

the positive screen and providing them with guideline-concordant treatment recommendations, screened patients do not fair better than those who were not screened.[8] Thus, screening is important to enhance the identification of mental health concerns within primary care, but screening alone is an insufficient intervention to improve outcomes for patients.

There are numerous barriers limiting the effectiveness of screening alone including the unavailability of mental health providers, cost of care, long delays for services, high no-show and drop-out rates, stigma around mental health conditions, limited training and comfort of PCPs, and poor communication between primary care and specialty mental health professionals.[9–11] Although the solution to this problem will need to be multifactorial, mental health registries have been a helpful solution to improve outcomes in adult populations.[6] Despite the increasing use of registries in adult care, they have been slow to develop in pediatrics. Bottino and colleagues[12] demonstrated that the use of clinical registries in pediatric primary care is feasible and effective to increase immunization rates, but there has been limited development and evaluation of registries for pediatric mental health conditions in primary care. Thus, the purpose of this article is to provide an overview of clinical registries as a needed measurement-based care tool in primary care, review the limited existing research on the use of registries to address mental health needs in pediatric primary care, identify current barriers to the use of pediatric registries, and to outline important steps to develop the use of registries in pediatric primary care.

WHAT ARE CLINICAL REGISTRIES?

Gliklich and colleagues[13] define health registries as "an organized system that uses observational study methods to collect uniform data (clinical or otherwise) to evaluate specified outcomes for a population defined by a particular disease, condition, or exposure, and that serves a predetermined scientific, clinical, or policy purpose." Health registries can be used for multiple purposes including clinical care, research, population monitoring, and health care policy development. Simply stated, clinical registries are databases that track clinically relevant data over time to monitor and improve clinical outcomes. The chronic care model[14] and collaborative mental health care models[15] cite the use of clinical registries as a core component of effective management of chronic health care needs including mental health needs. Clinical registries integrate principles of measurement-based care (MBC), population health, and clinical health informatics in order to collect and track data across multiple levels of analysis (eg, patient, provider, clinic, and population).

At the individual patient level, clinical registries use principles of MBC to track individual patient outcomes and guide treatment. The goal of MBC is "to enhance precision and consistency in disease assessment, tracking, and treatment to achieve optimal outcomes."[16] Clinical registries serve as the tool that collects and stores these clinically relevant data over time within an MBC framework. When using clinical judgment alone, mental health providers identify deterioration in approximately 1 in 5 patients who experience worsening symptoms[17] and are even poorer at identifying patients who are not worsening, but are not benefiting from treatment.[18] Frequently using rating scales to assess and track symptoms over time can prompt providers to change the treatment plan when patients are not appropriately responding to treatment and minimize the risk of clinical inertia.[19,20] Registries can also support referral tracking and identify patients who are lost to follow-up to ensure that patients do not fall through the cracks. When used in collaborative care or other integrated models, the registry can flag individual patients who are worsening or not responding within specific timeframes in order to alert the care team that consultation and support are indicated.

At the caseload level, clinical registries can track important program evaluation data including the average expected improvement for specific conditions, caseload size, clinical productivity, length of time in treatment, and average number of sessions until response or remission is achieved. If multiple providers or clinics are using the same registry, differences in treatment outcomes can be compared across users or groups to identify areas for further training and quality improvement for providers who are not achieving outcomes as well as others. Conversely, it is also helpful to identify emerging best practices when providers or clinics are able to achieve greater or faster treatment outcomes than other users within the registry.

Informed by principles of population health, clinical registries can also help identify, predict, and monitor treatment outcomes across defined populations. Population health focuses on the health outcomes of a group of individuals, including the distribution of such outcomes within the group.[21] Thus, health systems can use aggregated clinical registry data to monitor outcomes, compare outcomes across demographic groups, and create predictive analytics to better identify patients who will need care, at what level of care, and which treatment modality is best for which patients, and under what circumstances.[22] For example, clinical researchers can use the data to determine which patients are most and least likely to benefit from a particular treatment strategy, provider, or level of care. Predictive analysis using clinical registry data can also help stratify patient risk for important low incidence, population health outcomes such as youth suicide. At the population level, registries can also help to identify populations or geographic areas in need of further resources or support.

Although limited in the pediatric world, there are several examples of registries in the adult world.[23,24] Some of the technology and health informatics used in these adult registries can be helpful in the creation of youth registries; however, the measures included in adult registries typically are not validated or designed for pediatric populations. Further, because of important developmental differences between children and adults, predictive analytics derived from adult registries may not apply to youth. Thus, there is considerable value in understanding the ways in which pediatric-specific registries can be used to support the mental health of youth.

BARRIERS TO REGISTRIES IN PEDIATRIC PRIMARY CARE

There are several barriers to implementing mental health registries, and many are unique to pediatric populations. One major concern is that there are no widely distributed, commercially available clinical mental health registries for children. For example, the Advancing Integrated Mental Health Solutions (AIMS) Center, based at the University of Washington, offers a prepacked, "plug and play" type of registry for adults that can be used with adolescents. However, this registry only includes the Patient Health Questionnaire-9 item (PHQ9)[25] and Generalized Anxiety Disorder −7 items scale (GAD7),[26] and neither of these measures has been validated for children. Clinical mental health registries require significant complexity behind the scenes to make them user friendly. As such, even small modifications can require a significant amount of work, making customization difficult, time-consuming, and often cost-prohibitive on the rare occasion that organizations are willing to adapt or modify their registry programs to meet the needs of youth.[27] Thus, simply asking for new measures to be added to these commercially available adult mental health registries is often not an available solution at this time.

The fact that children are rapidly developing is another significant barrier to the creation of clinical pediatric mental health registries. Given this rapid development, registries need to include multiple versions of measures to assess the same condition over time. For example, a provider may need to use the preschool form of the Spence for children 3 to 6 years of age,[28] the school-age Spence[29] or SCARED[30] for school-aged children, and the GAD7[26] for adolescents and early adults. Although multi-informant assessment is often beneficial across the lifespan, it can be particularly important, and is often necessary, in the assessment of youth.[31] This adds another layer of complexity, as registries not only need to include multiple measures depending on age, but may also need to include measures for multiple informants including children, caregivers, and teachers. This compounds the amount of data that needs to be entered and stored, and makes the presentation and interpretation of registry data more complex.

These barriers are in addition to the general obstacles involved with developing and effectively using clinical behavioral health registries. For example, building, maintaining, and using a behavioral health registry typically requires technological, administrative, and clinical personnel.[32,33] Previous research supports the use of clinicians and care managers to effectively manage and use registries once they are developed.[23,34] However, steps need to be taken to ensure the quality of data, as input errors, inaccurate or incomplete data, and incorrectly registered patients can threaten the utility of the data.[32] Further, if the registry requires double documentation, this may be burdensome to clinicians and increase the probability of errors. To improve data quality, automated logic check algorithms can prevent out-of-range values and provide alerts for incomplete or outlying data.[33,35] Thus, clinical pediatric behavioral health registries can require a significant investment of time and money to develop and implement, and continued investment to maintain and troubleshoot technological and systems barriers.

WHAT IS KNOWN ABOUT BEHAVIORAL HEALTH REGISTRIES IN PEDIATRIC PRIMARY CARE?

There has been little published about pediatric behavioral health registries to date. Despite the importance of clinical registries in adult collaborative care for depression,[15] the pediatric collaborative care models developed for depression and anxiety have excluded the use of a formal clinical registry as part of their intervention.[36-38] However, there is increasing attention to the topic in recent years, particularly around the management of attention deficit hyperactivity disorder (ADHD). For example, Geltman and colleagues[39] found that when using a clinical registry to track administration of rating scales and frequency of visits, patients were 2 times more likely to have rating scale results documented in the medical record, and they observed a 29% increase in patients who attended the recommended number of visits during the project period. Similarly, Schwarzwald and colleagues[40] found that the use of an ADHD registry significantly increased the number of patients who followed up within 30 days of their initial prescription of ADHD medication. Although not a registry in and of itself, the ADHD Care Assistant includes an electronic survey tool to collect data from parents and teachers.[41] The ADHD Care Assistant also serves to facilitate communication between PCPs and schools and has an electronic health record module that tracks individual progress over time. Thus, the ADHD care assistant is a promising tool for obtaining ADHD data for the purpose of a registry, collaboration between professionals across settings, and tracking clinical outcomes over time.

One study was identified that included the use of 6 separate pediatric health registries in a pediatric setting (ie, ADHD, anxiety/depression, substance abuse, early intervention, and complex special health care needs [CSHCN] with a comorbid mental health diagnosis and a separate registry for CSHCN without a comorbid mental health diagnosis).[34] A licensed independent social worker (LISW) and parent partner/care coordinator provided intervention and managed the registry. The authors did not provide many specific details about how the registry was constructed and maintained. The registry used the Preschool Pediatric Symptom Checklist (P-PSC)[42] for children 1 to 3 years of age, Pediatric Symptom Checklist (PSC)[43] for children ages 4 to 13 years, the Patient Health Questionnaire-9 for Adolescents (PHQ9a)[44] to screen and monitor symptoms of depression for youth between 14 and 21 years of age, and the Vanderbilt[45] scales to diagnose and monitor treatment for ADHD. The authors found that use of the registry, colocated mental health provider, and parent partner/care coordinator resulted in significantly reduced total medical expenditures and emergency department visits. However, it is unclear the extent to which the registry or the in-clinic providers drove outcomes, and there was no counterfactual condition to attenuate the threat of history effects to internal validity. These emerging findings provide evidence that constructing and using a mental health registry is possible within primary care, and the initial evidence supports the utility; however, considerable more work is needed to understand how to build, use, maintain, and evaluate clinical registries for youth with mental health needs.

GETTING STARTED

Despite these barriers, there is significant promise in the application of clinical mental health registries to support behavioral health in pediatric populations. The authors recommend starting small, being strategic in the initial phases of development, and gradually building the complexity over time. There are comprehensive documents that describe the steps to designing and building a registry that provide details far beyond the scope of this article but serve as a good reference to guide development of pediatric mental health registries.[13] For the purposes of this article, the authors will synthesize these comprehensive documents into a useable framework for moving forward in deciding whether and how to develop clinical pediatric mental health registry.

The authors propose 5 general steps when considering and building a pediatric mental health registry. First, when planning a registry, it is important to articulate the reason for developing a clinical registry and the purpose it will serve. Although this step may seem obvious and be tempting to skip or quickly complete, it is important to be as specific and granular as possible, as this is the foundation from which everything else will be built. One should consider the broad range of conditions present in the youth served (eg, developmental, social determinants of health/ACEs, mental health, resilience, physical health) and the specific components of one's service delivery model or population that one wants to track. The authors also recommend thinking broadly about MBC to include not only clinical outcomes, but also important programmatic outcomes such as show rates, referral patterns, model fidelity metrics (eg, number of sessions attended if one is running a short-term intervention model), interventions used, as well as provider-level data to evaluate adoption and implementation fidelity metrics (eg, percent of possible patients seen or referred). A useful purpose goes beyond "to improve depression outcomes" to include definitions of which specific outcomes are important (eg, depressive symptoms on PHQ9, follow-through with referrals, number of depression-specific visits, and emergency room usage) and for whom (eg, the whole patient panel, those who screen positive on PHQ9, those with severe depression, patients with public insurance, or families with refugee status).

Second, it is important to determine if a registry is feasible and an appropriate method to achieve one's purpose. Determining whether the data needed already exists, whether there is already a method for collecting or storing this data from which one can extend, and whether the resources to not only build, but also maintain the registry are available. If one has a clear purpose and determines a clinical registry is both feasible and appropriate, step 3 is identifying key stakeholders and building a registry team. In pediatric primary care, the team may include a range of people including PCPs, integrated behavioral health consultants, care coordinators, nursing staff, check-in staff, family advisors, and informational technology support team members. This team will be essential in thinking through the needed data, efficient ways of collecting this data, and ongoing management and use of the registry.

Fourth, it will be important to develop an oversight plan and committee to ensure the quality and safety of the registry data and that the registry data is effectively being used only for its intended purpose (see Chorostowska-Wynimko and colleagues[33] for review of optimization of data quality and safety). Finally, the authors recommend using a quality improvement or implementation science approach to guide the development, maintenance, and use of the clinical registry such as the Plan-Do-Study-Act (PDSA)[46] approach.

It may be helpful to start with a simple, password-protected Excel documenting that tracks simple outcomes or focuses on one condition at a time. The AIMS center has a publicly available spreadsheet for the GAD7 and PHQ9 that can be used as-is or referenced as a model for the development of one's own registry (https://aims.uw.edu/resource-library/aims-caseload-tracker). Another option would be to leverage existing features in the EHR such as using flowsheets to track progress over time, creating patient lists, using searchable discrete data fields that can be systematically exported from EPIC, or built-in functions such as EPIC's Healthy Planet (https://www.epic.com/software#PopulationHealth). Health Insurance Portability and Accountability Act of 1996-compliant data capturing and storage systems such as REDCap can collect and store data in a secure way, include simple data summary tools, and can export into other types of files for more comprehensive analysis.[41] Using principles of MBC, one could include clinical decision-making support tools to increase fidelity to treatment standards.[24]

SUMMARY

Clinical registries are an important tool in the implementation of measurement-based care within primary care. Overall, there is limited information and evidence on the development and use of clinical registries for pediatric mental health care needs. However, there is a significant amount of evidence supporting their use in the adult world and with other pediatric chronic health conditions, and the evidence that does exist for pediatric mental health needs suggests that the use of clinical registries for youth may be feasible and improve outcomes. Although there is a significant need for future work in the development and evaluation of clinical registries for youth, they represent a powerful measure-based care tool for the advancement of pediatric mental health.

DISCLOSURE

The authors have nothing to disclose.

REFERENCES

1. Kessler RC, Berglund P, Demler O, et al. Lifetime prevalence and age-of-onset distributions of DSM-IV disorders in the National Comorbidity Survey Replication. Arch Gen Psychiatry 2005;62(6):593–602.
2. Wang PS, Berglund PA, Olfson M, et al. Delays in initial treatment contact after first onset of a mental disorder. Health Serv Res 2004;39(2):393–416.
3. Weitzman C, Wegner L. Promoting optimal development: screening for behavioral and emotional problems. Pediatrics 2015;135(2):384–95.
4. Sheldrick RC, Merchant S, Perrin EC. Identification of developmental-behavioral problems in primary care: a systematic review. Pediatrics 2011;128(2):356–63.
5. Zuckerbrot RA, Jensen PS. Improving recognition of adolescent depression in primary care. Arch Pediatr Adolesc Med 2006;160(7):694–704.
6. Roseman M, Saadat N, Riehm KE, et al. Depression screening and health outcomes in children and adolescents: a systematic review. Can J Psychiatry 2017;62(12):813–7.
7. Thombs BD, Ziegelstein RC, Roseman M, et al. There are no randomized controlled trials that support the United States Preventive Services Task Force guideline on screening for depression in primary care: a systematic review. BMC Med 2014;12(1):13.
8. Rollman BL, Hanusa BH, Lowe HJ, et al. A randomized trial using computerized decision support to improve treatment of major depression in primary care. J Gen Intern Med 2002;17(7):493–503.
9. Cunningham PJ. Beyond parity: primary Care Physicians' Perspectives on Access to Mental Health Care: more PCPs have trouble obtaining mental health services for their patients than have problems getting other specialty services. Health Aff 2009;28(Suppl1):w490–501.
10. Kolko D. Options for the delivery of mental health services. American academy of pediatrics textbook of pediatric care. Elk Grove Village (IL): American Academy of Pediatrics; 2009.
11. McMillan JA, Land M, Leslie LK. Pediatric residency education and the behavioral and mental health crisis: a call to action. Pediatrics 2017;139(1):e20162141.
12. Bottino CJ, Cox JE, Kahlon PS, et al. Improving immunization rates in a hospital-based primary care practice. Pediatrics 2014;133(4):e1047–54.
13. Gliklich RE, Dreyer NA, Leavy MB. Registries for evaluating patient outcomes: a user's guide. Rockville (MD): Government Printing Office; 2014.
14. Bodenheimer T, Wagner EH, Grumbach K. Improving primary care for patients with chronic illness: the chronic care model, Part 2. JAMA 2002;288(15):1909–14.
15. Ratzliff A, Unützer J, Katon W, et al. Integrated care: creating effective mental and primary health care teams. Hoboken (NJ): John Wiley & Sons; 2016.
16. Harding KJK, Rush AJ, Arbuckle M, et al. Measurement-based care in psychiatric practice: a policy framework for implementation. J Clin Psychiatry 2011;72(8):1136–43.
17. Hatfield D, McCullough L, Frantz SH, et al. Do we know when our clients get worse? An investigation of therapists' ability to detect negative client change. Clin Psychol Psychother 2010;17(1):25–32.
18. Hannan C, Lambert MJ, Harmon C, et al. A lab test and algorithms for identifying clients at risk for treatment failure. J Clin Psychol 2005;61(2):155–63.
19. Fihn SD, McDonell MB, Diehr P, et al. Effects of sustained audit/feedback on self-reported health status of primary care patients. Am J Med 2004;116(4):241–8.

20. Zimmerman M, McGlinchey JB. Depressed patients' acceptability of the use of self-administered scales to measure outcome in clinical practice. Ann Clin Psychiatry 2008;20(3):125–9.
21. Kindig DA. Understanding population health terminology. Milbank Q 2007;85(1): 139–61.
22. Lobb R, Colditz GA. Implementation science and its application to population health. Annu Rev Public Health 2013;34:235–51.
23. Unützer J, Choi Y, Cook IA, et al. Clinical computing: a web-based data management system to improve care for depression in a multicenter clinical trial. Psychiatr Serv 2002;53(6):671–8.
24. Fortney JC, Pyne JM, Steven CA, et al. A web-based clinical decision support system for depression care management. Am J Manag Care 2010;16(11):849.
25. Johnson JG, Harris ES, Spitzer RL, et al. The patient health questionnaire for adolescents: validation of an instrument for the assessment of mental disorders among adolescent primary care patients. J Adolesc Health 2002;30(3):196–204.
26. Mossman SA, Luft MJ, Schroeder HK, et al. The Generalized Anxiety Disorder 7-item (GAD-7) scale in adolescents with generalized anxiety disorder: signal detection and validation. Ann Clin Psychiatry 2017;29(4):227.
27. Durkalski V, Zhao W, Dillon C, et al. A web-based clinical trial management system for a sham-controlled multicenter clinical trial in depression. Clin Trials 2010; 7(2):174–82.
28. Spence SH, Rapee R, McDonald C, et al. The structure of anxiety symptoms among preschoolers. Behav Res Ther 2001;39(11):1293–316.
29. Spence SH. A measure of anxiety symptoms among children. Behav Res Ther 1998;36(5):545–66.
30. Birmaher B, Brent DA, Chiappetta L, et al. Psychometric properties of the screen for child anxiety related emotional disorders (SCARED): a replication study. J Am Acad Child Adolesc Psychiatry 1999;38(10):1230–6.
31. De Los Reyes A, Augenstein TM, Wang M, et al. The validity of the multi-informant approach to assessing child and adolescent mental health. Psychol Bull 2015; 141(4):858.
32. Arts D, de Keizer N, Scheffer G-J, et al. Quality of data collected for severity of illness scores in the Dutch National Intensive Care Evaluation (NICE) registry. Intensive Care Med 2002;28(5):656–9.
33. Chorostowska-Wynimko J, Wencker M, Horváth I. The importance of effective registries in pulmonary diseases and how to optimize their output. Chron Respir Dis 2019;16. 1479973119881777.
34. Yogman MW, Betjemann S, Sagaser A, et al. Integrated behavioral health care in pediatric primary care: a quality improvement project. Clin Pediatr 2018;57(4): 461–70.
35. Chalmers JD, Aliberti S, Polverino E, et al. The EMBARC European Bronchiectasis Registry: protocol for an international observational study. ERJ Open Res 2016;2(1):00081–2015.
36. Asarnow JR, Jaycox LH, Duan N, et al. Effectiveness of a quality improvement intervention for adolescent depression in primary care clinics: a randomized controlled trial. JAMA 2005;293(3):311–9.
37. Richardson LP, Ludman E, McCauley E, et al. Collaborative care for adolescents with depression in primary care: a randomized clinical trial. JAMA 2014;312(8): 809–16.

38. Weersing VR, Brent DA, Rozenman MS, et al. Brief behavioral therapy for pediatric anxiety and depression in primary care: a randomized clinical trial. JAMA Psychiatry 2017;74(6):571–8.
39. Geltman PL, Fried LE, Arsenault LN, et al. A planned care approach and patient registry to improve adherence to clinical guidelines for the diagnosis and management of attention-deficit/hyperactivity disorder. Acad Pediatr 2015;15(3): 289–96.
40. Schwarzwald M, Hernandez-Grande A, Chapman S, et al. Meeting the measure: improving ADHD care in the medical home. Am J Accountable Care 2017;5: 46–50.
41. Power TJ, Michel J, Mayne S, et al. Coordinating systems of care using health information technology: development of the ADHD care assistant. Adv Sch Ment Health Promot 2016;9(3-4):201–18.
42. Sheldrick RC, Henson BS, Merchant S, et al. The Preschool Pediatric Symptom Checklist (PPSC): development and initial validation of a new social/emotional screening instrument. Acad Pediatr 2012;12(5):456–67.
43. Jellinek MS, Murphy JM, Little M, et al. Use of the Pediatric Symptom Checklist to screen for psychosocial problems in pediatric primary care: a national feasibility study. Arch Pediatr Adolesc Med 1999;153(3):254–60.
44. Allgaier AK, Pietsch K, Frühe B, et al. Screening for depression in adolescents: validity of the patient health questionnaire in pediatric care. Depress Anxiety 2012;29(10):906–13.
45. Wolraich ML, Lambert W, Doffing MA, et al. Psychometric properties of the Vanderbilt ADHD diagnostic parent rating scale in a referred population. J Pediatr Psychol 2003;28(8):559–68.
46. Leis JA, Shojania KG. A primer on PDSA: executing plan–do–study–act cycles in practice, not just in name. BMJ Qual Saf 2017;26(7):572–7.

Regulators, Payors, and the Impact of Measurement-Based Care on Value-Based Care in Psychiatry

Alan Axelson, MD[a],*, David Brent, MD[b]

KEYWORDS

- Healthcare transformation • Value-based contracting • Measurement-based care
- Clinical data registry • Outcomes measurement
- Measuring health plan performance

KEY POINTS

- Health care is well along in the process of value-based transformation but still has a long way to go.
- Purchasers, both governmental and employer/commercial, are moving forward with organized and funded programs to implement their vision of value-based care.
- Psychiatrists, especially those who work with children, have a responsibility to assert themselves in the development and implementation of measures and processes that are scientifically valid and have a positive clinical impact.
- In this process of transformation, professionals must advocate for structures and processes that continue to support the clinician/patient engagement necessary for therapeutic progress.

INTRODUCTION

"The transition of the U.S. healthcare system from a volume-based fee-for-service system into an economic ecosystem that rewards the creation of value is a long game. Major economic systems require time for new competencies to replace legacy thinking and practices. Though it's a long game, it isn't a new game."

Michael Leavitt[1]

Dr A. Axelson has nothing to disclose. Supported in part by P50 MH115838; receives royalties from Guilford Press, UpToDate, and eRT; consultation fees from Healthwise.
[a] InterCare Solutions, LTD, 2370 Morrow Road, Pittsburgh, PA 15241, USA; [b] Department of Psychiatry, University of Pittsburgh School of Medicine, 3811 O'Hara Street, Pittsburgh, PA 15213, USA
* Corresponding author.
E-mail address: axelson@intercarehealth.com

Child Adolesc Psychiatric Clin N Am 29 (2020) 743–754
https://doi.org/10.1016/j.chc.2020.05.001   childpsych.theclinics.com

In this Guest Expert Comment, Leavitt asserts that the US health care system is approximately 25 years into what is likely a 40-year transition to a value-based care (VBC) system. He recounts the impact of the federal government as the driving force in this transition, referencing the universal adoption of diagnosis-related groups by Medicare in the late 1980s as the initiating event of "a continued drive toward a demonstrably better, safer and more consumer-friendly American healthcare system."

The Centers for Medicare & Medicaid Services (CMS) currently define VBC as paying for health care services in a manner that directly links payments to performance on cost, quality, and patient experience of care.[2] The CMS Web site lays out the full complex, multiyear program for the rollout of VBC, because it has an impact on physicians and health services organizations that are directly linked to Medicare reimbursement. The goal of this program is no less than the transformation of the health care delivery system.

Although the details of these CMS VBC programs may not connect directly to the practice of child and adolescent psychiatry, its principles are transforming the entire health care system in a way that ultimately also will affect the delivery of child psychiatric services. Although other articles in this issue deal with the clinical and quality aspects of measurement-based care (MBC), this article addresses how CMS, payors, purchasers, and nongovernmental organizations are encouraging the adoption of MBC as a core component of the transition to VBC. Child and adolescent psychiatrists, as individual clinicians, leaders in organized systems that provide care, and part of professional organizations, will encounter the VBC transition. To the extent that child and adolescent psychiatrists understand the forces that are driving and structuring this transformation, they may be able to exert influence or even become change agents to be sure the needs of children and families and those who treat them are recognized and supported.

HISTORY OF MEASUREMENT-BASED CARE AND VALUE-BASED CARE IN MENTAL HEALTH

In line with the focus of this article on the impact of MBC on VBC in psychiatry, a good place to begin is the establishment of the Kennedy Forum in 2013, with its goal of transforming the position of behavioral health treatment in the American health system. The Kennedy Forum publication, *Demanding Better Quality and Outcomes*,[3] stated that behavioral health providers severely lack the resources and tools to measure outcomes and service effectiveness. In a call for greater provider accountability, it established a work group to examine these issues, ultimately publishing a report with several key conclusions:

- Without systematic monitoring, providers miss opportunities to improve treatment quality and clinical practice over time.
- Aggregated measurement data can be used to demonstrate the value of behavioral health services, potentially having an impact on reimbursement.
- Failure to use systematic monitoring to demonstrate the value of behavioral health may contribute to the chronic underfunding of behavioral health services in the United States.

Members of this work group continued their efforts in 2016 with the publication of "A Tipping Point for Measurement Based Care,"[4] which reviewed 51 articles examining the theoretic and empirical support for MBC. Once again, the work group conclusions were unequivocal, stating, "The time is long overdue for the field of mental health (MH) to embrace MBC and live up to the medical testing and treat-to-target principles applied by other medical specialties. The cost of routinely administering symptom severity scales is minimal, yet the benefits of MBC accrue to all the stakeholders involved, including patients, providers, purchasers, and payers." Although the investigators acknowledge that practitioners cite time burden, lack of clerical support, and paperwork burdens as reasons for not engaging in MBC, they still insist that with minimal effort, it should be possible enact MBC in most clinical settings. Although MBC is a necessary component of VBC, it is not sufficient to fully effect this transition.

With this challenge as a backdrop, organizations with common value-oriented concerns began to develop a more focused plan. In May of 2018, at the annual meeting of the American Psychiatric Association (APA) in New York, the APA Foundation Center on Workplace Mental Health; the Northeast Business Group on Health, representing the National Alliance of Healthcare Purchaser Coalitions (NAHPC); leadership of the New York APA district branch; and representatives of several major health plans met to discuss proposed objectives related to addressing barriers to access MH care. They all agreed it was time to act, collaboratively producing a set of recommendations to improve access to care within a value-based framework.[5]

These recommendations include

- Promoting the use of evidence-based tools, like the Patient Health Questionnaire-9 (PHQ-9) to identify and treat depression, and MBC to improve the quality of care delivered and thus to improve treatment outcomes
- Promoting access to PsychPRO, a registry developed by the APA for psychiatrists and other practitioners to support the delivery of high-quality care, adherence to practice guidelines, and the tracking of performance and treatment outcomes
- Informing health plans that enrollees should be screened for depression, anxiety, psychosis, bipolar disorder, suicide, and substance use and assessed using standardized self-report measures; and health plans should track and report on treatment outcomes, providing aggregate-level data
- Payors should provide incentive payments and minimize administrative requirements to primary care, MH, and substance use providers who participate in network and in quality-improvement programs that require the use of standardized measurement tools (PHQ-9, Generalized Anxiety Disorder-7, and others) at regular intervals.
- Insist that plans require the measurement of outcomes for each behavioral health patient by the responsible clinician, whether primary care or behavioral health.
- Track and report on outcomes if accountable care organizations are providing the MH/substance use disorder (SUD) treatment.
- Ask plans to report how they provide feedback to clinicians and how those clinicians are using screening and Healthcare Effectiveness Data and Information Set and other MH/SUD performance results to make treatment decisions.

These recommendations promptly won the endorsement of the NAHPC, a nonprofit purchaser-led organization dedicated to driving health care policy and health care value for its 12,000 employers/purchasers connecting with 45 million Americans. The recommendations, listed previously, formed the basis of a 5-year action plan, "The Path Forward for Mental Health and Substance Use."[6] This action plan, a first-of-its-kind private sector approach to improving MH and substance use care, is a combined effort of the NAHPC, APA, the Meadows Mental Health Policy Institute of Dallas, Texas, and the APA Foundation Center on Workplace Mental Health.

Announced in November 2019, the Path Forward identified the following critical issues:

- Members are not able to consistently access behavioral health clinicians in their network in a timely fashion.
- Consistent use of MBC is not standard practice among primary care physicians or behavioral health specialists.
- Stigma and silence around behavioral health conditions remain prevalent and limit effective workforce performance and engagement.
- Escalating suicide and opiate-related death rates necessitate a vigorous institutional commitment.

The Path Forward identified 5 priority strategies that had the best chances of positively transforming behavioral health care. These best practices, derived from eValue8, an NAHPC tool that defines, measures, and evaluates health plan performance, are

1. Improve network access for patients to behavioral health specialists.
2. Expand use of collaborative care to integrate behavioral health into primary care.
3. Implement MBC to improve quality and outcomes.
4. Expand telebehavioral health.
5. Ensure MH parity compliance.

The progress of this effort will be measured by the NAHPC using their eValue8 platform that articulates expectations from purchasers and asks questions to determine what the health plans are doing to either impede or enhance the health of the covered population. The eValue8 performance reports allow participants to evaluate health plans on local, regional, and national levels. Plans and purchasers receive objective scores enabling comparison of plans against regional and national benchmarks and a roadmap for improvement. Plans learn what they need to do to align their strategies with purchaser expectations to maximize the value of the health care investment.[7]

As part of its new emphasis on behavioral health, NAHPC developed a special MH eValue8 module specifically to assess the performance of health plans and behavioral health organizations in key areas. The development of the eValue8 Mental Health Deep Dive engaged a diverse array of MH/SUD experts, coalition leaders, and purchasers and included members of the American Academy of Child and Adolescent Psychiatry (AACAP) Committee on Health Care Access and Economics in the development of its questions and benchmarks.

Thus, starting from Kennedy Forum in 2013, a place has been arrived at, where the power of major health care purchasers is being used to promote the quality and delivery of MH services, which in turn creates system-wide pressure on health plans to fold MH care into the VBC model and promote MBC techniques.

ORGANIZATIONAL INVOLVEMENT WITH MEASUREMENT-BASED CARE AND VALUE-BASED CARE

The American Psychiatric Association Position on Measurement-Based Care and Value-Based Care

"The American Psychiatric Association (APA) supports the use of Measurement Based Care (MBC) by psychiatrists in the evidence-based treatment of mental health conditions in a manner that is streamlined, efficient, and does not create a burden that can negatively impact clinical workflow. MBC can, when implemented appropriately, support clinical care, improve patient outcomes, and demonstrate the value of psychiatric care. Approved by the APA Board of Trustees, December 2018."[8] The APA has taken several steps to build and expand MBC in clinical practice in preparation for VBC. In 2016, the APA developed a PsychPRO mental health clinical data registry in order to provide clinician members with the infrastructure to meet the regulatory requirements of the developing Medicare value incentive programs and quality requirements. PsychPRO is a data collection tool that can aid behavioral health providers in implementing MBC, performing research, and transmitting data to CMS to meet quality data reporting requirements.[9] By early 2017, PsychPRO had enrolled enough participants to be certified as a CMS Qualified Clinical Data Registry for MH. Transmission of data from PsychPRO to CMS for enrolled Medicare practitioners avoided a 4% reimbursement penalty for under-reporting of quality data and was a first step to benefit from the Medicare Merit-Based Incentive Payment System (MIPS) value-based payment system. PsychPRO also currently is integrated with more than 50 electronic health record platforms, allowing these MIPS benefits to be accrued with minimal provider effort in participating systems. The APA is 1 of 7 organizations awarded a CMS grant to develop the PsychPRO Quality Measures Development Initiative, gathering meaningful input from clinicians across the country. Part of the grant includes incentives to encourage physicians to focus on quality, value of care, and patient health. Behavioral health providers of all discipline across the United States may be eligible to participate.

The APA, partnering with several entities, is involved in an Agency for Healthcare Research and Quality–funded Outcome Measure Harmonization and Data Infrastructure for Patient Centered Outcomes Research in Depression project. The partners are OM1, the American Board of Family Medicine PRIME Registry, Advocate Aurora Health, and Baystate Health. Currently implementing phase II (September 2019–May 2021), APA project staff are recruiting practices that utilize the PHQ-9 in the ongoing assessment of patient treatment. This initiative already has demonstrated that data

- Can be captured within the clinician workflow and directly from patients
- Can be exchanged seamlessly with multiple registries
- Provided back to clinicians in a useable format inform decision making

As of January 2020, the APA has more than 5 staff committed to the implementation of PsychPRO and these value-based contracting programs.

AMERICAN ACADEMY OF CHILD AND ADOLESCENT PSYCHIATRY WORK ON ENHANCING MEASUREMENT-BASED CARE AND VALUE-BASED CARE

The AACAP efforts to develop measures to enhance the precision and consistency of services coordination and outcomes began in 2001, when it worked collaboratively with the American Association of Community Psychiatrists (AACP) to develop the Child and Adolescent Level of Care Utilization System, using 6 interactive dimensions of assessment https://cchealth.org/mentalhealth/pdf/LOCUS.pdf, level of care determination criteria.[10] Subsequent refinement of training protocols moved the emphasis from the physical location of the level of care to a focus on service intensity that can be managed through the coordination of community-based services. This resulted in the renaming of the instrument to the Child and Adolescent Services Intensity Instrument (CASII) with training and management sponsored by AACAP. Because the service needs of infants and toddlers are fundamentally different from those of older children, in 2009 the AACAP developed the Early Childhood Service Intensity Instrument (ECSII).[11]

The CASII and ECSII are intended to provide validated and reliable measures to guide treatment needs and justify level-of-care decisions, which are at the very core of VBC. CASII/ECSII plays a role in the state child MH departments of Arizona, Hawaii, and Minnesota. It is designated by legislation as the authorized level of care criteria by the state of Connecticut. It also has the support of case law in at least 2 other states. Its traditional training program has been presented in more than 30 states.

To improve the access and efficiency of training, AACAP developed on-line training modules for both the CASII and the ECSII, supported by the AACAP Pathways Online Learning Portal www.aacap.org. The utilization of the assets of the Learning Portal are just beginning, but it clearly offers a new sophisticated tool for helping AACAP members incorporate new information into clinical practice.

INSURANCE AND PAYORS INTERFACE AND ENGAGE WITH MEASUREMENT-BASED CARE

Both commercial and medicare payors have now embraced MBC as a transition to VBC. For example, Optum, the largest behavioral health management company, emphasized the need for

1. Clinical consensus on appropriate measures
2. Ease of capturing and extracting data that are current, accurate, sensitive to changes, and nonburdensome to payors, providers, and consumers
3. Culture of measurement and transparency (Douglas Newton, MD, MPH, personal communication, 2020)

Optum's concerns are similar to the results of the 2018 OPEN MINDS Performance Management survey of behavioral health specialty provider organization executive teams,[12] listing the top 3 challenges to managing value as

1. Data management and reporting
2. Building needed information technology infrastructure
3. Lack of clarity about performance requirements from payors

The overarching support for MBC but with concern about barriers to implementation is similarly expressed in the APA MBC position statement, "Psychiatrists utilizing MBC use standardized, objective measurements at regular intervals in the assessment and treatment of patients to inform clinical decision-making and provide tangible evidence of treatment benefits across a variety of settings and psychiatric conditions...However, consistent implementation of valid and reliable measurement tools has not yet become universal in mental health care."[8]

The Affordable Care Act established that access to MH care must be a component of the standard insurance benefit. Using standard measures to screen for the presence of early symptoms of psychiatric illnesses, including SUD, was introduced as part of primary care visits to facilitate access to MH treatment services. CMS established CPT code 96 127—brief emotional/behavioral assessment limited (eg, Pediatric Symptom Checklist [PSC], Vanderbilt ADHD Diagnostic Rating Scale, Screen for Child Anxiety Related Emotional Disorders PHQ-9, depression inventory, and attention-deficit/hyperactivity disorder scale), with scoring and documentation, per instrument.[13]

Medicare policy pays for the use of up to 4 assessment tools in a primary care assessment visit. Policies for specific payment for the use of these tools in specialty psychiatric visits are unclear. Collaborative action on this issue may be a good first step forward in promoting MBC.

Behavioral health leaders in major health plans all support the adoption of MBC and, like Optum, are implementing plans to expand its adoption. For the most part, current plans are focused on the programs that provide higher intensity services, such as hospitals, residential centers for the treatment of SUDs and eating disorders, and day treatment programs. Health care expenditures in these areas and the readiness of the organizations, which already are responding to the MBC requirements of other payment sources and regulators, support this focus. In the outpatient treatment services sector that claims 60% of the behavioral health medical spend, network participation and access are such big problems that the encouragement of MBC by outpatient practitioners is a lower priority. Despite years of effort to effect change, prompt reliable access to outpatient psychiatric treatment by in-network psychiatrists, especially for children and adolescents, remains elusive. Health plans also are focusing on expanding telepsychiatry opportunities, particularly to rural areas where physical access is a significant barrier to care. Behavioral health treatment, informed by sophisticated measurement tools that are integrated into easily accessible platforms that also present relevant treatment protocols and efficiently tract patient engagement, will be required to make these innovative systems work, demonstrating the value and quality of these new service delivery models. Thus, although MBC is not an outpatient focus of health plans in general, the integration of MBC with health plans' current outpatient priorities remains highly relevant. Furthermore, given the focus on expanding access and network coverage, there is a clear opportunity to connect access to MBC value initiatives and allow child and adolescent psychiatrists to have significant influence in the processes that are promoting the growth of VBC going forward.

The Challenge of Measuring Value Through Measurement-Based Care

As this discussion demonstrates, major institutions across the country from payors to regulators to professional associations all are moving to establishing a measurement-based structure for VBC care. Research into which measures are most effective and how to deploy them, however, provides a cautionary tale. In 2012, the California legislature charged the Department of Health Care Services (DHCS) to develop a performance measure system for MH that could inform fiscal decisions and the purchase of services.[14] Despite this legislative mandate, there was no development of the robust data infrastructure for quality monitoring or standardized approach for measuring child outcomes to meet this requirement.[15] In this context, DHCS contracted with a major university to address the question, "What is the best statewide approach to evaluate functional status for children and youth that are served by the California public specialty mental health service system?"[16]

In a 2019 *Psychiatric Services* article, Zima and colleagues[17] describe the process of evaluating and recommending measures for this mandated statewide performance outcome system. Of the 15 rating scales currently utilized by different states and agencies, only the Achenbach System of Empirically Based Assessment, the Strengths and Difficulties Questionnaire, and the PSC were rated in the high-equivocal to high range on effective care, scientific acceptability, usability, feasibility, and overall utility. The 14-member expert rating panel found that only the PSC met all 9 criteria identified as priorities for adopting a state wide measure—"it covers broad age range; captures a wide breadth of symptoms; is available in California's top three threshold languages; is easy to use; is brief and consumer centered; and has acceptable evidence strength, moderate to high overall utility, and an assesses a time period that can align with the child's unique episode of care" resulting in its recommendation for statewide use. In its final decision, the California DHCS mandated use of the PSC and the Child and Adolescent Needs and Strengths scale.

This comprehensive scientific review of current rating scales concluded that there is a lack of capacity to compare child clinical outcomes across states and California counties and that frequently used outcome measures often were not supported by scientific evidence. The investigators identified that to reach the goal of high-quality care at lower cost through improved quality, policy action is required to promote a standard outcome and measurement methodology and noted that quality measurement of MH care, particularly in child MH outcomes, had lagged far behind other health care sectors. All the instruments under consideration used a traditional fixed-item, fixed-length structure with origins more than 20 years old.

It also is particularly important for child psychiatrists to consider that, as discussed previously, if the AACAP advocates the use of CASII/ECSII as an outcome measure and commits to a supporting education and consultation program, it must address the fact that the CASII instrument did not fare well in the California evaluation process. Although its use in 3 states supported its inclusion as 1 of the 15 measurement tools initially considered, its evaluation, according to the Oxford Center for Evidence-Based Medicine protocol rating category 4, corresponding to poor-quality cohort study, did not permit its inclusion in the list of 11 candidate measures evaluated by the UCLA Delphi panel.[17]

The California outcomes study highlights problems using legacy instruments to drive value in the emerging large-scale digitally managed health care system. As in other specialties, accessibility, user interface, interoperability, and data management are starting to be addressed in behavioral health. Multiple Web-based platforms are being developed to support MBC in clinical practice and reduce administrative and workflow burden. Examples include Owl Insights (https://www.owlinsights.com), Mirah (https://www.mirah.com), and CNS Vital Signs (https://www.cnsvs.com). Adaptive Testing Technologies (https://adaptivetestingtechnologies.com) offers perhaps the next generation of these systems, using the concept of multidimensional item response theory to deploy a Computer Adaptive Testing suite that can rapidly and simultaneously evaluate and score symptoms across a broad range of psychopathology. The recently published validation study of adaptive measurement tools for children, the K-CAT, may set a benchmark for the scientific rigor required to qualify the measurement instruments needed for widespread implementation of VBC.[18]

Next Steps for Child Psychiatry

Psychiatric training programs and the directors that lead them need to candidly evaluate if their programs and faculty, who are bringing training and clinical experiences from another era, are implicitly fostering a negative bias against health care management, network participation, and the tools needed to support value-based contracting. Health plans have a legitimate mission to improve the quality, accountability, and efficiency of behavioral health care, appropriately managing overtaxed resources. This generation of trainees, who have been reared with a whole different digital experience, needs to be engaged through shared learning experiences—trainees and their supervisors learning from each other. Physician leaders must be trained who are comfortable with technology and innovation, capable of working with teams. Innovative, learning focused organizations will be attracted to theses graduates and to the extent the organizations are living their corporate mission statements, new graduate clinicians will be attracted to these clinical settings.

There are very real financial and resource considerations. Working out the economics of the necessary transformation is not clear. Commercial health plans are market based and are listening to their customers, in particular the large self-insured companies, where they supply the administrative and management services. To claim the increased reimbursement needed to support more effective care, the contribution of MBC must truly and demonstrably improve the value of the health care delivered. Demonstrating a positive impact on general health spending, where much of the savings may be realized, is a continuing challenge.

Adding new approaches to insuring value must be accompanied by stopping approaches that have high cost, low value, and unintended negative consequences. The AACP makes this point in their November 27, 2018 position statement: "The AACP is concerned that treatment plan documentation in its current state, creates unnecessary administrative burden for physicians, without evidence of benefit for patients, reducing direct patient contact time, thereby negatively impacting quality of care."[19]

Collectively, child and adolescent psychiatrists have special responsibilities and opportunities. They encounter children at the very origins of behavioral health problems that may lead to serious illnesses that result in chronic morbidity and even death. Because they may not need to fall in line with the financial and regulatory pressures of Medicare and The Joint Commission, they still have time to experiment with different approaches to MBC and the transition to VBC. They should not squander this brief reprieve to inertia and unfocused action.

There are important lessons in the review of Zima and colleagues,[17] discussed previously. There is the explicit finding, "there is a lack of capacity to compare child clinical outcomes across states and California counties. Frequently used outcome measures often were not supported by scientific evidence or Delphi panel ratings. Policy action is needed to promote the selection of a common clinical outcome measure and measurement methodology for children receiving publicly funded mental health care."[17] It also strongly implies that MBC influenced by political process does not support good science, transparency, and the continuing innovation necessary to sustain an evolving behavioral health care system.

Existing outcome measures for children's services lack clinical consensus and do not meet the Optum MBC requirement of ease of capturing and extracting data that are current, accurate, sensitive to changes, and nonburdensome to payors, providers, and consumers.

There is no question that the use of sensitive measurement tools effectively integrated with treatment decision protocols is essential to support the innovation necessary to deliver appropriate care to the enlarging population of children and adolescents in need of psychiatric treatment. Not only do child and adolescent psychiatrists need to advocate for new ways to deliver care but also they must work to change a regulatory environment that forces using valuable resources to meet regulations based in the 1970s and 1980s as well as health care interventions that are low value. Care needs to be taken that, in a rush to provide a rating scale to everyone, expensive systems that do not improve care are not put in place.

System leaders with a clear organized plan and the allocation of sufficient resources from various sources can take advantage of the momentum of this tipping point to be sure the needs of children are adequately addressed in emerging systems of care. In a recent review, *Implementing Measurement Based Care in Behavioral Health: A Review*, the investigators opine, "although decades of research have elevated MBC as an evidence-based practice, research is needed to explore mechanisms of MBC to better understand the components of MBC associated with effectiveness."[20]

Components of their agenda are relevant to the development of systems sufficiently robust to shift the payment structures toward value-based contracts and diminish reliance on regulatory compliance as a means of controlling waste and spending on low value activity:

1. Develop criteria for monitoring fidelity and reporting quality of implementation.
2. Develop brief and psychometrically strong measures.
3. Streamline measurement feedback systems to include only key ingredients and enhance electronic health record interoperability.
4. Identify discrete strategies to support implementation.

5. Make evidence-based policy decisions
6. Align reimbursement structures.

It is likely that the lack of clarity regarding the value formula, the economic incentives and operational trade-offs related to implementing MBC, will persist for some time. To truly incorporate MBC into most of the settings where treatment is delivered each day, to every patient, child psychiatrist leaders must convince clinicians that it improves the effectiveness, quality, and safety of the care they are providing and that the organizations promoting the MBC process have a value focus, relating payment to quality of service with full recognition of the implementation burden. If this is the clear purpose, psychiatrists may embrace these organizations. If they experience MBC as an increase in administrative burden that is compliance driven, they will avoid systems that incorporate the use of measures, further complicating the problem of access.

To effect real change, Clayton M. Christensen and colleagues' principles of disruptive innovation need to be applied. Their 2009 publication, *The Innovator's Prescription*,[21] makes specific observations and recommendations directly related to psychiatric care that now, 10 years later, are being manifest in organizations committed to solving problems through innovation and transparency.

To truly to have a value focus, VBC should be implemented as a component of a Learning Organizations, following the principles presented by Peter M. Senge in *The Fifth Discipline: The Art & Practice of the Learning Organization.*[22] He warns that if pursuing measurement as an end in itself, risks of falling into a negative trap of focusing on what is easy to measure rather than what is important… Senge writes, "I believe that, the prevailing system of management is, at its core, dedicated to mediocrity. It forces people to work harder and harder to compensate for failing to tap the spirit and collective intelligence that characterizes working together at their best."

Tapping into the wisdom of W.E. Deming, the grandfather of quality management, in a statement made late in his career, critical of certain management approaches of existing organizations, "Management by measurement, focusing on short-term metrics, devalues intangibles. You can only measure 3 percent of what matters."

To address the health care delivery problems that at times seem overwhelming, not only are sophisticated measurement tools needed but also sophisticated tools for learning and change. Such resources are described and available through the Society for Organizational Learning North America, https://www.solonline.org.

Child and adolescent psychiatry with its collaborative and systems focused perspective, is uniquely equipped to make important contributions. It should

1. Thoughtfully establish a clearly stated position and strategy on MBC and the transition of the health care system to VBC, promoting initiatives that reflect the needs of children and families. This can be done in individual clinical practices, treatment organizations where child and adolescent psychiatrists have leadership responsibility, and the AACAP, their professional organization.
2. Integrate MBC and VBC principles into training programs and continuing education.
3. Partner with the APA Foundation Center on Workplace Mental Health, to become an active part of the behavioral healthcare transformation initiative.

REFERENCES

1. Leavitt M. Playing the long game in the journey toward a truly value-based U.S. healthcare system. Modern Healthcare 2019.

2. Center for Medicare & Medicaid services CMS definition of value-based care: CMS value based programs - Affinity group. Available at: www.cms.gov. Accessed March 6, 2020.
3. Demanding Better Quality and Outcomes, Fixing Behavioral Health Care in America - A National Call for Measurement-Based Care in the Delivery of Behavioral Health Services. Available at: https://thekennedyforum-dot-org.s3.amazonaws.com/documents/KennedyForum-MeasurementBasedCare_2.pdf. Accessed March 6, 2020.
4. Fortney JC, Unützer J, Wrenn G, et al. A tipping point for measurement-based care. Psychiatr Serv 2017;68(2):179–88.
5. Recommendations for improving access to mental health and substance use care. Available at: http://workplacementalhealth.org/Mental-Health-Topics/Improving-Access-to-MH-and-Substance-Use-Care. Accessed March 6, 2020.
6. The path forward for mental health and substance use - improving access to effective treatment. Available at: https://www.nationalalliancehealth.org/www/initiatives/initiatives-national/workplace-mental-health/pathforward. Accessed March 6, 2020.
7. Achieving value in mental health support – a Deep dive powered by eValue8 - 2018. Available at: https://www.nationalalliancehealth.org/initiatives/initiatives-national/workplace-mental-health/evalue8-deepdive. Accessed March 6, 2020.
8. APA position statement on utilization of measurement based care, approved by the APA board of trustees. 2018. Available at: https://www.psychiatry.org/home/policy-finder. Accessed March 8, 2020.
9. PsychPRO CMS- Qualified clinical data Registry (QCDR) for mental health. The APA website. Available at: https://www.psychiatry.org/psychiatrists/registry/about-psychpro. Accessed March 8, 2020.
10. American Association of Community Psychiatrists AACP - CA-LOCUS Child Adolescent – Level of Care Utilization System LOCUS. Available at: https://cchealth.org/mentalhealth/pdf/LOCUS.pdf. Accessed March 8, 2020.
11. AACAP Child and Adolescent Service Intensity Instrument© (CASII). Available at: https://www.aacap.org/AACAP/Member_Resources/Practice_Information/CASII.aspx. Accessed March 8, 2020.
12. 2018 OPEN MINDS Performance Management Survey of Behavioral Health Specialty Provider Organization Executive Teams Challenges to Managing Value. 2019. Available at: https://www.openminds.com/market-intelligence/executive-briefings/what-are-health-plans-doing-about-vbr/. Accessed March 8, 2020.
13. American Academy of Pediatrics - Standardized Screening/Testing Coding Fact Sheet for Primary Care Pediatricians - Developmental/Behavioral/Emotional. Available at: https://www.aap.org/en-us/Documents/coding_factsheet_developmentalscreeningtestingandEmotionalBehvioraassessment.pdf. Accessed March 8, 2020.
14. Performance outcomes system statute: welfare and institutions code, section 14707.5. Available at: https://codes.findlaw.com/ca/welfare-and-institutions-code/wic-sect-14707-5.html. Accessed February 7, 2019.
15. Marks M. Promises still to keep: a decade of the mental health services act. Sacramento (CA): Little Hoover Commission; 2015. Available at: https://lhc.ca.gov/report/promises-still-keep-decade-mental-health-services-act. Accessed March 8, 2020.
16. California Department of Health Care Services. Performance outcomes system plan for Medi-Cal specialty mental health services for children and youth. Sacramento (CA): Department of Health Care Services; 2015. Available at: https://www.

dhcs.ca.gov/individuals/Documents/POS_LegReport_05_15.pdf.   Accessed March 8, 2020.

17. Zima BT, Marti FA, Lee CE, et al. Selection of a child clinical outcome measure for statewide use in publicly funded outpatient mental health programs. Psychiatr Serv 2019;70:381–8.

18. Gibbons RD, Kupfer DJ, Frank E, et al. Computerized adaptive tests for rapid and accurate assessment of psychopathology dimensions in youth. J Am Acad Child Adolesc Psychiatry 2019. S0890-8567(19)31466-2.

19. Dragatsi D, Norian I, Minkoff K. American Association of Community Psychiatrists Position Statement: putting patients first by improving treatment planning and reducing administrative and clinical burden of treatment plan documentation. Community Ment Health J 2019;55(1):4–8.

20. Lewis CC, Boyd M, Puspitasari A, et al. Implementing measurement based care in behavioral health a review. JAMA Psychiatry 2019;76(3):324–35.

21. Christensen CM, Grossman JH, Hwang J. The innovator's prescription: a disruptive solutions for health care. McGraw-Hill; 2009.

22. Peter M. Senge: the fifth discipline: the Art & practice of the learning organization. Revised edition. Currency Doubleday a Division of Random House, Inc; 2006. p. xviii.

Integrating Measurement-Based Care into Trainee Education

Cristen Collins, MD[a,b], Sarah Mohiuddin, MD[c],
Anna Kerlek, MD[a,b],*

KEYWORDS

- Measurement-based care • Training programs
- Child and adolescent psychiatry fellowship • Rating instruments • ACGME
- Quality improvement

KEY POINTS

- There is no published literature on the use of rating scales in child and adolescent psychiatry fellowships, although there is literature describing use in other residency programs, such as general psychiatry, pediatrics, and family medicine.
- Survey to American Association of Directors of Psychiatric Residency Training (AADPRT) listserv indicated rating scales are used in several child and adolescent psychiatry training programs across the country, although they vary in the use of specific rating scales, if they are optional or required, presence or absence of didactics on their use, perception of rating instruments by fellows and faculty, integration with quality improvement projects, and use in practice after graduation.
- Using measurement-based care (MBC) for quality improvement data could satisfy an Accreditation Council for Graduate Medical Education requirement as well as promote learning how rating scales impact current patient care.
- The use of MBC in fellowship training may influence graduates' decision to continue to use this in their own practice as early career child psychiatrists, and further into their careers.

INTRODUCTION

There is increasing emphasis on the use of standardized measures in the field of child psychiatry. In child psychiatric research, use of standardized instruments for both diagnostic assessment and treatment response play an integral role in the care of

[a] Department of Psychiatry and Behavioral Health, Nationwide Children's Hospital, 700 Children's Drive, Columbus, OH 43205, USA; [b] Department of Psychiatry and Behavioral Health, The Ohio State University Wexner Medical Center Harding Hospital, 1670 Upham Drive, Columbus, OH 43210, USA; [c] University of Michigan Medicine, 4250 Plymouth Road, Ann Arbor, MI 48109, USA
* Corresponding author. Department of Psychiatry and Behavioral Health, Nationwide Children's Hospital, 700 Children's Drive, Columbus, OH 43205.
E-mail address: Anna.Kerlek@nationwidechildrens.org

Child Adolesc Psychiatric Clin N Am 29 (2020) 755–762
https://doi.org/10.1016/j.chc.2020.05.002
1056-4993/20/© 2020 Elsevier Inc. All rights reserved.

patients. Despite the widespread use of these tools in clinical research, the use of objective measurement tools in clinical practice remains limited and inconsistently used. This may in part be because of lack of standardization in child and adolescent psychiatric fellowship training regarding the use of objective instruments in diagnostic assessment and treatment planning. The addition of systematic training during graduate medical education may be of particular importance as training experiences remain an important determining factor of postgraduate behavior.[1] The purpose of this article was to review literature in psychiatric and nonpsychiatric training programs using measurement-based care (MBC), review benefits and barriers to MBC in training programs, provide data on the use of MBC across child and adolescent psychiatry fellowships, and offer recommendations for those wishing to implement MBC into their programs.

Accreditation Council for Graduate Medical Education and Milestones

Both the Accreditation Council for Graduate Medical Education (ACGME) Psychiatry Residency Program Requirements and the Psychiatry Milestone Project encourage the systematic use of assessment tools and rating scales. There are a number of milestones that require competency with clinical application of objective rating scales including milestones for patient care (PC1), requiring fellows to be able to "select and use appropriate diagnostic tests (rating scales, psychoeducational testing)" as well as milestones specific to medical knowledge (MK3) specific to "neurodiagnostic testing and its application in clinical settings."[2,3]

Measurement-Based Care in General Psychiatry Residency Programs

Although there is no published literature to our knowledge on the use of rating scales in child and adolescent psychiatry fellowships, there is literature describing their use in general psychiatry residency programs. Arbuckle and colleagues[4] reported that before implementation of a curriculum in MBC, nearly half of the residents in their academic training program reported they were not encouraged by supervisors to regularly use standardized assessments to monitor treatment response. This academic general psychiatry training program developed a curriculum to educate their third-year residents in MBC and quality improvement methodology.[5,6] The trainees received interactive sessions providing information on the availability, evidence, and approaches to using these measurements in their clinical care. Simultaneously, they were involved in a year-long Quality Improvement (QI) project with the purpose of applying the Patient Health Questionnaire-9 (PHQ-9) in patient care settings. Findings revealed residents were able to increase the use of depression screening as well as monthly monitoring of outpatients with a diagnosis of depression. Trainees found the rating scales useful when it was challenging to assess clinical improvement within session. Ultimately, trainees who used the PHQ-9 had increased likelihood to use additional assessments than their colleagues who did not.

In another study assessing the use of the Quick Inventory of Depressive Symptoms-Self Report (QIDS-SR) in clinic, residents' Quality Improvement Knowledge Assessment Tools (QIKAT) and QI Self-Assessment Survey scores were both significantly higher following the intervention.[5] The investigators concluded that combining educational sessions with QI approaches can significantly impact residents' use of standardized assessments in the outpatient setting.

Another publication described Rush University Medical Center's interprofessional child community fellowship for psychiatry residents and psychiatric nurse practitioners that concentrated on competencies including evaluation of services, client outcomes, and implementation of MBC.[7] The investigators specifically noted the use of the Screen for Child Anxiety and Related Emotional Disorder (SCARED) as a way to measure treatment response.

Measurement-Based Care in Nonpsychiatry Residency Programs

Nonpsychiatric training programs have also recognized the value of identification and monitoring of emotional and behavioral disturbances by using rating scales; several examples follow.

In a pediatric residency program, 4 interns provided parents with a Pediatric Symptoms Checklist (PSC) to be completed in the waiting room before the appointment, and the Patient Satisfaction Questionnaire to be completed in the examination room after the child's visit.[8] The investigators concluded that the use of rating scales in pediatric ambulatory clinics may increase discussions about emotional and behavioral issues between parents and residents. In addition, they found that rating instruments may increase the number and variety of behavioral health-type discussions.

Pediatric residents at Wake Forest received a curriculum consisting of interactive didactics and experiential clinic sessions on the use of screening instruments and interview techniques in routine follow-ups with the goal of determining if the patient was experiencing an emotional or behavioral problem.[9] The investigators examined the following through electronic chart review of nearly 2 years of data from 62 residents' continuity clinics: presenting problem, mental health diagnosis, use of rating instrument, intervention, and referrals. Because of data suggesting that internalizing disorders were not being recognized at the expected rate during clinic, the Children's Depression Inventory and the Multidimensional Anxiety Scale for Children were provided for trainee use. The review also signaled the need for additional training in recognition of depression and anxiety including increased use of screening instruments. Furthermore, the program instituted revisions of the behavioral health curriculum, specifically in the education of the use of screening measures including how to score and interpret results.

The 35th Forum for Behavioral Sciences in Family Medicine provided a workshop titled "Teaching Child Psychiatric Assessment Skills: Using Mental Health Screening Instruments" for educators in family medicine residencies.[10] The goal was for the family medicine educators to implement a variety of mental health screening tools with residents as part of the ACGME requirement for behavioral and mental health experience. The mental health screening tools included Pediatric Symptom Checklist (PSC-17), National Institute for Children's Health Quality (NICHQ) Vanderbilt Assessment Scale, SCARED, PHQ-9 for teens, and Retrospective-Modified Overt Aggression Scales. The founders of the workshop suggested that the content could be replicated by educators who wanted to teach about the use of screening instruments in training programs.

Benefits and Barriers with Measurement-Based Care

There are several well-documented benefits of implementation and utilization of MBC in mental health services.[11] Not only do these benefits increase the likelihood of more quickly recognizing deterioration or lack of progress with the current interventions, but MBC could further facilitate fellows' therapeutic relationships with patients and their parents. In addition, the use of measurement tools enhance patient outcomes, as demonstrated in major clinical trials, such as the Clinical Antipsychotic Trials of Intervention Effectiveness and Sequenced Treatment Alternatives to Relieve Depression.[12]

A survey of general psychiatry residents cited barriers to using standardized patient assessments.[4] Residents reported limited formal training as the most common barrier (31%), as well as lack of time (19%), limited access to these assessments (16%), and lack of consensus on which instrument to use (9%). Residents generally reported that these assessments could help them monitor symptoms, develop a diagnosis and treatment plan, communicate with patients about their symptoms, as well as involve them in monitoring their own symptoms. These trainees reported neutrality on the overall workload as well as efficiency. Overall, the residents felt positively about the potential value of these assessments in clinical practice. This signifies the need for practical barriers to be addressed so as not to hinder the use of these assessments. Likewise, a survey about the use of rating scales administered to practicing psychiatrists attending a continuing medical education conference in California, Massachusetts, New York, or Wisconsin in 2006 or 2007, reported similar results.[13] Namely, these psychiatrists noted multiple reasons for not using standardized scales to measure treatment outcomes in the treatment of depression. These included the belief they would not be clinically helpful, consuming too much time, too disruptive to clinical practice, uncertainty on which instrument to use, and lack of training on their use.

METHODS

The authors posted questions on the American Association of Directors of Psychiatric Residency Training (AADPRT) listserv, which includes the directors of 140 accredited child and adolescent psychiatry training programs as of 2019. These questions inquired about specific rating scales fellows use to monitor psychiatric symptoms, if they are optional or required, presence or absence of didactics on their use, perception of MBC by fellows and faculty, integration with quality improvement projects, and if fellows plan on using rating scales in their own practice on graduation.

RESULTS

Eleven of the 140 child and adolescent psychiatry program directors responded to the survey. In addition, the 2 institutions represented by the authors were also included to total 13 responses. Program directors reported a wide variety of rating instruments used to measure patient symptoms (**Box 1**).

All the programs used rating scales during intake assessments with follow-up use dependent on specific diagnosis. Programs differed with regard to the rating scales being required or optional for patient assessments. In the informal survey, 3 of the 11 programs cited rating scales as being optional, 7 required them, and 1 program did not report either. Use of rating scales were taught through a variety of methods; during orientation, didactics (including online teaching), ongoing supervision, and in the moment teaching. Use of rating scales were perceived positively by 7 of the programs. A few programs reported that when the rating scales extended clinic time, their use was perceived negatively. Notably, 1 program reported that the Child and Adolescent Needs and Strength (CANS) is required by the state for all new Medicaid intakes; however, this rating instrument was perceived as lengthy, time-consuming (15–30 minute period), and may detract from the therapeutic alliance. The CANS is proprietary and required a full day of instruction and certification, thus potentially limiting its use. Notably, across the listserv response, the CANS is not as routinely used as more commonly recognized, less time-consuming and free rating scales such as the PHQ-9.

The most commonly reported challenges included limited staff available to administer rating scales, perception of them extending clinic time, and detracting time with patients. One program reported significant challenges in administering rating scales on electronic devices (such as iPads) due to poor WiFi connection and resistance from staff in monitoring the device. One program specifically reported front desk staff

Box 1
General rating scales

- Pediatric Symptom Checklist-17 (PSC-17) and the Pediatric Symptom Checklist-35 (PSC-35)
- Child Behavior Checklist (CBCL)
- Child Symptom Inventory (CSI)
- Columbia Impairment Scale (CIS)
- Child and Adolescent Needs and Strength (CANS)

Rating Scales Measuring Depressive Symptoms:
- Patient Health Questionnaire-9 (PHQ-9)
- Mood and Feelings Questionnaire (MFQ)
- Center for Epidemiologic Studies – Depression Child (CES-DC)
- Preschool Feelings Checklist (PFC)

Rating Scales Measuring Anxiety Symptoms:
- Screen for Child Anxiety Related Disorders (SCARED)
- Preschool Anxiety Scale (PAS)

Rating Scale Measuring Mania Symptoms:
- Parent Young Mania Rating Scale (P-YMRS)
- Child Mania Rating Scale-Parent (CMRS-P)

Rating Scale Measuring Psychotic Symptoms:
- Prodromal Questionnaire-Brief (PQ-B)

Rating Scales Measuring Attention-Deficit/Hyperactivity Disorder Symptoms and Behavior Disturbance:
- Conners Comprehensive Behavior Rating Scale
- Vanderbilt Assessment Scale
- Swanson, Nolan and Pelham Questionnaire (SNAP)
- Retrospective Modified Overt Aggression Scale (R-MOAS)

Rating Scales Measuring Autism Symptoms:
- Social Communication Questionnaire (SCQ)
- Modified Checklist for Autism in Toddlers (M-CHAT)

Rating Scale Measuring Substance Use:
- The CRAFFT Screening Test for substance use

Rating Scale Measuring Obsessive Compulsive Symptoms:
- Children's Yale-Brown Obsessive Compulsive Scale (CY-BOCS)

Rating Scale Measuring Tics:
- Yale Global Tic Severity Scale (YGTSS)

Rating Scales Measuring Posttraumatic Stress Disorder (PTSD) Symptoms:
- Unspecific various Post Traumatic Stress Disorder scales including Child PTSD Symptoms Scale (CPSS)

did not want to be held responsible for making sure the iPads were returned, charged, did not get broken, and not being used for other purposes such as playing games or using the Internet. Despite their additional ideas to minimize front desk staff concerns, such as sturdy iPad cases or docking them such as in a store, unreliable WiFi became such an issue that the clinic did not continue this pilot program.

Five of the programs reported QI projects regarding the use of rating scales at their institutions. These included projects examining tools associated with social media use, sleep, extrapyramidal symptoms, the feasibility of using rating scales in clinic, and the use of CANS or PSC. One program used the results of rating instruments to increase shared decision making in the form of option grids for treating complex behavior problems. Option grids are tools that psychiatrists and families can use together in discussing multiple possible treatment recommendations.

Furthermore, 6 of the programs that replied reported that graduated fellows routinely used rating scales in their own practice after graduation, whereas the others either were unsure or did not respond. Specifically, 1 program created a packet of readily available nonproprietary rating scales for use in the fellow clinic and then encouraged to continue to use this packet in their practice following fellowship. Graduating fellows shared they continue to use these in a variety of settings, including both private practice and hospital-based settings.

The investigators of the paper work at institutions and in fellowship programs that support the use of MBC in child psychiatric clinics. Nationwide Children's Hospital uses rating scales at every outpatient psychiatry appointment in both the fellow and faculty clinic. Patients are instructed to arrive 45 minutes before the initial appointment and 15 minutes before subsequent appointments to complete tools that are administered on iPads. These are pulled into the patients' electronic medical chart for psychiatrists to access immediately (both the raw data and the scored final measures). Diagnostic appointments require PHQ-9, SCARED, Child Mania Rating Scale-Parent, and Vanderbilt, in addition to short-response questions. All follow-ups include PHQ-9 but the clinician may elect which additional measures to administer on the iPad. Fellows and faculty generally perceive these as helpful for patient care. As patients and their families are typically compliant in completing questions in the time allotted before scheduled appointments with the psychiatrist, they do not tend to extend appointment times. A current fellow QI project is examining serial changes in PHQ-9 scores and their association with demographic and clinical features.

At the University of Michigan, objective measurement tools are used in Department of Psychiatry outpatient clinics, including adult psychiatry, child and adolescent psychiatry, and addiction psychiatry for both clinical care as well as training and education. All patients are enrolled in the program at the first visit and complete initial instruments online 30 minutes before their scheduled appointment. Rating scales assigned to patients are individualized based on general clinic versus subspecialty clinic appointments. Similar to Nationwide Children's Hospital, results are immediately available to clinicians and can be auto-populated into the electronic medical record. Patients can then be assigned specific rating scales to be completed at specific time points over a designated period of time. From an education perspective, use of objective rating tools are covered in a 3-part didactic series covering developmental testing, neuropsychological testing, speech and language testing, and use of diagnostic tools in a variety of psychiatric disorders including attention-deficit/hyperactivity disorder, aggression, depression, anxiety, posttraumatic stress disorder, and autism spectrum disorders. In addition to the use of objective rating scales in the outpatient clinic over an 18-month outpatient rotation, fellows are also trained more extensively in the interpretation of neuropsychological testing. This includes approximately 24 patient encounters and observation of formal neuropsychological testing over 8 sessions. This experience includes use of these results in diagnostic and treatment planning, as well as training in the discussion of results with patients and families.

DISCUSSION

The response rate to the informal AADPRT survey was low (less than 10%) despite 3 separate inquires across a 3-month span, so it remains difficult to fully understand the use of MBC in the vast majority of fellowships in the country. However, of those who did respond, program directors reported their fellows were using a variety of rating scales, and often had specific curricula to address medical knowledge and use of these scales. The reported challenges and barriers to the use of rating instruments were consistent with previous literature on barriers to implementation. A specific challenge to using MBC noted in the survey was related to technological problems. Ensuring adequate WiFi connection by potentially involving hospital IT services and increasing staff buy-in would be vital in administering rating scales on electronic devices. Nationwide Children's Hospital and University of Michigan provide examples of patients' self-reporting data and fellows' ability to immediately see the results. This provides a more seamless review of MBC for fellows to integrate patients' symptom evaluation and treatment planning.

Similar to current evidence of general psychiatry training in MBC, our survey demonstrated training and clinical use of objective rating instruments in child psychiatry training programs. Half of the directors reported their fellows were using MBC for QI data. This is important as the ACGME requires that child and adolescent psychiatry fellows "demonstrate the ability to investigate and evaluate their care of patients, to appraise and assimilate scientific evidence, and to continuously improve patient care based on constant self-evaluation and lifelong learning." Previous publications have also demonstrated models for integrating QI and MBC into a training program.[5,6] The longitudinal outpatient clinical experiences in the last year of training would provide a timely opportunity for such integration, and the project could be ongoing with tasks continued year to year.

An additional benefit to providing training during fellowship in the use of rating instruments would be optimization of coding and billing. Child and adolescent psychiatrists may bill for the use and review of rating scales. Thus, promoting use of MBC in training additionally has the benefit of teaching fellows real-life practice and systems-based care competencies.

FUTURE DIRECTIONS

One of the authors of the paper is a PGY-5 child and adolescent psychiatry fellow at Nationwide Children's Hospital. Trainees at this program report the use of rating scales increases efficiency due to having readily available information before entering the examination room, thus targeting reported symptoms from the beginning. Literature reports that use of self-report data can increase patient and family understanding of care, as well as enhance communication between psychiatrist and family.[11] From a trainee perspective, this is particularly impactful during the steep learning curve of fellows' training in their final years before graduation as they are trying to refine their skills and individualize their practice. Therefore, we recommend implementation of MBC into child and adolescent fellowship programs.

Dollar and colleagues[11] provide steps and concrete guidance for practices wishing to adopt MBC. The investigators use the implementation guide as part of a QI process to enhance buy-in "through a straightforward linear sequence of activities." The investigators detail a 13-step plan that outlines how to engage and train staff in measurement based care, determine measures and frequencies, method of documentation and how data will be collected, as well as how to identify and sustain a similar successful program. Training programs wishing to implement MBC into fellows' practice could use this article as a guide.

In conclusion, use of rating scales in fellowship training will not only improve care at the individual patient level, but the training curricula may be enhanced by the integration of MBC and QI projects, serving to also support ACGME requirements. The use of

MBC in fellowship training may additionally influence graduates' decision to continue use in their own practice as early career child psychiatrists, and further into their careers.

DISCLOSURE

The authors have nothing to disclose.

REFERENCES

1. Cheng TL, DeWitt TG, Savageau JA, et al. Determinants of counseling in primary care pediatric practice: physician attitudes about time, money, and health issues. Arch Pediatr Adolesc Med 1999;153:629–35.
2. Accreditation Council for Graduate Medical Education. The Child and Adolescent Psychiatry Milestone Project. Available at: https://www.acgme.org/Portals/0/PDFs/Milestones/ChildandAdolescentPsychiatryMilestones.pdf?ver=2015-11-06-120533-753. Accessed November 30, 2019.
3. Accreditation Council for Graduate Medical Education. ACGME Program Requirements for Graduate Medical Education in Child and Adolescent Psychiatry (Subspecialty of Psychiatry). Available at: https://www.acgme.org/Portals/0/PFAssets/ProgramRequirements/405_ChildAdolescentPsychiatry_2019.pdf?ver=2019-06-19-091518-287. Accessed November 30, 2019.
4. Arbuckle MR, Weinberg M, Harding KJK, et al. The feasibility of standardized patient assessments as best practice in an academic training program. Psychiatr Serv 2013;64:209–11.
5. Arbuckle MR, Weinberg M, Cabaniss DL, et al. Training psychiatry residents in quality improvement: an integrated, year-long curriculum. Acad Psychiatry 2013;37:42–5.
6. Arbuckle MR, Weinberg M, Kistler SC, et al. A curriculum in measurement-based care: screening and monitoring of depression in a psychiatric resident clinic. Acad Psychiatry 2013;37:317–20.
7. Delaney KR, Karnik NS. Building a child mental health workforce for the 21st century: closing the training gap. J Prof Nurs 2019;35:133–7.
8. Applegate H, Kelley ML, Applegate BW, et al. Clinical case study: pediatric residents' discussions of and interventions for children's behavioral and emotional problems. J Pediatr Psychol 2003;28:315–21.
9. Williams J, Klinepeter K, Palmes G, et al. Use of an electronic record audit to enhance mental health training for pediatric residents. Teach Learn Med 2007;19:357–61.
10. Hargrave TM, Arthur ME. Teaching child psychiatric assessment skills: using pediatric mental health screening tools. Int J Psychiatry Med 2015;50:60–72.
11. Dollar KM, Kirchner JE, DePhilippis D, et al. Steps for implementing measurement-based care: implementation planning guide development and use in quality improvement. Psychol Serv 2019. https://doi.org/10.1037/ser0000368.
12. Baker M. Measurement-based care and psychiatric education: are we doing enough? Psychiatric News 2015. Available at: https://doi.org/10.1176/appi.pn.2015.5a18. Accessed October 31, 2019.
13. Zimmerman M, McGlinchey JB. Why don't psychiatrists use scales to measure outcome when treating depressed patients? J Clin Psychiatry 2008;69:1916–9.

Health Information Technology Resources to Support Measurement-Based Care

John Torous, MD, MBI[a],*, Adam C. Powell, PhD[b],
Elena Rodriguez-Villa, BS[a]

KEYWORDS

- Apps • User-centered design • Measured based care

KEY POINTS

- Smartphones are ubiquitous and offer unprecedented opportunity to reach underserved populations suffering from mental illness.
- Smartphone applications are uniquely positioned to help patients access and inform their own care through collecting a combination of active and passive data.
- Health information technology that uses smartphone applications for accessible infrastructure offers the potential of scaling measurement-based care.
- Health information technology can only be converted into measurement-based care if interest is drawn on, engagement is consistent, smartphone applications are specific and simple, and patients are supported.

INTRODUCTION

Health information technology (IT) can reinvent health care delivery. The health IT sector has produced offerings targeted to patients, health care providers, and managed care organizations, each with the potential to impact the cost and quality of care.[1] Collectively, these offerings were projected to constitute more than an $80 billion market in the United States in 2020, with mobile health solutions and applications (apps) accounting for $14 billion.[2] The US market for apps is but 1 component of a far broader global market. Numerous apps to address mental and physical illness are available in China and India, and the apps pursue a broad variety of monetization strategies.[3,4]

The wide adoption of smartphones across all demographic segments has facilitated the creation of digital biomarkers: electronic measures of behavior, cognition, socialization, and physical state captured through electronic means.[5] The ubiquity of mobile

[a] Department of Psychiatry, Beth Israel Deaconess Medical Center, Harvard Medical School, 330 Brookline Avenue, Boston, MA 02115, USA; [b] Payer+Provider Syndicate, 11 Beach Street, Ste. 4E, Boston, MA 02111, USA
* Corresponding author.
E-mail address: jtorous@bidmc.harvard.edu

Child Adolesc Psychiatric Clin N Am 29 (2020) 763–773
https://doi.org/10.1016/j.chc.2020.06.011
1056-4993/20/© 2020 Elsevier Inc. All rights reserved.

devices, paired with the scalability of digital tools and resources, offers unprecedented opportunity to reach and evaluate the health of underserved populations around the world, including children and adults suffering from mental illness. Cross-sector, international interest, and investment in health care technology illustrate the promise of mobile health to increase access and quality of care and facilitate measurement-based care.

Integration of data from apps with electronic health records, save for a few notable examples, such as Apple HealthKit's integration with the Epic system, has proven to be a challenge to the widespread use of digital biomarkers to empower measurement-based care.[6] Part of the problem stems from the fact that different health IT vendors have built their businesses around serving consumers, health care providers, and managed care organizations, and many vendors do not cross over with offerings for multiple segments of the industry.[1] Thus, actually leveraging health IT resources to support measurement-based care for youth mental health remains difficult. In part, the cost and variance in health IT have led to a heterogeneous landscape with impressive efforts, but few national or global programs that leverage the scalability and true potential of health IT. One challenge has been that nations have taken a scattershot approach to reimbursing for the costs of digital health interventions, with many currently being paid for directly by patients and their employers, rather than by insurers.[7] To help encourage the development and reimbursement of digital health tools that foster measurement-based care, the role that the smartphone is currently playing in the care process and how its impact could be increased going forward are discussed.

The understanding of smartphones for mobile technology as an agent, accelerator, or supplement to mental health care is restricted to the last 10 years. There is no precursor to the prevalence of devices that can measure heart rate, detect movement, and track location all at once. The adoption of mobile technology is already the fastest spread of any technology in human history. In 2018, smartphones accounted for 60% of connections made to the Internet around the world.[8] From a health IT perspective, smartphones represent an unparalleled opportunity to connect care to those who need it. However, without a roadmap to follow or a model to base outcomes on, mobile mental health resources are often evolving efforts toward realizing what will be most effective, efficient, or engaging for a patient rather than finished and final products. A recent review of mobile health apps to support the detection, management, and maintenance of youth mental health revealed only 6 published studies meeting inclusion criteria.[9] In light of the billions of smartphones and seemingly boundless enthusiasm for digital health, why has the impact of smartphones in mental health for measurement-based care been so limited to date? A critical appraisal and review of these efforts, a compilation of recent studies, app store ratings, and app reviews, can provide developers, health care providers, and patients with critical insight. Successes and failures combined draw a blueprint for future technologies and health IT to be built on.

Most patients today, especially youth, are willing to use smartphones to understand or monitor their behavior and symptoms. Mobile apps are uniquely positioned to help patients access and inform their own care. This article outlines patterns in features and design that distinguish effective mobile mental health apps and interventions that support measurement-based care. It denotes recurring themes and qualities in apps across topic and intended audiences. The authors suggest that with the right support from peers and clinicians, mobile mental health apps that are simple, specific, and smart can engage patients and enhance treatment through measurement-based care.

Effective measurement-based care hinges on access to accurate data points. The more statistics available to a clinician, the more informed and impactful measurement-based care can be. Mobile mental health apps with low user engagement hinder useful or meaningful information being collected. Engaging users is a common roadblock, and even some of the most popular and downloaded mobile mental health apps reveal considerably low utilization.[10,11] To increase utilization and convert health IT into measurement-based care, this article highlights 4 criteria and actions that help distinguish successful mobile mental health interventions (**Fig. 1**):

1. Interest: Draw on pervading interest in mobile mental health
2. Engagement: Offer personalized design features and recommendations
3. Specificity and simplicity: Provide simple, specific, and timely feedback
4. Support: Incorporate support from peers, family and friends, and caregivers

Throughout the article, the authors explain how mindLAMP, an open-source and free digital mental health tool, offers a tangible example of combing health IT into measurement-based care. Drawing on the principles that demarcate effective digital mental health tools, mindLAMP captures the lived experience of patients to inform recovery and enhance treatment. Readers can learn more about mindLAMP, running it themselves, or adapting it to their local needs at digitalpsych.org/lamp. As free software created by two of the authors of this article (E.R.-V., J.T.), the goal of mindLAMP is to offer a useful and free resource to the community toward increasing access to and advancing care.

INTEREST: SMARTPHONE INTERVENTIONS ARE FEASIBLE BECAUSE USERS ARE OPEN TO TRYING THEM

Technology pervades daily living. It touches on routine health-related practices from tracking steps taken walking to work to making an appointment with a primary care physician. Exposure to technology, across age groups, geographies, and income brackets, results in increasing comfort with digital tools and the breadth and depth of their capabilities. This comfort with digital devices, added to by the perceived time they save and the information they connect people to, builds trust. Widespread ownership and growing confidence in smartphones open a window of opportunity for caregivers to reach populations in need.

Surveys to date show that smartphones are prevalent among individuals living with mental illness. Results from a survey distributed at 4 distinct settings across the United States: a state-run outpatient clinic in Massachusetts, a country-run community outpatient clinic in California, a hybrid clinic that treats patients with public and private insurance in Louisiana, and a university outpatient clinic in Wisconsin, found that 62.5% of patients across sites owned a smartphone, exceeding the national average

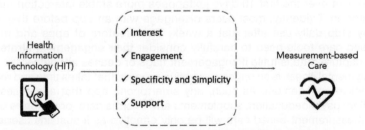

Fig. 1. Health IT can only be converted into measurement-based care if interest is drawn on, engagement is consistent, smartphone apps are specific and simple, and patients are supported.

at the time by a small margin, and 70.6% of owners would be willing to use smartphones to monitor symptoms.[12] A similar survey was administered in India and showed that 31.8% of a patient population surveyed owned a mobile device, mirroring India's reported national ownership average at 30%, and 60.2% of smartphone owners reported they were also open to using a mobile device to monitor their symptoms.[13] These findings suggest that across countries, smartphone ownership among mentally ill patients is representative of the larger population, and that interest in using mobile devices to improve conditions is high.

Smartphone owners are open to using mobile devices to supplement mental health care as a means to better understand their condition or behaviors.[13] Surveys gauging which features individuals are excited to use as a means to monitor symptoms show that individuals are interested in comparing their mood against activities or external factors, and that overall, they would like to feel more in control and aware of their mood.[14] This form of measurement-based care may also offer therapeutic potential. Emotional self-awareness has been shown to be inversely related to reported symptoms of depression.[15,16] Recording feelings and contextualizing them encourage reflection. Through collecting both passive and active data, mobile mental health apps are uniquely capable of offering patients insight into behavioral patterns. They can increase emotional awareness and help patients and draw connections to their actions. However, interest in using mobile technology to learn about oneself is not enough. For interest to incite change, patients need to be engaged.

ENGAGEMENT: USERS WANT TO INTERACT WITH TECHNOLOGY AND TOOLS THAT MATCH THEM

High levels of smartphone ownership and interest in using digital tools for mental health favor the continued build and distribution of smartphone interventions. However, excitement from patients or clinicians does not promise engagement in practice. More often than not, mobile apps, across industries, regardless of content, and despite diverse features, idle on a device without regular use as reflected in the low engagement rates with most measurement-based care apps. Attracting users and drawing initial enthusiasm are a challenge, but growing and sustaining interest might be an even greater one.

The challenge of engagement is daunting. A recent study that reviewed data on the use of mobile mental health apps found that only 4% of these apps downloaded are actually opened.[11] In an effort to improve their well-being, users may be motivated to browse for and select an app, but this does not indicate whether or how often they will open it. App-open rates drop 80% between days 1 and 10 after an app is downloaded, compared with only 20% between days 15 and 30.[11] The marked decrease in engagement over the first 10 days juxtaposes more stable interaction that users exhibit later on. Evidently, most users disengage with an app before they open it, and many stop daily use after just a week. The creators of apps and measurement-based care tools need to carefully consider their engagement strategy. The ability to capture data is futile if engagement flags or ceases altogether.

Treating mental illness is an ongoing, iterative process that takes time and requires a level of active engagement. As such, any smartphone app that addresses mental health, offers psychoeducation, supplements and informs care, or performs other aspects of measurement-based care will be only effective as it sustains user engagement. The more data points technology collects around a user, the better able it is to offer relevant information and resources. In this case, regular patient activity helps to inform how and which mental health interventions are offered to them. A recent study assigned 301 people with mental illness to 1 of 4 treatments that used Intelli-Care, a mobile platform for mental health interventions that offers a suite of apps that target focused outcomes.[17] Participants who were offered suggestions on specific new apps to try out used the app more frequently than those who were not.[17] Engagement is more likely if and when content is or feels customized.

Although apps today are not able or designed to replace care, they can augment care through offering information and activities that are relevant and customized to the patient. Treatment, education, and tools for recovery need to meet needs and match interest. mindLAMP, a digital platform designed to support recovery for patients with serious mental illness, is built as an example of a measurement-based care tool.[18–20] The mindLAMP app offers users education and activities based on algorithms that are fed real-time data. The content, design, time, and delivery of 3 mindLAMP interventions are detailed in **Table 1** to highlight their responsivity. By using smartphones and sensors to assess patient activity and understand their needs, unprecedented opportunities for customization are possible today.

Customization extends beyond features and functionality. People maintain their own set of preferences and carry their own biases when it comes to design. Through understanding how a user likes to consume content and by catering an aesthetic they are most comfortable with, developers are more likely to engage users over time. A study gauged the preferences and ways a group of 58 young adults used their mobile devices and found that overall design preferences varied and that the adolescents surveyed favored different features.[21] Four categories of smartphone users emerged from the study, however, depicting some patterns in how age and illness informed preference. In order to understand and ultimately meet a patient's long-term treatment needs and support measurement-based care, an effective smartphone intervention must first cater to their likings or existing biases to facilitate engagement. Fortunately, health IT tools, and especially smartphone apps, are easily able to change their interface and form. Customization and personalization capabilities that are inherent to smartphones, however, have not yet been fully used to advance measurement-based care in child and adolescent psychiatry.

SPECIFICITY AND SIMPLICITY: SMARTPHONE INTERVENTIONS ARE MOST EFFECTIVE IF AND WHEN THEY FOCUS ON A SINGULAR OUTCOME

Smartphones are by definition portable. They are on-the-go devices designed and marketed for regular bursts of short activity. Users engage with their smartphone in transit, mid conversation, and alongside peers. Smartphones make multitasking possible. Users are able to consume information and share media all the while completing a separate activity. Smartphone apps support transient interactions because they can be opened, closed, and opened again at the user's convenience. Although this can facilitate measurement-based care, it also presents a trap because such measurement can quickly become too intensive, complex, and invasive. Rather, mobile mental health measurements and interventions are most effective if and when they are simple, specific, and brief.

Many medical apps available today are not easy for users to navigate. A study focused on the practicality of mobile health apps for measurement-based care illustrated irritation and confusion among users trying out new apps.[22] Frustration with technology, whether it stems from insufficient instruction or unfamiliarity, does not inspire confidence. Smartphone apps need to be intuitive and focused in order to build user confidence and encourage utilization. Games or features without an obvious purpose may interfere with usability and are superfluous to many users.[7]

Table 1
mindLAMP interventions

Dimension	Trigger	Intervention	Content	Design	Time (s)	Delivery
Anxiety	Spike in heart rate	Inhale-exhale	Audio-guided breathing exercise of long inhalations and exhalations. Emphasis is placed on long breaths consistent in duration	Single-touch "Go" to begin. Can be put on repeat	30	Notification on home screen that slides to open. Also available in repository of *Guided Meditations* after first use. Option to record your own
Mood	Daily. Preset time determined by user	Short self-report survey	5 statements related to mood. User decides the degree to which they agree with the statement	Single-touch "Go to begin." One tap to select a response to each question. Likert scale	60	Notification on home screen that slides to open. Also available in repository of *Mood Surveys* after first use
Unusual thoughts	Change in distress levels detected by phone	Scratch card	Covered image of nature. User swipes finger continuously over image to uncover it	Single-touch "Go to begin." User can preselect images from their photo library to be covered	30–60	Notification on home screen that slides to open. Also available in repository of *Activities*

The IntelliCare suite previously mentioned consists of apps with activities and information that take less than 30 seconds to complete or review.[17] Out of 301 participants, 253 continued to use IntelliCare apps for a median 92 days after a study that prescribed them concluded.[17] That most users used the mobile mental health apps offered for an additional 3 months indicates perceived value and ease of use. Brief interventions make engagement more likely because they do interrupt or interfere with patients' lives. Time and attention are limited, and as such, users want near instantaneous feedback or information. Smartphone users expect speed and responsivity.[23] To meet these expectations, digital mental health measurements, interventions, and education should be delivered in such a way that is succinct and reactive, making daily, lasting use more plausible.

The mindLAMP platform, introduced earlier in this article, offers complex customizations, but in clinical use it has been also found that simple uses are often just as effective. Data are categorized and depicted in graphs that can be arranged to highlight patterns or understand behaviors over time. Patients, their family and friends, and clinicians have access to this dashboard. During therapy sessions, clinicians are able to pull up graphs that make it easier for patients to recall their feelings and consider them in the context of life events. Most prominently, the graphs create a visual diary for patients. As shown in **Fig. 2**, some of mindLAMP's simpler features, such as comparing physical activity to mood symptoms, are also the most impactful in informing treatment.

SUPPORT: LASTING CHANGE IS A COLLABORATIVE EFFORT

Living with mental illness is more challenging alone. Support from peers with lived experience, family and friends, and clinicians make recovery possible. Positive interactions build confidence, and strong relationships offer accountability and context for treatment. Interventions for behavioral change or symptom improvement are most effective when a patient is supported and their support system is aware and engaged in their efforts.[24] Measurement-based care can offer the right data and support the right triggers to help guide, launch, and support the right interventions for patients. Separating measurement from intervention defeats not only the entire purpose of measurement-based care but also the true potential of smartphones to connect patients to systems of support. Mobile mental health apps, therefore, can provide an

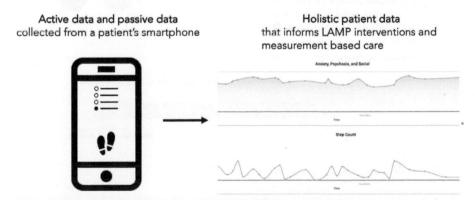

Active data and passive data
collected from a patient's smartphone

Holistic patient data
that informs LAMP interventions and
measurement based care

Fig. 2. Passive data (eg, step count from the phone) and active data (eg, surveys from the phone) combine to create a holistic view of patient information. These aggregated data inform LAMP app interventions as well as ongoing treatment.

opportunity to open lines of communication. Through avenues such as social media, young adults are already accustomed to using their smartphone to connect with friends. Not surprisingly, they express interest in smartphone features that allow them to interact with peers with lived experience.[25] Moderated chat features on apps for adults with mental illness show similar popularity. Smartphone apps that have included opportunities and functions for peer support have retained higher daily open rates than mindfulness, mood tracking, and breathing exercise apps.[11]

Despite how accessible and available smartphones make communication, they do not replace face-to-face human connection.[26] Relationships built offline with friends, family members, and clinicians are invaluable. They are crucial in offering stability and insight, building trust over time that can be drawn on to facilitate recovery. A recent study found that most university students and community members surveyed, across all ages, preferred face-to-face treatment over online care.[27] Digital solutions for mental health treatment do not eliminate the need or value of a caregiver or provider. Instead, they offer novel avenues to inform and enhance the kind of personalized care a clinician provides.

Patients appreciate the role of a clinician in supporting recovery. Of survey respondents open to using a mobile application to improve their mental health, 86.2% would give their clinician access to data collected on their mood or related to their behavior.[14] This overwhelming majority indicates that patients trust their care providers and that they value their insight and acumen. Smartphone data, extracted from mobile apps, can paint clinicians a fuller picture of a patient's illness. Patients recognize the value this may add in determining treatment and adapting it over time. Mobile mental health apps present clinicians with an unprecedented opportunity to supplement care with a holistic and more complete understanding of a patient's lived experience.

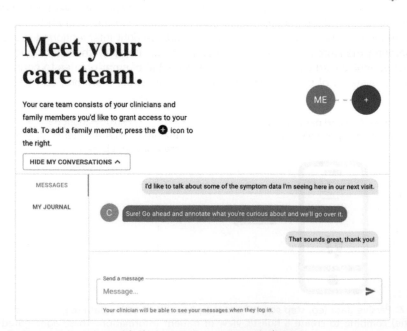

Fig. 3. Patients can connect with their care team using mindLAMP.

mindLAMP offers an example of how measurement-based care tools can support such collaborative efforts. Although the app can be used for self-help by a patient or as a registry by a clinician, mindLAMP can also further the therapeutic alliance between a patient and their provider. Offering tools that facilitate communication about data appeals to patients, although often clinicians are hesitant to receive such real-time data.[18] However, by establishing guidelines that determine or limit when messages will be read and responded to, it is possible to create safe and effective means for collaboration around measurement-based care with clinicians or trusted peers (**Fig. 3**).

SUMMARY

Smartphone apps are a form of accessible infrastructure that offers the potential of scaling measurement-based care. As an example, LAMP harnesses health IT to inform measurement-based care through a customizable design that features straightforward interventions and a platform that engages patients and support systems to collect and understand data. Given high interest and comfort levels across ages and around the world, a holistic mobile mental health intervention is uniquely positioned to connect measurement-based care to those who need it.

DISCLOSURE

A.C. Powell reports employment by Payer+Provider Syndicate and stock ownership of Berkshire Hathaway, Community Health Systems, CVS Health Corp, HCA Healthcare, Payer+Provider Syndicate, Quorum Health Corp, and Tenet Healthcare Corp and serves paid positions on the Scientific Advisory Board of PsyberGuide and on the Expert's Council of the Mary Christie Foundation. E. Rodriguez-Villa has nothing to disclose.

REFERENCES

1. Powell AC, Glaser J. The healthcare information technology sector. In: Burns LR, editor. The business of healthcare innovation. 3rd edition. Cambridge (UK): Cambridge University Press; 2020. p. 435.
2. Markets and Markets. Healthcare IT market by product (EHR, RIS, PACS, VNA, CPOE, mHealth, telehealth, healthcare analytics, supply chain management, revenue cycle management, CRM, claims management, fraud management) by end user (provider, payer) – global forecast to 2020. 2015. Available at: www.marketsandmarkets.com/Market-Reports/healthcare-it-252.html. Accessed February 16, 2020.
3. Powell AC, Yue Z, Shan C, et al. The monetization strategies of apps for anxiety management: an international comparison. J Technol Behav Sci 2019;4(2):67–72.
4. Powell A, Singh P, Torous J. The complexity of mental health app privacy policies: a potential barrier to privacy. JMIR Mhealth Uhealth 2018;6(7):e158.
5. Torous J, Rodriguez J, Powell A. The new digital divide for digital biomarkers. Digit Biomark 2017;1(1):87–91.
6. Powell AC, Torous.JB, Firth J, et al. Generating value with mental health apps. BJPsych Open 2020;6(2).
7. Olschesky M. How the Epic/Healthkit integration actually works. Datica. 2014. Available at: https://datica.com/blog/how-the-epic-healthkit-integration-actually-works/. Accessed March 12, 2020.

8. The mobile economy 2019. The GSM association. Available at: https://www. gsmaintelligence.com/research/?file=b9a6e6202ee1d5f787cfebb95d3639c5& download. Accessed December 27, 2019.

9. Punukollu M, Marques M. Use of mobile apps and technologies in child and adolescent mental health: a systematic review. Evid Based Ment Health 2019; 22(4):161–6.

10. Torous J, Staples P, Slaters L, et al. Characterizing smartphone engagement for schizophrenia: results of a naturalist mobile health study. Clin Schizophr Relat Psychoses 2017.

11. Baumel A, Muench F, Edan S, et al. Objective user engagement with mental health apps: systematic search and panel-based usage analysis. J Med Internet Res 2019;21(9):e14567.

12. Torous J, Chan SR, Tan SYM, et al. Patient smartphone ownership and interest in mobile apps to monitor symptoms of mental health conditions: a survey in four geographically distinct psychiatric clinics. JMIR Ment Health 2014;1(1):e5.

13. Deb KS, Tuli A, Sood M, et al. Is India ready for mental health apps (MHApps)? A quantitative-qualitative exploration of caregivers' perspective on smartphone-based solutions for managing severe mental illnesses in low resource settings. PLoS One 2018;13(9):e0203353.

14. Proudfoot JG, Parker GB, Pavlovic DH, et al. Community attitudes to the appropriation of mobile phones for monitoring and managing depression, anxiety, and stress. J Med Internet Res 2010;12(5):e64.

15. Caldeira C, Chen Y, Chan L, et al. Mobile apps for mood tracking: an analysis of features and user reviews. In: American Medical Informatics Association, editor. AMIA Annual Symposium Proceedings, vol. 2017. Bethesda (MD): American Medical Informatics Association; 2017. p. 495.

16. Kauer SD, Reid SC, Crooke AHD, et al. Self-monitoring using mobile phones in the early stages of adolescent depression: randomized controlled trial. J Med Internet Res 2012;14(3):e67.

17. Mohr DC, Schueller SM, Tomasino KN, et al. Comparison of the effects of coaching and receipt of app recommendations on depression, anxiety, and engagement in the IntelliCare Platform: factorial randomized controlled trial. J Med Internet Res 2019;21(8):e13609.

18. Torous J, Wisniewski H, Bird B, et al. Creating a digital health smartphone app and digital phenotyping platform for mental health and diverse healthcare needs: an interdisciplinary and collaborative approach. J Technol Behav Sci 2019; 4(2):1–13.

19. Liu G, Henson P, Keshavan M, et al. Assessing the potential of longitudinal smartphone based cognitive assessment in schizophrenia: a naturalistic pilot study. Schizophr Res Cogn 2019;17:100144.

20. Wisniewski H, Henson P, Torous J. Using a smartphone app to identify clinically relevant behavior trends via symptom report, cognition scores, and exercise levels: a case series. Front Psychiatry 2019;10:652.

21. Fleming T, Merry S, Stasiak K, et al. The importance of user segmentation for designing digital therapy for adolescent mental health: findings from scoping processes. JMIR Ment Health 2019;6(5):e12656.

22. Sarkar U, Gourley GI, Lyles CR, et al. Usability of commercially available mobile applications for diverse patients. J Gen Intern Med 2016;31(12):1417–26.

23. Aji M, Gordon C, Peters D, et al. Exploring user needs and preferences for mobile apps for sleep disturbance: mixed methods study. JMIR Ment Health 2019;6(5): e13895.

24. Mueser KT, Torrey WC, Lynde D, et al. Implementing evidence-based practices for people with severe mental illness. Behav Modif 2003;27(3):387–411.
25. Aschbrenner KA, Naslund JA, Tomlinson EF, et al. Adolescents' use of digital technologies and preferences for mobile health coaching in public mental health settings. Front Public Health 2019;7:178.
26. MHealth design toolkit. The GSM association. Available at: https://www.gsma.com/mobilefordevelopment/wp-content/themes/theme_mobilefordevelopment/mhealth/GC_GSMA_FinalBooklet.pdf. Accessed December 27, 2019.
27. March S, Day J, Ritchie G, et al. Attitudes toward e-mental health services in a community sample of adults: online survey. J Med Internet Res 2018; 20(2):e59.

Counterpoint
Risks of Implementing Measurement-Based Care in Child and Adolescent Psychiatry

Andrew S. Lustbader, MD[a,b,]*, Mark S. Borer, MD[c]

KEYWORDS

- Measurement-based care (MBC) • Clinical rating scales • Symptom reduction
- Root cause • Psychiatric screening measures • Dignity • Suffering

KEY POINTS

- There are benefits and risks of using measurement-based care in different clinical settings.
- Psychiatry must ensure that sound clinical judgment not be overtaken by measurement-based care in clinical decision making.
- There is a substantial risk of psychiatry systematizing measurement-based care, paving the way for third-party payers to use measurement-based care as the overriding basis for mental health care reimbursement.
- There are developing models to work with third-party payers where they will develop payment schedules integrating reasonable psychiatric input.

INTRODUCTION

Measurement-based care (MBC), coined by Trivedi in 2006 and defined by Fortney as "the systematic administration of symptom rating scales and use of the results to drive clinical decision making at the level of the individual patient," has a number of benefits in clinical settings.[1] Tools are usually patient- (or parent-) reported outcome measures focusing on identifying and measuring severity of symptoms and/or functioning. These tools are meant to help inform decision making in 2 possible ways: assisting in deciding on which interventions to use with a patient (eg, what form of therapy, what kind of school, medications if necessary, what form of family and community engagement, etc); and assisting in analyzing the efficacy of a given treatment.

[a] Yale Child Study Center, New Haven, CT, USA; [b] Therapeutic Center for Children and Families, 215 Main Street, Westport, CT 06880, USA; [c] Psychiatric Access for Central DE, 846 Walker Road Suite 32-2, Dover, DE 19904, USA
* Corresponding author. 215 Main Street, Westport, CT 06880.
E-mail address: Andrew.Lustbader@yale.edu

Child Adolesc Psychiatric Clin N Am 29 (2020) 775–782
https://doi.org/10.1016/j.chc.2020.06.012
1056-4993/20/© 2020 Elsevier Inc. All rights reserved.

Abbreviations	
CDI	Children's Depression Inventory
MBC	measurement-based care

Sometimes these instruments may also be used to qualitatively inform clinicians about specific symptomatology.

Psychiatric MBC tools should be used as screening measures as part of every nonpsychiatric medical and surgical, general, and subspecialty practice. The usefulness of identifying underlying and/or comorbid psychiatric illness has been well established.[2–4] Cassidy and Jellinek indicate that "as many as half of all pediatric office visits reflect behavioral, psychosocial, and educational concerns."[3] Many primary care and medical/surgical subspecialty practices screen for depression (often using the Patient Health Questionnaire-9), but usually not using a general screening measure that could pick up other significant psychiatric issues that could impact clinically relevant physical symptoms. Other articles in this issue of *Child and Adolescent Psychiatric Clinics of North America* discuss the importance of using psychiatric screening measures in nonpsychiatric settings. However, in the various types of psychiatric specialty settings, we believe the way forward is not so clear.

DISCUSSION
Should Measurable Psychiatric Symptom Reduction Be the Overriding Method of Driving Clinical Decision Making and Understanding Patient Outcomes?

When further working definitions of MBC are examined, commonalities can be identified. Aboraya and colleagues write that, "Our working definition of MBC in psychiatry is 'the use of validated measurement instruments to objectify the assessment, treatment, and clinical outcomes, including efficacy, safety, tolerability, functioning, and quality of life, in patients with psychiatric disorders.'"[5] Trivedi and associates define MBC as "the routine measurement of symptoms and side effects at each treatment visit and the use of a treatment manual describing when and how to modify medication doses based on these measures."[6] The implication of these 2 definitions, as well as the one used by Fortney as mentioned elsewhere in this article, is that a direct correlation exists between the extent to which measurements guide care in psychiatric settings and improved patient outcomes. All 3 definitions also operate under the logical assumptions of physical medicine: that a psychiatric diagnosis will have a homogenous treatment response with a fairly similar course of action across patients and time. However, there are several logical fallacies in this argument.

The first issue is that measurements and tools used to guide decision making operate under the assumption that the etiology of each group of symptoms is the same; put differently, these measures do not assess whether a disorder or set of symptoms is caused by biological, social, and/or physical factors. Although some patients may present with similar symptoms, the root cause(s) of their disorder(s) may be quite different from one to the next, and thus treatment options must be assessed separately. For example, a patient may have symptoms that could be interpreted as a mild heart attack or a panic attack. Obviously, the treatments would be vastly different. Furthermore, if the patient had both, then each problem would require treatment on its own, but within the context of the other diagnosis.

Although most medical and surgical specialties and subspecialties usually deal with physically verifiable disorders that can be observed independently, psychiatry's diagnostic entities are generally theoretic conceptions which encapsulate complex cognitive, behavioral, and emotional processes.[7] Thus, most psychiatric disorders cannot be independently confirmed through tests that prove their biological etiology through discrete outputs (eg, positive or negative laboratory numerical values, or imaging studies) for which the parameters are based on data from published randomized placebo-controlled clinical trials with homogenous populations.

The second issue is that psychiatric diagnoses and expected treatment responses do not have the homogeneity of those that are studied in randomized clinical trials. Patients in community settings are more commonly heterogeneous, with high rates of comorbidity with a complex interplay of personality, behavioral, social, family systemic, and biological factors influencing their symptoms. MBC does not assess the meaning and context of each presenting symptom—a critical part of professional relationship-based Hippocratic medical care—but rather examines each symptom in a vacuum. If MBC becomes the central focus of treatment (eg, if it becomes the sole form of decision making for ongoing reimbursement by third-party payers), it could have the potential for a harmful impact on patient care. It undermines the doctor–patient relationship as the therapy becomes geared toward alleviating symptoms as described in MBC-approved routine symptom checklists rather than focusing on underlying illness. Not only do weekly sessions become encumbered by lengthy progress measurements, but the focus of the therapy itself is both consciously and unconsciously geared toward the "outcome metrics," not on ensuring that the underlying issues are addressed so that they do not continue to hamper patients' lives.

For example, a cardiologist would not discharge someone from treatment after they have had a myocardial infarction purely on the basis of whether or not they are able to walk up a flight of stairs pain free. The patient would be assessed for an underlying cause of the myocardial infarction (eg, cardiovascular disease, blockage of certain arteries, etc), and given medications, recommendations for lifestyle changes in nutrition and exercise, and then be closely monitored. By the same standard, when patients who suffer from panic attacks and agoraphobia have diminished panic enough to leave the house under certain circumstances, treatment should clearly not end there; the root cause of the anxiety, as well as relational, emotional, intellectual, moral, and environmental factors, must be addressed. If these factors are not addressed, as might be the case on a treatment wholly dependent on MBC-based symptom reduction, life for such a person could be routinely quite painful. Symptom reduction must be a goal, but only within the context of the meaning and suffering of a person's complex life.

Furthermore, MBC only measures snapshots in time. Children and adolescents especially have a poor sense of time, usually only best able to access the immediate present. Frequently, they do not recall difficult emotional and/or behavioral responses a week or even a few days before a session without some prompting. Metrics would therefore likely reflect the young patient's report of relative well-being expressed in that session. Clinicians, in contrast, have a trained sense of the arc of treatment with regular attention being paid to conscious and unconscious processes and reflected in clinical notes. Progress would be assessed by emotional and behavioral data obtained by the clinician from family, schools, and other community sources, and would not be persuaded solely by the metrics of a current session.

MBC also has limitations reflected in other clinical situations. For example, as part of the therapeutic process, patients face aspects of their lives that can be shameful or painful to explore; as a result, they decompensate before showing improvement. They can have unrealistic expectations of treatments that are deflating when not met quickly. Moreover, treatment that maintains the status quo is often the best that can be done psychiatrically for some patients, much the same way a diabetic will attempt to keep their hemoglobin A1C stable, which is still likely to be well above normal.

To further accentuate the point that most MBC-approved metrics do not capture quality of life and sense of wellbeing, we examine the Recovery Assessment Scale, recently discussed by Benedict Carey in the New York Times:

> In... the first study of its kind,[8] Dutch researchers tested a standard life-quality measure, the Recovery Assessment Scale, that is typically used to rate an individual's confidence, hope, sense of purpose, willingness to ask for help, and other features of a full, stable life. The team administered the 24-item questionnaire to three groups of people: one with a diagnosis of a psychotic disorder, like schizophrenia; the siblings of members of this first group, who had no such diagnosis; and a control group of unrelated people who had no history of mental-health problems. The scale found little detectable differences between the groups. The widely used R.A.S., as the scale is known, is "of questionable usefulness," the authors concluded. If everyone looks roughly the same on the scale, then how can the scale be used to measure improvement?[9]

Carey goes on to say:

> The R.A.S., and many similar scales, amount to little more than symptom checklists, in the end not much different from those used to track the short-term effects of a drug...The scales originated decades ago with mental-health consumers, or "survivors," who saw the usual clinical definitions of symptoms relief, like the Hamilton Depression Scale, as unable to capture the fullness of personal recovery...Responses [to scales] can vary by the day, or even the hour, depending on what insults or encouragements hold sway in the moment. People who find a way to move on with their lives after receiving a psychiatric diagnosis—depression, anxiety, bipolar disorder, schizophrenia—generally must do so the hard way: gradually, by fine-tuning some combination of personal rituals, social connections, work demands, therapy and, when necessary, medications. And these idiosyncratic regimens of self-care are not easily captured by the measures currently available to researchers.[9]

Clinical Vignette: An Example of Qualitative Psychiatric Use of Measurement-Based Care Instruments in Routine Care

A gregarious and smiling 16-year-old girl presented as anxious with some panic at the beginning of her junior year in high school. Before meeting her, a parental and family history were taken and an SNAP-IV (90 questions, routinely given) was given to the parents to check to see if there were any diagnostic categories that needed to be further explored. In this particular case, there were no diagnostic areas that the history and mental status did not reveal, but during the initial mental status examination with the adolescent, she filled out a 27-question, Children's Depression Inventory (CDI) together with the psychiatrist. Although the overall score was significant—it fell into the moderate to severe range—what was more useful for ongoing treatment was the idea that her responses to many of the questions were reviewed as she was taking the screening measure, leading to fruitful discussions about aspects of her mental status that might have taken longer to uncover. It also provided a mild sense of relief as she realized what she was experiencing was more common than she had imagined.

As the treatment progressed, the depressive and panic symptoms and issues (some that were raised by the CDI) were discussed in ongoing sessions in an organic way— bypassing the need for MBC measuring improvement—permitting the psychiatrist to assess her improvement during the natural evolution of her therapy. Many of her issues had not registered on the CDI, however, because they were related to her situation at home, to some social concerns, and to some cognitive difficulties, which had become evident after the first weeks of therapy.

During those first weeks of therapy, she had continued to decline, as she had hoped that starting treatment would instantly cause her symptoms to dissipate. Her constant need to seem to be well (and smiling) was in part generated by her parents getting angry with her when she expressed any sad or vulnerable feelings of her own. Treatment had therefore included parent and family work as well as individual work and medication (a selective serotonin reuptake inhibitor). Yet the pace of progress was slowed by the father's lack of insight, some social challenges, and some difficulties in school.

Cognitive testing was recommended, which revealed some difficulty with processing. Consequently, her school was notified and began to provide support by working with her parents to create an individualized education plan. As she began to understand how her processing abilities and emotions played a role in her learning—both academically and socially—she was able to better temper her expectations of herself and accept a more accurate view of herself. She also permitted herself to join group therapy at school.

Another CDI was completed with the psychiatrist for qualitative purposes, approximately 4 months into the treatment. Symptoms discussed during the taking of the CDI were again useful in the therapeutic discussions that followed. Although the metrics indicated her depression had diminished, she clearly remained in a constant level of distress. With the individual, family, and group therapies, as well as the school modifications and the use of the medication, she was markedly better by the eighth month and remained well with medication checks for the next 8 to 9 months later, when the selective serotonin reuptake inhibitor was discontinued. As of the writing of this article, she continues to thrive In her third year of college and checks in 2 to 3 times a year when she is home.

Had the therapy depended on symptom reduction reflected in MBC, it would have likely been terminated much before she was able to get such marked and lasting improvement. Because the therapist was responsive to her emotional distress, and understood the meaning of her symptoms—symptoms, in part, qualitatively highlighted by the CDI's—the correct treatments were initiated and improvement was marked and lasting.

Should Measurable Psychiatric Symptom Reduction Be the Basis for Third-Party Payers to Reimburse Psychiatric Treatment?

One of the greatest risks of implementing MBC in psychiatric settings is that psychiatrists and mental health professionals may be hindered by insurance incentives created to reward and/or reimburse only those patients with certain outcomes as defined by approved measures and tools. They would be asked to translate into numbers and statistics patients' experience and feelings, such as degree of suffering. These efforts to manage care would minimize, perhaps to the point of elimination, one of the essential aspects of healing: the critical relationship between the doctor and the patient. Additionally, by using these measurements, psychiatrists would be permitting these third-party payers to use statistics and numbers to direct interventions to the detriment of patients, define limited services that can be covered, limit reimbursements, and expand the need to focus on the nonrelational aspects of care delivery.

Health insurance companies have a financial incentive to minimize costs to increase profits, which may frequently lead to underpayment for clinically determined care. The mental health field suffers more than other medical and surgical specialties owing to a lack of enforcement of parity. Quality mental health care often involves frequent sessions over a long duration, and progress can often be uneven and slow.

In a ruling from a class action lawsuit from March of 2019 (*Wit v UBH*), the court decided that parity laws must be enforced. In that ruling, Judge Spero states, "It is a generally accepted standard of care that effective treatment requires treatment of the individual's underlying condition and is not limited to alleviation of the individual's current symptoms."[10a] Therefore, psychiatrists cannot be content to measure patient success solely by an amelioration of symptoms as evidenced by MBC. Doing so would represent an abdication of their role as treaters of the mental illnesses that underlie patients' distress. If established as the way of measuring treatment outcomes by the health insurance industry, MBC runs the risk of being used as a tool to limit necessary forms of talk therapy, often creating temporary improvements and not sufficiently

---

[a] Private email correspondence from lead counsel Meiram Bendat includes key points summarizing some of the judge's findings of *Wit v. UBH*, March 5, 2019:, "In his detailed ruling, Chief Magistrate Judge Joseph Spero found the following to be the generally accepted standards for behavioral healthcare from which UBH's guidelines deviated:, 1. It is a generally accepted standard of care that effective treatment requires treatment of the individual's underlying condition and is not limited to alleviation of the individual's current symptoms;, 2. It is a generally accepted standard of care that effective treatment requires treatment of co-occurring behavioral health disorders and/or medical conditions in a coordinated manner that considers the interactions of the disorders and conditions and their implications for determining the appropriate level of care;, 3. It is a generally accepted standard of care that patients should receive treatment for mental health and substance use disorders at the least intensive and restrictive level of care that is, safe and effective – the fact that a lower level of care is less restrictive or intensive does not justify selecting that level if it is also expected to be less effective. Placement in a less restrictive environment is appropriate only if it is likely to be safe and just as effective as treatment at a higher level of care in addressing a patient's overall condition, including underlying and co-occurring conditions;, 4. It is a generally accepted standard of care that when there is ambiguity as to the appropriate level of care, the practitioner should err on the side of caution by placing the patient in a higher level of care;, 5. It is a generally accepted standard of care that effective treatment of mental health and substance use disorders includes services needed to maintain functioning or prevent deterioration;, 6. It is a generally accepted standard of care that the appropriate duration of treatment for behavioral health disorders is based on the individual needs of the patient; there is no specific limit on the duration of such treatment;, 7. It is a generally accepted standard of care that the unique needs of children and adolescents must be taken into account when making level of care decisions involving their treatment for mental health or substance use disorders;, 8. It is a generally accepted standard of care that the determination of the appropriate level of care for patients with mental health and/or substance use disorders should be made on the basis of a multidimensional assessment that takes into account a wide variety of information about the patient., The court acknowledged that accreditation by organizations such as URAC and NCQA does not entail substantive review of medical necessity criteria developed by insurers. Therefore, such accreditation does not guarantee use of medical necessity criteria that are consistent with generally accepted standards for behavioral healthcare or with the terms of insurance policies or any laws., In light of the court's findings, including that UBH's experts (comprised of several of its own medical directors) "had serious credibility problems" and "that with respect to a significant portion of their testimony each of them was evasive – and even deceptive," robust safeguards against abuses by managed behavioral healthcare organizations are clearly warranted, such as:, 1. Legislation mandating **exclusive** adherence to medical necessity criteria developed by nonprofit, clinical specialty organizations such as the American Society of Addiction Medicine (ASAM), American Academy of Child and Adolescent Psychiatry (AACAP), and the American Association of Community Psychiatrists (AACP);, 2. Formal recognition by the American Psychiatric Association that managed care psychiatric reviewers owe a primary ethical obligation to insureds, consistent with:, 1. AMA Principles of Medical Ethics: I,III,VII and AMA Code of Medical Ethics Opinion E-10.1.1 (https://www.ama-assn.org/delivering-care/ethical-obligations-medical-directors) and , 2. *Their fiduciary duties under ERISA* (https://www.dol.gov/general/topic/retirement/fiduciaryresp)."

addressing underlying causes; this can ultimately hamper remission, cause relapse and/or more serious problems, and prolong morbidity.

Additionally, third-party payers may prioritize medication treatment over psychotherapy or other psychosocial interventions much earlier in the arc of a treatment, before these other effective treatments may even be attempted. This could occur in children and adolescents as well as in adults and the elderly, many of whom would then be subjected to unnecessary risk of harmful side effects of the medications. Requiring medications to be used as an early line of treatment, in adolescents and children as well as adults, would effectively leapfrog therapies that may be superior to medication, and could also render the medications less effective.

Other scenarios include situations in which third-party payers deny care because there has not been sufficient positive change in MBC metrics; however, the reasons that the individual has not improved may be environmental (such as illness or death of family members, changing jobs or schools, or other changes in a person's life). Care has also been denied when enough positive change has been determined by MBC metrics, despite the fact that the patient may still be in distress and the underlying problems still exist. In the clinical vignette presented in this article, both of these scenarios could have played out in the second and fourth months, respectively, had third-party payers used MBC as their sole rationale for reimbursement.

Hence, in 3 of the most common types of clinical psychiatric outpatient settings— individual or group-based private practice, freestanding public not-for-profit clinics, and larger hospital-based organizations that often have multiple types of psychiatric settings, including outpatient departments—if MBC is used as the measurement for reimbursement, psychiatric care could be sorely hampered. Psychiatry cannot succumb to the concept that reimbursement will exclusively be tied to measurable goals, without substantive critical clinical input of treating mental health providers.

SUMMARY

There is clear and convincing value in the use of clinical measurement tools for screening and assessment of mental health needs in the primary care and subspecialty medical and surgical setting to identify psychological factors that have a role in physical illnesses, many of which will impact the medical or surgical treatments. Therefore, despite some difficulties with implementation described elsewhere in this journal, these measures are critically important tools for the early identification of mental health issues.

In clinical psychiatric practice, quality of life and what is meaningful to each individual is significantly more challenging to measure than functionality. Clinical care must be guided by a more nuanced and comprehensive assessment of progress than can be generated by standardized questionnaires. Therefore, in most psychiatric settings, the use of MBC as a qualitative tool can enhance clinical practice; however, as a quantitative tool, it would be counterproductive for it to be used as the predominant driver of clinical decision making.

If psychiatry accepts MBC as a simple and nearly exclusive way to measure patient improvement and if the managed care industry were to rely more heavily on MBC for reimbursement standards, we believe that the overall quality of mental health treatment would be jeopardized.

ACKNOWLEDGMENTS

The authors acknowledge Barry Sarvet, MD, and Susanna Lustbader, Research Associate.

DISCLOSURE

The authors have nothing to disclose.

REFERENCES

1. Fortney JC, Unutzer J, Wrenn G, et al. A tipping point for measurement-based care. Psychiatr Serv 2017;68(2):179–88.
2. American Academy of Pediatrics. Committee on psychosocial aspects of child and family health and task force on mental health. The future of pediatrics: mental health competencies for pediatric primary care. Pediatrics 2009;124(1):410–21.
3. Cassidy LJ, Jellinek MS. Approaches to recognition and management of childhood psychiatric disorders in pediatric primary care. Pediatr Clin North Am 1998;45(5):1037–52.
4. Costello EJ. Primary care pediatrics and child psychopathology: a review of diagnostic, treatment, and referral practices. Pediatrics 1986;78:1044–51.
5. Aboraya A, Nasrallah HA, Elswick DE, et al. Measurement-based care in psychiatry-past, present, and future. Innov Clin Neurosci 2018;15(11–12):13–26.
6. Trivedi MH, Rush AJ, Wisniewski SR, et al. Evaluation of outcomes with citalopram for depression using measurement-based care in STAR*D: implications for clinical practice. Am J Psychiatry 2006;163:28–40.
7. Cooper R. What is Wrong with the DSM? Hist Psychiatry 2004;15(1):5–25.
8. van der Krieke L, Bartels-Velthuis A, et al. Genetic risk and outcome of psychosis investigators. Psychiatr Serv 2019;70(12):1123–9.
9. Carey B. Mental health researchers ask: what is 'recovery'? New York Times 2020.
10. United States District Court Northern District Of California David Wit, et al., Plaintiffs, V. United Behavioral Health, Defendant. GARY ALEXANDER, et al., Plaintiffs, v. United Behavioral Health, Defendant. Case 3:14-cv-02346-JCS Document 418 Filed 03/05/19 Page 1-106.

UNITED STATES POSTAL SERVICE® Statement of Ownership, Management, and Circulation
(All Periodicals Publications Except Requester Publications)

1. Publication Title	2. Publication Number	3. Filing Date
CHILD AND ADOLESCENT PSYCHIATRIC CLINICS OF NORTH AMERICA	011 – 368	9/18/2020

4. Issue Frequency	5. Number of Issues Published Annually	6. Annual Subscription Price
JAN, APR, JUL, OCT	4	$335.00

7. Complete Mailing Address of Known Office of Publication (Not printer) (Street, city, county, state, and ZIP+4®)

ELSEVIER INC.
230 Park Avenue, Suite 800
New York, NY 10169

Contact Person: Malathi Samayan
Telephone (Include area code): 91-44-42994507

8. Complete Mailing Address of Headquarters or General Business Office of Publisher (Not printer)

ELSEVIER INC.
230 Park Avenue, Suite 800
New York, NY 10169

9. Full Names and Complete Mailing Addresses of Publisher, Editor, and Managing Editor (Do not leave blank)

Publisher (Name and complete mailing address)

DOLORES MELONI, ELSEVIER INC.
1600 JOHN F KENNEDY BLVD. SUITE 1800
PHILADELPHIA, PA 19103-2899

Editor (Name and complete mailing address)

LAUREN BOYLE, ELSEVIER INC.
1600 JOHN F KENNEDY BLVD. SUITE 1800
PHILADELPHIA, PA 19103-2899

Managing Editor (Name and complete mailing address)

PATRICK MANLEY, ELSEVIER INC.
1600 JOHN F KENNEDY BLVD. SUITE 1800
PHILADELPHIA, PA 19103-2899

10. Owner (Do not leave blank. If the publication is owned by a corporation, give the name and address of the corporation immediately followed by the names and addresses of all stockholders owning or holding 1 percent or more of the total amount of stock. If not owned by a corporation, give the names and addresses of the individual owners. If owned by a partnership or other unincorporated firm, give its name and address as well as those of each individual owner. If the publication is published by a nonprofit organization, give its name and address.)

Full Name	Complete Mailing Address
WHOLLY OWNED SUBSIDIARY OF REED/ELSEVIER, US HOLDINGS	1600 JOHN F KENNEDY BLVD. SUITE 1800 PHILADELPHIA, PA 19103-2899

11. Known Bondholders, Mortgagees, and Other Security Holders Owning or Holding 1 Percent or More of Total Amount of Bonds, Mortgages, or Other Securities. If none, check box ▶ ☐ None

Full Name	Complete Mailing Address
N/A	

12. Tax Status (For completion by nonprofit organizations authorized to mail at nonprofit rates) (Check one)
The purpose, function, and nonprofit status of this organization and the exempt status for federal income tax purposes:
☒ Has Not Changed During Preceding 12 Months
☐ Has Changed During Preceding 12 Months (Publisher must submit explanation of change with this statement)

PS Form 3526, July 2014 [Page 1 of 4 (see instructions page 4)] PSN: 7530-01-000-9931   PRIVACY NOTICE: See our privacy policy on www.usps.com.

---

13. Publication Title		14. Issue Date for Circulation Data Below
CHILD AND ADOLESCENT PSYCHIATRIC CLINICS OF NORTH AMERICA		JULY 2020

15. Extent and Nature of Circulation			Average No. Copies Each Issue During Preceding 12 Months	No. Copies of Single Issue Published Nearest to Filing Date
a. Total Number of Copies (Net press run)			148	144
b. Paid Circulation (By Mail and Outside the Mail)	(1)	Mailed Outside-County Paid Subscriptions Stated on PS Form 3541 (Include paid distribution above nominal rate, advertiser's proof copies, and exchange copies)	89	84
	(2)	Mailed In-County Paid Subscriptions Stated on PS Form 3541 (Include paid distribution above nominal rate, advertiser's proof copies, and exchange copies)	0	0
	(3)	Paid Distribution Outside the Mails Including Sales Through Dealers and Carriers, Street Vendors, Counter Sales, and Other Paid Distribution Outside USPS®	25	26
	(4)	Paid Distribution by Other Classes of Mail Through the USPS (e.g., First-Class Mail®)	0	0
c. Total Paid Distribution (Sum of 15b (1), (2), (3), and (4))		▶	114	110
d. Free or Nominal Rate Distribution (By Mail and Outside the Mail)	(1)	Free or Nominal Rate Outside-County Copies included on PS Form 3541	17	16
	(2)	Free or Nominal Rate In-County Copies included on PS Form 3541	0	0
	(3)	Free or Nominal Rate Copies Mailed at Other Classes Through the USPS (e.g., First-Class Mail)	0	0
	(4)	Free or Nominal Rate Distribution Outside the Mail (Carriers or other means)	0	0
e. Total Free or Nominal Rate Distribution (Sum of 15d (1), (2), (3) and (4))		▶	17	16
f. Total Distribution (Sum of 15c and 15e)		▶	131	126
g. Copies not Distributed (See Instructions to Publishers #4 (page 3))		▶	17	18
h. Total (Sum of 15f and g)		▶	148	144
i. Percent Paid (15c divided by 15f times 100)			87.02%	87.3%

* If you are claiming electronic copies, go to line 16 on page 3. If you are not claiming electronic copies, skip to line 17 on page 3.

16. Electronic Copy Circulation		Average No. Copies Each Issue During Preceding 12 Months	No. Copies of Single Issue Published Nearest to Filing Date
a. Paid Electronic Copies	▶		
b. Total Paid Print Copies (Line 15c) + Paid Electronic Copies (Line 16a)	▶		
c. Total Print Distribution (Line 15f) + Paid Electronic Copies (Line 16a)	▶		
d. Percent Paid (Both Print & Electronic Copies) (16b divided by 16c × 100)	▶		

☒ I certify that 50% of all my distributed copies (electronic and print) are paid above a nominal price.

17. Publication of Statement of Ownership

☒ If the publication is a general publication, publication of this statement is required. Will be printed in the OCTOBER 2020 issue of this publication.   ☐ Publication not required.

18. Signature and Title of Editor, Publisher, Business Manager, or Owner		Date
Malathi Samayan - Distribution Controller *Malathi Samayan*		9/18/2020

I certify that all information furnished on this form is true and complete. I understand that anyone who furnishes false or misleading information on this form or who omits material or information requested on the form may be subject to criminal sanctions (including fines and imprisonment) and/or civil sanctions (including civil penalties).

PS Form 3526, July 2014 (Page 3 of 4)   PRIVACY NOTICE: See our privacy policy on www.usps.com